Introducing User-friendly Family Therapy

Introducing User-friendly Family Therapy fills an important gap in the literature of family therapy by examining users' experiences of therapy. This book reports some original research which documents users' views about therapy and argues that family therapists, in emphasizing technique and expert interventions to bring about change, frequently underestimate the centrality of users' own experiences, and in the process recapitulate the negative aspects of the medical model. Although it may be claimed that such approaches are effective, they often fail to empower users to deal with their problems on their own terms. User-friendly approaches to therapy adopt a different stance – they attempt to create a therapeutic climate which encourages therapists to work closely with users in jointly creating ideas and solutions which are not only effective but also make sense to users themselves.

The first part of the book critiques the historical development and current practice of family therapy and gradually introduces the reader to a user-friendly approach. The second part presents an action research project and reviews consumer studies of therapy, including social work, marriage guidance and family therapy research before concluding with guidelines for putting a user-friendly perspective into practice. Thought-provoking and practical in emphasis, this book places the user at the centre of the stage and insists that family therapy has now reached a stage where it needs to concentrate on becoming more genuinely empowering and user-friendly.

Introducing User-friendly Family Therapy will stimulate professionals working with families, managers and policy makers to reassess their ways of thinking and working.

Sigurd Reimers is family therapist with the Bath Mental Health Care NHS Trust and Training Officer with Somerset Child Protection Committee. **Andy Treacher** is clinical tutor to the Doctorate in Clinical Psychology course and co-director of the Diploma Course in Family and Marital Therapy at the University of Exeter. He is based at the Department of Clinical and Community Psychology, Royal Devon and Exeter Hospital, Wonford, where he works as a family therapist.

Introducing User-friendly Family Therapy

Sigurd Reimers and Andy Treacher
with the collaboration of Carolyn White

Foreword by Lynn Hoffman

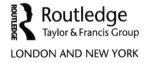

Routledge
Taylor & Francis Group

LONDON AND NEW YORK

First published 1995
by Routledge
27 Church Road, Hove, East Sussex, BN3 2FA

Simultaneously published in the USA and Canada
by Routledge
270 Madison Ave, New York NY 10016

Routledge is an imprint of the Taylor & Francis Group, an informa business

Transferred to Digital Printing 2010

Typeset in Times by LaserScript, Mitcham, Surrey

British Library Cataloguing in Publication Data
A catalogue record for this book is available from the British Library

Library of Congress Cataloging in Publication Data
A catalog record for this book has been requested

ISBN 978-0-415-07431-5 (pbk)

Publisher's Note
The publisher has gone to great lengths to ensure the quality of this reprint
but points out that some imperfections in the original may be apparent.

Contents

Illustrations

Foreword

Lynn Hoffman

'*In order to discover whether professed benevolence is really independent, ask the beneficiary rather than the benefactor.*'
(R. B. Perry, quoted in Mayer and Timms, 1970)

This quote should be on the marquee of the huge entertainment park that has been known as Family Therapy. Sigurd Reimers and Andy Treacher have compiled a landmark study of the attention – or lack of it – that has characterized family therapy inquiries into the nature of the therapeutic experience *for the therapeutees*. As in the case of hearing-impaired people before Sign was accepted as a formal language, our own clients have seemed to be dumb, in the sense of being both mute and without knowledge. So why bother to ask them what they think about therapy of any kind?

The title of this book is acknowledged by its authors to be both flip and ironic, but the deeper message is not lost. How can you say that family therapy is like the unfriendly computer with which so many of us have struggled? Are we really talking about the sacred art of healing? Reimers and Treacher have pulled the rug out from under us and told us (or their users' responses have) some plain truths. In most of the user reaction studies discussed in this book, depending on the circumstances and the model used, the users' discomfort with some or all aspects of family therapy has hit high percentiles.

However, Reimers and Treacher have been fair in pulling the rug out from under themselves too. They are perhaps getting on the side of the angels by being part of the first wave of repenters, but the fact that they were among the family therapy faithful for so long softens what could be (and may still be felt as) a blameful tirade. Also, unlike many of the studies of user reactions they summarize, these two put their own studies to work. They changed what they were doing in an effort to become more congruent with what their users were saying they did or did not like.

The choice, of course, of what to replace 'client' or 'patient' with is an interesting one. In the USA, 'user' is a term for 'drug taker' or someone who takes advantage of people, so it has some unfriendly connotations. As an

American, I alternately use 'consumer' or 'customer', which of course goes with our well-known emphasis on commerce. A German friend, writer/consultant Jürgen Hargens, in a letter that impressed me very much, said he uses the word 'KundIn' in describing the people he sees and explains to them why he uses it. Since the word not only means customer but expert person, they are pleased. It is too bad that in English there is no equivalent. But 'user-friendly' is a nice start.

These authors also get good marks for writing with a personal imprint. They use the 'I' instead of the more formal 'we' or the impersonal 'It is felt'. Chapters are clearly identified with the names of the authors, and sections within chapters are also marked. This honouring of a subjective position tends to move the writer from a written kind of language to a spoken one, and is itself user-friendly to the reader. I enjoyed reading about the steps both authors went through in their respective educations and early apprenticeships, from initial enthusiasm for family therapy to questioning the assumptions about users held by the entire field. By being story-tellers of their own struggles, they have not lost the sense of wonder of the little boy who commented that the emperor had no clothes.

However, the emphasis of this book is naturally on the British scene, which differs greatly from the American one. The chapter on the relationship between social policy and the way families are seen and treated is most interesting. Despite regressive tendencies due to 'Thatcherism' it seems that there are some progressive advances, like a *Patient's Charter* for users' rights coming under the National Health Service, or the Access to Health Records Act (1990). This latter rule may begin to make a dent on what I call psychiatric hate-speech, the impenetrable clinical language that demeans people without saying so. It would be a good rule for the US to adopt too.

But family therapy (or family intrusion, depending how you look at it) is an international product. It is a growth industry in our country and has just been recognized at the Federal level as a legitimate profession. Hence this book could hardly come at a better (or worse) time to highlight our own dilemmas. Managed care is sweeping over the mental health profession like a selective weedkiller. Some people are saying that family therapists have little option but to medicalize or die. In a current debate in one of our family therapy magazines, the psychiatrist Lyman Wynne and colleagues commiserate with MFTs (the acronym for Marriage and Family Therapists) because they will end up marginalized unless they get better training in psychopathology or partner up with someone from the major disciplines (i.e. the ones who got legalized first: psychiatry, psychology and social work).

As if this challenge wasn't enough, the new Bible ordaining the standards for true mental conditions, *DSM IV*, is about to come out. Within this diagnostic system, only heavy-duty afflictions like the major psychoses, particularly if they call for medication by a psychiatrist, warrant recognition by insurance companies – mere relationship problems have no currency. A person needs a psychiatric epithet to qualify for reimbursement. Thus software becomes destiny. And family therapists, perhaps, could become history.

But now comes this book! Beset from above, family therapists could always say, 'But our clients, those who come to us privately or are sent at an agency's expense, they at least will appreciate us.' Reimers' and Treacher's research throws that idea into the myth bin. In family systems therapy, at least, love of therapy seems to be as much the exception as the rule. So it makes sense that the authors have set up a defence of the ideas of that much maligned psychologist, Carl Rogers, and use the term 'family-centred' as an appreciative description of the kind of family therapy they believe in.

Reimers and Treacher not only hold up Rogers as one possible model for a user-friendly therapy (although his approach is different in many aspects of practice and theory), but describe some hopeful evidence of change already happening in family therapy. They do not give up on the field, as Jeffrey Masson seems to do in his equally courageous (some would say outrageous) book *Against Therapy*. They give due credit to the growing group of people who are really trying to hear the voices of the people who are their customers. And they also give credit to the one consumer group, the National Alliance for the Mentally Ill, that has organized against family systems therapy, mainly because of its parent-blaming approach to schizophrenia.

In distributing praise for therapists who have become more family- or person-centred, the authors cite the work of Harlene Anderson and the late Harry Goolishian, who have taken a radical position in saying that the person who meets with someone with a complaint should come from a position of 'not knowing' rather than the more expected 'all knowing'. The authors also praise the outstanding feminists who have criticized the people-as-machine-parts aspect of systems theory and its remoteness. They admire the work of Michael White who allies with people against their troubles, and the communitarian 'Just Therapy' group in New Zealand. I also thank them for noting some of my own recent stirrings of unease.

Reimers and Treacher also point out that we need to develop trainee-friendly approaches to supervision as well. I couldn't agree more. I instituted reflecting conversations in supervisory settings that were based on what I call, following Rogers, a 'mirror of positive regard'. Not only did I want to create an atmosphere of safety but I had noticed that people in seminars or classes, which are small authoritarian states no matter how democratic the teacher tries to be, are apt to become either lions or lambs. Lions raise their hands all the time, get called on by the teacher or supervisor, and feel smarter and smarter. Lambs raise their hands timidly, then not at all and feel more and more stupid. My reflecting format cut into that vicious cycle amazingly quickly.

But, to go back to Reimers and Treacher again – they point out how great has been the influence of the pioneers in the field: all medically trained, and many of them child analysts. Distance from the family was in their life blood. Virginia Satir was a major exception. She came from social work and was far from distant with her families, but at the Mental Research Institute one psychiatrist once said to me that the other researchers there were a little embarrassed by her, the way you might feel about a child who goes outside without her clothes on. In general, the use of technology has fostered in family therapy, as it has in hi-tech medicine, an illusion of objectivity and professionalization that is anything but warm.

Reimers and Treacher also made me reflect that the use of the one-way screen, the audiotape and then the videotape, while excellent for wider dissemination of knowledge that wasn't going to make it to the academies for at least ten years, was not only user-unfriendly but user-oblivious. The real clients of the early family therapists were the audiences behind the screen: the trainees, the supervisors, the visitors sitting in the bleachers. Or the people who later saw an edited tape at one of the larger and larger conferences on family therapy that began to dominate the field. The family was usually only considered once, when they were asked to sign a release which was frequently used for purposes of which they never dreamed.

Even while agreeing with their position, however, Reimers' and Treacher's book has reminded me with great force of how hard it will be to get changes on the profound level they recommend. The whole idea goes against the practice of turning neophytes into professionals. Schools of psychology or social work are mostly technique factories, like medical schools, with a spoonful of 'client empowerment' thrown in to sweeten the brew. This situation is amplified in our country by the need of managed care for clear and simple diagnoses. In fact, one can hardly envision increased respect for users given the new mental health picture. Psychiatrists will become the kings (joined maybe by a few queens), psychologists the knights and social workers the pawns. It will be up to us 'marginal' family therapists, who have little to lose as long as we are outside the main game, to adopt the user-friendly attitudes or do the unconventional research that this study so keenly endorses.

An image comes to mind of a river dividing into two streams around a piece of land which may or may not be an island. One stream flows past cultivated countryside, towns and cities; the other disappears into an area of uncharted wilderness. There are two groups of explorers, one going up each branch of the stream. One group represents the more established professions and they are going up the settled branch. The other group is a more ragged band, representing the late-comer professions such as family therapy. The first group, setting out with modern boats and accessories, will probably find some version of their longed-for promised land. As for the wilderness people, they will survive with their funny backpacks, well-used binoculars, nondescript gear and patched up boats, because they are visionaries whose forays into uncharted futures have brought many useful discoveries back into the present time.

This image brings me to the ideas of what at least two wilderness visionaries think a more user-friendly therapy would look like. Reimers and Treacher do not offer new techniques so much as therapeutic guidelines that are based on a much stronger ethical practice. As far as which approaches to family therapy they prefer, they do not choose favourites so much as disfavouring some in particular.

They mainly voice a wish for 'integrated' or 'eclectic' styles within a user-friendly framework.

Here is one place where I question their ideals. Eclectic or integrated models aren't real models. They usually mean that everyone is allowed to do their own thing. Often, in a family agency or training centre, the word 'eclectic' has been used to protect more individual-oriented practitioners who don't want to let go their way of working but don't want to be blamed for it. Also, these terms are seen as a way to paper over turf battles or possible wars between models. There are always many loyalties involved, based on what Carl Whitaker used to call 'the fight among the grandfathers'. I would say that a tolerance for 'multiple voices' might be a better way to put it. That would offer shelter to the many good paths that have been discovered within the larger territory of 'user-friendly' country.

Research is another tricky place to institute change. A user-friendly research would more often take users' opinions of therapy at face value. Reimers and Treacher more or less advocate this approach, admittedly qualitative and flawed though it is. As far as research on family therapy effectiveness goes, they do not feel there is much out there that proves anything conclusively, except for the more educational or behavioural approaches which limit themselves to quantifiable goals. Maybe the user research method will turn out to be the best after all: just ask the people themselves what they thought worked or didn't.

My own feeling is that we have been barking up the wrong tree, in the wrong wood, with the wrong dog. I sometimes wish we could admit that psychology as we have known it is a flawed field. This is first and foremost due to the fact that we ourselves are the field that we are trying to explore. We ourselves are a continual and unavoidable source of experimenter bias and the reflexivity implicit in this situation offers an impenetrable barrier to confirming any guess. This is why I find social construction theory (Gergen, 1991) comforting; it tells me that the source of what I thought was a problem is simply the condition of being another human being.

Reimers and Treacher tackle this issue with a wonderful quote from Søren Kierkegaard (1974) who says that a deluded person builds a beautiful palace even though an outside observer can only see a dog kennel or at best a porter's lodge. He adds that for the observer to try to correct the false idea would only offend the person: 'For he [sic] has no fear of being under a delusion, if only he can get the system completed by means of a delusion.' If we could accept the fact that we all live in delusions, and that these delusions, such as they are, contain the only grounds for our connectedness, we might do better.

However, let me throw in a more practical idea for addressing this predicament. John Shotter's inspired concept 'Knowing of the Third Kind' is based on the observation that psychology (and philosophy before it) have always divided the field into two parts. There is inside psychology (the mind, the psyche, the soul) and outside psychology (the world, behaviour, events). He and Don Schön, whose influential book *The Reflective Practitioner* was published in 1983, seem to be pioneering another version of psychology. It refers to the back and forth interaction between people as they negotiate the simplest tasks of living. They study communications like: Go here, Stand still, What is it? and so forth. These exchanges have been so native to our operations in the world that they have been invisible to us. But it is this joint action, as John Shotter calls it, that is the essence of what teachers, parents, therapists, playmates, friends, and most other people do most of the time. I feel that this sort of psychology probably should get a different name: human studies, or relational studies, or communication studies. But within such a 'joint action' approach, there is finally room for not only user-friendliness, but user-inclusion.

In sum, Reimers' and Treacher's achievement is a first-of-its-kind, head-on attack on a central ethical problem in our field. The book's value is not so much in its aesthetics – it seems more like an archipelago sprawled about in islands rather than a country with nice, neat borders – but its value exceeds the sum of its parts. By selecting out and naming one of family therapy's best kept secrets – our collective disinterest in our customers' thoughts and feelings about therapy – and putting together all the disparate bits of research that have tried to break through to that secret, it is a stunning success. Even though I thought I too was on the side of the angels, I feel I have not gone far enough. Reimers and Treacher are saying: 'Give back therapy to the people you serve.' I commend them for their honesty and hard work and plain stubborn disinclination to accept the status quo. Their beliefs bear out those expressed in another passage from Kierkegaard (brought to my attention by my Norwegian friend Finn Wangberg) on what it is to help:

> The relationship between the helper and the one to be helped must be such that, if one shall really succeed in leading a person to a certain place, one first has to make sure one finds where the other is, and start there. This is the secret of the art of helping. Anyone who cannot do that, suffers from a delusion, thinking she can help another person. [Thus] . . . all true help starts with a humiliation. The helper must first subordinate herself to the one she wishes to help, and thereby understand that helping is not to rule but to serve; that to help is not to be the most power seeking, but the most patient; that to help is to be prepared to accept that you are wrong when you do not understand what your neighbour understands.
>
> (Søren Kierkegaard, 1948)

REFERENCES

Gergen, K. (1991) *The Saturated Self*, New York: Basic Books.

Kierkegaard, S. (1948) 'The viewpoint for my authorship' (*Synspunktet for min Forfatter-virksomhet*) Finn Wangberg (tr.).

Mayer, J. and Timms, N. (1970) *The Client Speaks: Working Class Impressions of Casework*, London: Routledge and Kegan Paul.

Rogers, C. (1961) *On Becoming a Person*, Boston: Houghton Mifflin.

Schön, D. (1983) *The Reflective Practitioner: How Professionals Think in Action*, Hants: M. T. Smith.

Acknowledgements

This book, and the ideas behind it, have a large cast. We wish to acknowledge with gratitude the help of a number of people. First our colleagues in Western Wiltshire who contributed in a variety of ways to the three user surveys: Barbara Cotterell, Brenda Davis, Sally Everett, Paula Ford, Rosemary Hamley, Rose Hull, Linda Masters, Trevor Morkham, Sally Noble, Clare Roys, Margaret Sykes and Mark Weekes. Richard Velleman, Donna Smith, Pam Pimpernell, Eddy Street and John Carpenter have also made important contributions to developing the idea of user-friendliness.

Second, a number of secretaries and typists have been involved in typing the survey reports and various parts of the book: Edith Bass, Hilary Chamulewicz, Linda Coles, Joyce Cooper, Sheila Kilmurray, Liz Mears, Marilyn Parfitt, Jane Smith and Sybil Townsend. A special thank you also to Cally Pettit and Tracey Hart who shared the typing of most of the manuscript.

The material used in Chapter 10 on the effects of social policy on family life is widely available. However, the Open University course D311, Family Life and Social Policy, has brought together some crucial source material and ideas which have been of great help to us. We would also like to thank the *Journal of Family Therapy* for giving us permission to include extracts from the following pages: vol. 8 pp. 267–306, vol. 10 pp. 1–8 and vol. 12 pp. 59–72.

Last, but not least, we thank the users who have generously shared their ideas and experiences of therapy with us. Our one regret (and we would hope not to repeat this mistake in the future) is that we have not offered to keep in touch with them during the writing of the book.

Although we have been greatly influenced by many people, the responsibility for the book remains firmly with us.

Chapter 1

Introducing user-friendly family therapy

Andy Treacher and Sigurd Reimers

It is genuinely difficult to establish whether family therapists take much interest in how their clients (users) experience being in family therapy with them. Maybe they do take an interest on a day-to-day basis but, if so, this interest is rarely reflected in family therapy publications. As we will demonstrate in a later chapter, the number of publications which actually attempt to give users a voice by recording their thoughts and feelings about being in therapy is remarkably small.

To illustrate this lack of interest, it is worth turning to the massive (715-page) Volume 2 of the *Handbook of Family Therapy*, edited by Alan Gurman and David Kniskern (1991). Its index contains no mention of 'client', 'clients, perceptions of' or any related item. Looking under the broader topic of 'family' proves slightly more fruitful since there are two references to 'family – goals of and therapist's goals' and 'family – goals of individual members'. Both items give a hint that users may have a point of view that needs to be considered but the first reference is particularly poignant. It concerns a controversial facet of structural family therapy practice which involves therapists being invited to challenge users' goals, on the basis that users only want to achieve symptomatic change, whereas structural family therapists are concerned with achieving deeper (structural) change in the family so that the symptoms are eradicated at a more basic level. Consulting Volume 1 (796 pages) of the same book (Gurman and Kniskern, 1981) also yields an interesting finding. There is, indeed, one reference to 'client' ('client-centred therapy') but ironically there is no such reference in the second volume, as we have already pointed out.

It is ironic and perplexing that family therapists have neglected their users in this way. Systemic theories, after all, stress such notions as feedback and circularity, and often take other forms of theorizing to task because they are considered to be 'linear' (unidirectional) in their thinking. The allegedly superior interactional theorizing of family therapy is assumed to be more sophisticated than other models which are dismissed because they concentrate on intrapsychic phenomena. Many theories of psychotherapy do suffer from major inconsistencies but we believe that this particular inconsistency has had, and still has, enormous implications for the development of the family therapy movement.

Anne Rogers, David Pilgrim and Ron Lacey (1993) in their pioneering book *Experiencing Psychiatry – Users' Views of Services*, provide us with some important clues, which help explain such a startling gap between theory and practice. They point out, in discussing related examples, that there are several reasons why psychiatric patients' views about their experience of therapy tend to be disregarded by the professionals who work with them. Since family therapy, as a movement, was initially dominated by psychiatrists, it is safe to assume that some of the movement's basic attitudes towards users were introduced through the back door. There is no reason to believe that the professionals who initially developed family therapy ideas changed their basic attitudes to users. These would have reflected their class background and initial professional training and practice. Medical practitioners are traditionally drawn from a very narrow class base and medical training inculcates hierarchical attitudes, so it is not surprising that we discover that family therapists have consistently disregarded users' views. Many of the original powerful opinion-makers within the movement brought a range of unchallenged reactionary assumptions and opinions into the movement. These key figures have influenced subsequent cohorts within the movement who have tended, in turn, to idealize them as 'founding fathers' (term used advisedly).

We would argue that family therapy research has been equally dominated by ideas that militate against researchers having a prime interest in the experience of therapy from the user's perspective. This argument is supported by evidence from the work of Rogers and her colleagues. Taking the crucial area of schizophrenia research as an example, they point out that research priorities are upside-down from a user's point of view. The Medical Research Council (a key funding agency in this country) has a list of priorities for research that totally ignores users' perspectives. Their list of priorities is headed by 'genetic investigations' followed by 'neuropathological studies of post-mortem brains'. Evaluation of services *to* users comes a poor eighth out of the ten cited priorities but *user* evaluation of services and treatment receives no mention whatsoever and yet approximately 1 per cent of British people are likely to suffer from schizophrenia in the course of their lifetime.

According to Rogers and her colleagues, there are four major reasons that explain why users' views have been traditionally disregarded within the mental health services:

1 Professionals feel entitled to disregard users' views when they do not coincide with their own.
2 Psychiatric users are viewed as continually irrational and hence incapable of giving a valid view.
3 Patients and relatives are assumed to share the same interests and, where they do not, the views of the former are disregarded by researchers.
4 Professionals give partial credence to the clients' perspectives provided that they fit in with their (expert) view.

We know of no specific research that has investigated family therapists' underlying attitudes to their users but unfortunately the prima-facie evidence all points to the fact that family therapists, despite pretensions to the opposite, are just as likely to neglect user perspectives as any of their professional colleagues. Most models of family therapy try not to pathologize users' behaviour but there are often striking contradictions within such models that create genuine uncertainty about their basic user-friendliness. For example, strict adherence to the original formulations of systems theory led to the neglect of the role of consciousness (and self-reflexivity) in determining behaviour. Users' experiences could therefore be ignored as epiphenomena that were of little importance to therapists intent on achieving change at a systemic level.

In Chapter 9 we will explore research that has attempted to correct this major weakness in the development of family therapy. In fact our computer search of the literature produced a remarkably small catch. The studies we discovered were interesting and important but there is no coherent body of research which can be safely mobilized in order to answer many of the tantalizing questions that a user-friendly approach would want answered.

Many of the studies we will review hark back to John Mayer and Noel Timms's classic study *The Client Speaks: Working Class Impressions of Casework* (1970). Significantly Mayer and Timms's book contains the following salutary quotation which is used as an epigraph:

> The confusion between the interest which a person himself has or takes, and the interest which a second person has or takes in him, is one of the pitfalls of parentage, teaching, religion and all varied forms of professed benevolence. In order to discover whether professed benevolence is really independent benevolence, ask the beneficiary rather than the benefactor.
>
> R. B. Perry, *Realms of Value*

In our view, the family therapy movement is dominated by the views of the benefactors not the beneficiaries. There is, as yet, no sign of an organized user movement which could articulate the views of users and ex-users of family therapy and hence redress the balance. And yet the family therapy movement, in professional terms, goes from strength to strength. In Britain there are now about 1,400 members of the Association for Family Therapy but in America, where the movement is particularly strong, there are now 17,000 therapists affiliated to the American Association for Marriage and Family Therapy. The majority of practitioners work in private practice. Family therapy is highly commercialized and family therapy ideas and methods are often sold like any other product.

Against this background it is timely to attempt to redress the balance and to attempt actively to counter the 'invisibility' of the users of family therapy. The primary aim of our book is, therefore, to help to contribute to a perspective in the family therapy movement that has been largely ignored because of the impact and fashionableness of models which too readily absorbed the alienating and dehumanizing facets of systems theorizing. This alternative perspective insists that therapy needs to be viewed as a co-operative project between user and therapist which takes seriously users' experience of family therapy.

As John Carpenter and Andy have pointed out in a previous book, some models of family therapy have tended to adopt approaches to therapy that stress the exact opposite:

> One common way to think about therapy is to consider it as a form of combat. Thus, the therapist, an heroic figure, pits himself (the pronoun is always male) against the many-headed monster 'resistance' and, by dint of subtle strategy and tremendous technique, eventually succeeds in becoming its master. Alternatively, it is like a game of chess, of move and counter-move, in which one side attempts to outwit the other and so force surrender.
>
> (Carpenter and Treacher, 1989, p. 1)

Models of therapy that adopt these types of metaphor have naturally contributed to a tradition in family therapy which has ignored users' experiences of therapy. Fortunately changes are continuing to occur within the family therapy movement so that theorizing of this type is clearly on the wane, but it is curious how little attention the newer models of family therapy (like the 'second-order approaches') have paid to users' opinions about therapy.

The basic ideas that prompted us to write this book are quite simple – as family therapists we became increasingly aware that our own day-to-day practice still reflected many of the weaknesses of the original models (structural and strategic family therapy) which our original trainers had taught us. What we lacked was any basic understanding of how users experienced therapy.

We had first met because we were both members of the Bristol branch of the Association for Family Therapy and the Bristol-based Family Therapy Co-operative. By happenstance we also briefly worked together (1986–1987) because we were both part-time members of the Chippenham Child and Family Guidance Clinic. While working together we were able to share a lot of ideas about developing a new approach, but since we also worked in other clinics (Andy at the Department of Child and Family Psychiatry at the Royal United Hospital, Bath; Sigurd at the Trowbridge Child and Family Guidance Clinic), it was difficult to collaborate regularly.

In October 1986, Carolyn White joined Andy, in Bath, in order to undertake nine months' work experience (as part of her degree in social studies). Carolyn was also very interested in users' views and was keen to undertake a project in Wiltshire. It was this project that really made the writing of this book possible. Carolyn was able to gain the co-operation of both teams (at the Chippenham and Trowbridge Clinics), but the two teams were themselves then prompted to carry out further studies which meant that the research eventually became more action-orientated as the teams became interested in applying the lessons they learnt from the users who participated in the surveys.

The results of the Wiltshire project are reported in Chapters 6 and 7 of this book, but it is important now to introduce you, the reader, to the overall structure of the book, which reflects the slightly differing paths that we have taken to develop our notions of user-friendliness. Andy has tended to develop his ideas largely because of his unhappiness with systemic models of family therapy that have tended to recapitulate many of the more problematic factors of the medical model. Sigurd, on the other hand, as a social work team leader charged with contributing to the running of a service, had been more preoccupied with the necessity of developing a service that was more in tune with users' needs. These different paths to developing ideas of user-friendliness have resulted in a division of labour as far as the book is concerned. Some chapters have been written conjointly but others could only have been written by us singly because our involvement with the issues concerned has been quite different.

The next section of this chapter is a reader's guide, which we hope will help you make some decisions about how to read our book. Like many other books, it is not necessarily best read from cover to cover. You may find that after reading this chapter and the next, you want to branch out and perhaps read the research survey chapters before returning to the more theoretical chapters (Chapters 3, 4 and 5).

READER'S GUIDE

Chapter 2 of our book paints a kaleidoscopic picture of contemporary family therapy. We argue that the overall picture is far from rosy and that there are many facets of family therapy that require urgent attention if the reputation of the movement is not to suffer.

This theme is discussed in sharper detail in Chapter 3. Andy reviews Jeffrey Masson's swingeing criticism of psychotherapy and concludes that he is essentially correct in including family therapy in his criticisms. We personally believe that family therapists (ourselves included) have persistently neglected to focus attention on the importance of ethical issues and have, in particular, been extremely complacent about the extent of abusive behaviour by therapists towards their users.

Chapters 4 and 5 are linked chapters which attempt to provide some explanations as to why users have been rendered invisible as far as family therapy theorists are concerned. In these chapters Andy uses a personal account of his own development as a therapist to explore how systems theory frameworks can seduce a well-intentioned therapist into neglecting the humanistic aspects of therapy. The pursuit of efficacy, the desire to be professionally powerful and the fascination of technically sophisticated interventions can combine to create a heady mixture which can intoxicate the therapist and seriously distort therapy as far as the user is concerned.

Chapter 6 by Sigurd and Carolyn is a pivotal chapter in the book since it reports the results of the initial survey we have already discussed. In this chapter we begin to move away from our own professional preoccupations to listen more carefully to what users think and feel about being in therapy.

In Chapter 7, Sigurd discusses how the results of the initial survey were translated into a form of action research which encouraged the therapy teams to begin to modify their practice on the basis of the feedback provided by users.

Chapters 8 and 9 (by Andy) review the remarkably small number of studies that have directly addressed users' experiences of marital and family therapy. The studies reviewed are very variegated and are difficult to summarize but nevertheless there are a number of important themes that emerge. For example, the importance and significance of the role of the therapeutic alliance, a corner-stone of user-friendliness, clearly emerges from this review.

Chapter 10 (by Sigurd) takes a wider-angle approach to user-friendliness by examining how changes in social policy have influenced family life and struc-ture. User-friendliness necessarily insists that therapists must be sensitive to the wider, societal pressures which impinge on families. The current moral panic about single-parent families is but one example of how societal attitudes towards particular minorities can be manipulated for political gains. Needless to say, the felt experience of such families (who are picked out for attack) is very complex, with families feeling distraught and victimized because of the basic de-humanization and unfairness of the attack to which they have been subjected.

Chapter 11 (by Sigurd and Andy) returns once again to the more narrow concerns of family therapy as a developing body of knowledge and practice. The chapter reviews the very different contributions that second-order thinking and feminism have made to modifying the original systemic formulations that formed the bedrock of many of the major models of family therapy. We conclude that both approaches have made contributions that can, with some modification, be absorbed by a user-friendly approach.

Chapter 12 (by Andy) is concerned with spelling out the major parameters of user-friendliness. Andy discusses a number of guidelines which provide a frame-work that can help practitioners maintain a more user-friendly, user-centred approach.

In Chapter 13 (by Sigurd), Sigurd illustrates how user-friendly ideas can change day-to-day practice. Often the changes suggested by him may seem relatively minor to you as a reader but he believes that our basic shift in emphasis is significant and contributes to creating a new context for therapy. Users are able to co-operate in 'constructing' therapy in ways that are hopefully less driven by our needs and our understandings of what therapy is about and more driven by users' needs and understandings.

In concluding our introduction it is necessary for us to make one or two points about our policy on citing other writers' work and referring to our users. When-ever possible we have tried to refer to other authors by their first names. This enables you, as a reader, to identify the gender of the writers – an important issue in a movement which has, unfortunately, been seen to be dominated by men (and yet a clear majority of practitioners are women). In some cases we do not identify the authors by first name either because we have used a review article as a source of our citation (and review articles typically do not cite authors' first names) or we have just not been able to trace the first name. In quoting users' experiences of being in therapy we have made sure to change names and details so that identification is impossible.

We also need to mention briefly the word 'user'. This is perhaps not an ideal term but we believe that it is preferable to 'client' (which has such commercial overtones) and 'patient' (a term whose original meaning of 'sufferer' has been obliterated by association with medicine). Within the medical model, the term 'patient' has associations with passivity and non-involvement in deciding the progress of therapy. More importantly, however, it is clear that the term 'user' has been embraced by many people who have experienced therapy or are currently experiencing therapy. Anne Rogers and her colleagues (1993) have carefully documented the growth of the user movement in this country, particularly in relation to mental health services.

Finally, having explored the use of the term 'user', we must also comment on our use of the term 'user-friendly'. We could perhaps have chosen the term 'user-centred' but we finally opted for user-friendly, although we have to admit that there is a slight tongue-in-cheek element in our using it. We use it in order to draw attention to the fact that many models of family therapy developed therapeutic methods that were basically user-unfriendly.

For a variety of reasons, which we will explain later, we have become aware of how vulnerable users often feel in therapy. The family therapy movement has recently developed an increasing awareness of users' vulnerability within their own families, wider networks and communities. However, users' felt experiences of therapy itself have tended to remain invisible and yet such experiences are crucial to therapists if they are concerned with developing therapies that are both effective (and satisfying) to users and ethically defensible. Without a greater awareness of these felt experiences we worry that family therapy will fail through failing to focus on what is going on under its very nose.

Chapter 2

Family therapy

A cause for concern?

Sigurd Reimers and Andy Treacher

Our book is primarily concerned with evaluating contemporary family therapy from a user's perspective. In order to begin this task we will start by exploring a fictitious example – this may seem at first sight to be an odd place to begin but we believe, nevertheless, that important lessons can be drawn from it. Our invitation to you as a reader is to pay attention particularly to the style of the therapist as you read the transcript. It may be helpful for you to keep one question in mind as the session unfolds – what would be my experience of working with this therapist if I had problems within my family that needed professional help?

THE 'B' FAMILY

Our example concerns the 'B' family. Frank (a middle-aged publican), his second wife Pat (roughly the same age) and two of his children, Ricky (who is in his late teens) and Janine (who has just started school), have turned up for their first appointment at a child guidance clinic with Carol N (a psychiatric social worker) and her colleague, Dr O'B, who remains behind the one-way screen throughout the session. The session begins with everybody seated except Ricky, who prowls round the interview room inspecting the video camera and the large mirror set into one of the room's walls.

Ricky: Here, Dad, you seen this camera?
Carol: If it's all right, we'll record you all – say if you're not happy, but we do find it useful.
Frank: Useful for what? Video nasties!
Ricky: (clutching his throat) Arghhh: 'Butchers Three'!
Frank: (laughing) 'The Final Conflict'!
Carol: Some people like looking at the tape 'cause it gives them a bit of distance on everything. You know, when they've cooled off. It can be quite a good way of getting things sorted out.
Frank: Listen, love, let's get this clear from the beginning; my daughter is not a 'thing'; all right?
Ricky: (at the two-way mirror) Mirror, mirror on the wall . . . who's the nuttiest of us all? (Pulls a face in the mirror).

Pat: Come and sit down, Rick . . .

Frank: (cutting in) Pat, the boy's only having a laugh. What's the matter with you?

Carol: I should take your mother's advice, Ricky. Well, that's a two-way mirror.

Ricky: Eh?

Frank: Look, what is this? *Candid Camera* or something?

Pat: Frank, she explained . . .

Frank: (cutting in) I thought your job was to get us to relax up a a bit: make us feel at home. Well, at this precise moment, I feel about as relaxed as a goldfish in a bowl.

Carol: Maybe you'd be a bit more comfortable if you let Janine go for a minute. (Janine is sitting on Frank's lap but is held closely by him.)

Frank: Who's behind the peep-hole then – or don't we get to know that?

Pat: My husband didn't . . . well, none of us really knew what to expect, like. We just . . .

Frank: I knew what I expected, Pat.

Janine: Daddy . . .?

Frank: (pulling her tightly to him) Yes, all right sweetheart, I won't let no one . . .

Carol: You are not unique, people do find it all a bit odd at first.

Pat: Well, I expect we'll get used to it. Have to, I suppose.

Frank: We don't have to do nothing, Pat. We don't even have to be here.

Carol: No. No, you don't. But I would like it if you'd stay Mr B. If only for me to get to know you all a bit better. Now I wonder if there's anybody you think should be here that isn't? You know, anyone important who's missing.

Frank: No.

Pat: I was hoping that mo – Frank's mother, that is – could've come but . . . well, she was a bit too busy in the end.

Frank: (holding Janine) Look at her now – good as gold.

Carol: (to Pat) And what does she do when she isn't?

Frank: Well, she did push a teacher into the swimming pool once. (Ricky laughs, Frank smiles.)

Carol: What did you do about that?

Frank: Well, Pat went down the school . . .

Carol: (to Pat) Did you punish her at all?

Frank: I never hit my kids. That's one thing you can't get me on.

Pat: She didn't say hit, Frank.

Frank: I know what the lady said, Pat.

Carol: But she does get told off?

Frank: Of course. When she deserves it.

Carol: And who decides that?

Frank: What d'you mean?

Janine: Daddy?
Frank: All right, babe. We're going in a minute.
Carol: (noticing Pat's glance) Yes, I think she wants to play for a bit . . .
Frank: (cutting in) She doesn't . . .
Carol: . . . Mrs B. Mrs B?
Pat: Yes?
Carol: D'you think you could ask your little girl if she wants to play? Well, I think she's probably a bit scared of me. You know, 'cause I'm a stranger and everything.
Pat: Oh, yes. Right. Janine? Janine, darling: D'you want to do a nice drawing for the lady here? Mmm?
Frank: Yes, go on then babe. Go on. Do a picture for daddy. (Janine climbs down from Frank's lap on to the floor.)
Carol: (to Frank) Thank you.
           I was just wondering if there's anything that any of you are worried about at the moment. You know, that's getting to you and might be having a knock-on effect on Janine?
           (Silence. Pat is unwilling to bring up any problems which might reflect badly on Frank.)
Frank: Well, I can't think of nothing.
Carol: Mmm. Mrs B?
Pat: No. Nothing. Nothing at all.
Ricky: Oh, I don't believe this.
Carol: What?
Ricky: Well, ask them about Diane; then you'll . . .
Frank: (cutting in) Ricky! Just button it, all right?
Pat: Diane – Janine's older sister – well, she's run off, hasn't she?
Carol: How long's she been gone?
Frank: Look, love, can we just drop it, all right?
Ricky: But Dad, that's what . . .
Frank: (cutting in) Ricky, we'll talk about it when we get home.
Ricky: Yes, but we won't, will we? That's the whole point.
Carol: What d'you mean?
Ricky: Well, we never talk about nothing.
Frank: We talk, we talk. We talk all the time.
Carol: Mrs B?
Pat: Well, sometimes it's a bit difficult. You know, Frank works that hard and, well, I'm in the pub a lot of the time . . .
Frank: No-one makes you go out to work, Pat.
Pat: We need the money, Frank, don't we?
Frank: We manage.
Ricky: It'd be a lot easier if you didn't spend so much dosh on Janine.
Frank: I treat you both the same; now don't you start that.
Pat: Well, whether we need the money isn't the point, is it?

Carol: (cutting in) Go on.

Pat: Well, it's like . . . it's like he's buying her off.

Frank: What?

Pat: It is, Frank. It gets back to the whole thing about me telling her off. Whenever I do and Janine gets upset, Frank doesn't, like, back me up – you don't, Frank – he just goes out and buys her a present.

Carol: (to Pat) And is that all part of why you're here, d'you think?

Frank: Listen, love, there's only one reason we're here and that's so that you can do some sort of tests . . .

Carol: (interrupting) Mr B – whenever I try to talk to your wife, I find you jumping in to answer for her, but I am asking you just to stop. All right: just for a moment. Because I do want to listen to your wife. Mrs B, can you tell me what made you get in touch with us in the first place?

Pat: Well, I wanted to help Janine . . .

Carol: Mmm?

Pat: And me. Yes. Well, it's not nice, you know. Living with a kid that hates you. It's true, Frank. She does. Well, the truth is I hate her as well, sometimes, that is. And I feel like, well, what I am I suppose. The horrible old stepmother. Because I'm not her real mum, am I? With the best will in the world I could never be that. And we both know it. Me and Janine.

(Janine smiles.)

Frank: We came here to sort out Janine! When's she going to get a bit of attention, eh? Why don't you tell us that, instead of keeping firing questions at us?

(The phone rings. Carol answers it.)

Carol: (phone) Yes? Yes, fine. Oh, has she? Thank you. (Hangs up.) Excuse me. I've just got to pop out for a moment.

(Carol leaves the room. Silence. Pat gets up, awkward now with Frank – paces about.)

Frank: Look at us, Pat – just look at the row we're into. And you say you're trying to help? And how old is she, eh? Young enough to be my daughter, that's what! And she sits there, all textbook and holier-than-thou, telling me how to bring up my kids?

Ricky: (gesticulating towards the mirror) Dad!

Frank: She's hardly out of the cradle herself; and don't go flapping your hands at me, Ricky, 'cause I don't care who's watching!

(He looks at the mirror and then at Pat.)

Frank: Oh, I've had enough of this!

(He snatches up Janine, she screams, and he makes for the door.)

Pat: Frank . . .

(As he reaches the door, it opens and his mother enters.)

Frank: What're you doing here?

Mo: Arriving just in time, by the look of things.

Frank: Too right, Mum. Let's get everybody home – come on Ricky, Pat . . .
             Mum?
Mo: Sit down, son. We're here to talk – so let's talk.
             (Carol follows Frank's mother into the room.)
Carol: I don't think there's anything wrong with Janine at all. Oh, she's playing
             up a bit, but no more than any other normal seven-year-old would, given
             the same circumstances.
Frank: So it's us what's mad then, is it? Me and Pat?
Carol: Nobody's mad, Mr B. But yes, I think there are things you could all
             probably do with sorting out.
Pat: How?
Carol: Well, what I'd like to suggest is something called family therapy. It means
             that we all meet again a few more times; just the same as today, and we try
             to sort things out. Together. Now it's not going to be easy, but I do think if
             you can just stay with it . . . I do think it'll help. So, it's up to you now, have
             you had enough, or shall I book you in for next week?
             (Pat glances at Frank. Frank looks at his mother. Pat looks at Carol.
             Frank's face shows that he is not happy with the outcome of the session.
             They agree to come back for another session but they fail to turn up.)

If you have not already guessed, it is important for us to let you into the secret of
this session. The 'B' family is the Butcher family from BBC Television's soap
opera *EastEnders*. The programme (episode 523) was broadcast in 1990 to an
estimated audience of 20 million viewers. The BBC and the episode's scriptwriter, Paul Doust, have kindly given us permission to reproduce the script here.

As a reader you may think that our examination of a fictitious example is
pointless but we would defend our decision to include it because we feel that art
often can reflect life. Obviously the transcript has many limitations because it
does not record either a real or a full session but we would, nevertheless, insist
that many families are currently being exposed to family therapy as disrespectful
as this. To help demonstrate this point we will just focus on two issues for the
moment: the issues of informed consent to undertake videotaping and to have an
observer behind a screen. A recent survey by Gregory Brock and Jeanette Coufal
(1989), members of the American Association for Marriage and Family Therapy
(AAMFT), included a question about client (user) consent. In answer to the
question, 'Do you get your client to *consent* to tape the session or have an
observer?' 3.8 per cent of respondents replied 'never', 13.4 per cent 'rarely', 30
per cent 'sometimes', 14.5 per cent 'often' and 38 per cent 'always'.

We would argue that gaining permission in the way modelled by Carol N, is
indefensible because it overlooks the fact that families at first interview are
usually extremely vulnerable and very suggestible. To gain informed consent
requires the therapist to inform users more fully of the reasons for taping and of
the safeguards that can be utilized in order to protect confidentiality (signing a
confidentiality form is an essential part of this procedure). From an ethical point

of view we believe that users need to be given a message that the use of taping and screens are issues to be discussed and negotiated. If the family or individual members of the family feel that they do not want the videotape or the screen to be used, then they have every right to say so. If a therapist uses his or her professional power to coerce a family into acceptance, then the so-called therapeutic 'victory' won by overcoming their 'resistance' may be an entirely Pyrrhic one, with the family either not turning up for the next session or attending but continually feeling uneasy because their wishes have been ignored. We make no apology for the military metaphors, which have been very prevalent in family therapy literature. We were particularly thinking of Carl Whitaker's idea of 'the battle for structure' (Napier and Whitaker, 1978).

There are many other features of the transcript that also require discussion. It is not possible to pick up the non-verbal communication involved but nevertheless it is clear from the transcript that Carol's style is extremely one-up, cold and confrontational. She has little insight into the family's reluctance to be with her and is quite prepared to confront Frank before she has built up any sort of relationship with him. Her 'know-it-all/I've-seen-it-all' style is particularly risky and user-unfriendly. She makes no attempt to give the family any guidance about how the session could be organized – she feels free to pace the session as she wants and makes no attempt to put the family at ease. There is no discussion of any contract between her and the family and she feels able to confront Frank so early on that she prompts him to think of leaving.

The session is potentially a rich source of user-friendly ideas. For example, a genuinely user-centred therapist would have noted a number of very important issues that could have been used for building a working alliance with the family. For instance, there is a clear disagreement between Pat and Frank as to why they should be in therapy. Classically Frank is troubled by the issue of whether Janine's behaviour will be labelled as mad. Pat feels very vulnerable because she is a stepmother to Janine; Frank feels vulnerable because he wants to cover up his heartbreak of his eldest daughter Diane going missing. Clearly the parents' quickly disclosed vulnerabilities could have been sensitively registered by the therapist but Carol's style of therapy is clearly antipathetic to such an approach.

From the evidence of the transcript (and the television episode) it seems that her style is a caricature of structural family therapy (a model which was quite fashionable in child guidance centres in the 1980s). It is therefore not surprising that the scriptwriter chose to depict the therapist as he did. Unfortunately, we have certainly met families whose experience of therapy has been every bit as user-unfriendly as this. By examining such worst-case scenarios we believe we can gain crucial insights about what needs to be changed in order to make family therapy much more helpful to users. As a reader you may well want to argue (despite what we say) that such bad therapy could not occur in everyday life but this is the point at which we need to broaden our argument in order to introduce some very worrying research findings that indicate that family therapy can be as user-unfriendly as the fictional session we've just explored.

RESEARCHING FAMILY THERAPY

David Howe's book *The Consumers' View of Family Therapy* caused considerable controversy in family therapy circles when it was first published in 1989. Howe's small-scale study is to be numbered amongst literally a handful of studies that have actually been interested in finding out how families feel about being on the receiving end of family therapy. Howe's book has been reviewed both positively and negatively by leading family therapists. In fact the response to the book is as interesting as the book itself. Before examining the findings in detail it is worth juxtaposing quotations from two, almost diametrically opposed, reviews of the book:

> The study makes fascinating reading as Howe, using well-chosen extracts from verbatim interviews with the families, reveals to us what they made of the therapists, their methods and their assumed purposes. The verdict of the families is depressingly negative and whilst Howe valiantly struggles to offer possible mitigating interpretations, he finally concludes that the field of family therapy as a whole stands indicted. But here lies the fatal flaw which mars the study but redeems its conclusion, so far as the practitioner is concerned. Howe strongly equates systemic family therapy with two specialized approaches only – the strategic and structural. He erroneously overlooks the equally systemic but antitechnological methods of experiential, contextual and dynamic workers. Howe's study is fascinating, thought-provoking but very partial. I challenge him to conduct a parallel investigation into the rich, non-behavioural interventions of the other approaches in the field!
>
> (Sue Walrond-Skinner, 1990, in the *Journal of Family Therapy*)

> David Howe's book is a great disappointment – an opportunity lost to tackle the subject of consumer views usefully. I am reluctant to labour the negatives but something must be said if only to warn prospective purchasers that they are unlikely to consider it worth the price. The book describes the work of six social workers . . . using a family therapy approach. . . . Given the very poor results of their therapy (and my guess is that the workers were at the time relatively inexperienced) they are, at least, to be commended for their courage. . . . Howe gives no details of any research instruments, any standardized questionnaire or any precaution against questioner subjectivity or bias. Indeed it is all presented as an amateurish attempt to gather disorganized data and one looks in vain for any of the usual underlying foundations expected of any sound piece of research . . .
>
> The book overflows with minor and major inaccuracies, all of which would undermine the experienced therapist's confidence in the author's knowledge of the current field and, worse, mislead the beginner. . . . But his confusion and muddling of theoretical models – especially his lack of clarity between structural and Milan systemic frameworks – is more serious. Much of the negative feedback from the families . . . seems fairly obviously to arise from

the inexperience of the therapy team and some basic errors made by them, but Howe has chosen to present his information as if all the comments are valid criticisms of family therapy as an approach.

Through his own lack of experience he describes the work of this particular team as being generally applicable in the field. Howe says, for instance, 'Instead of helping families change meaning in order to alter experience, families are encouraged to change their experience in order to alter meaning' and his conclusion is all family therapists are behaviourists.

The book is full of such misunderstandings. Conclusions are drawn unjustifiably and generalizations are made which are not borne out by a number of other follow-up studies with which I am familiar.

(Philippa Seligman, 1989, in *Community Care*)

Seligman's summary dismissal of the book is a pity – we believe she throws the baby out with the bath water. Many of her points about methodological weaknesses, including Howe's failure to clarify differences between models, are, we think, correct but she makes no reference to what clients actually said about their experience of therapy. She stresses the inexperience of the therapists but she does not report that the team had been working together for three years at the time of the study, and had regular consultancy input from a consultant psychiatrist. No doubt therapist inexperience could be postulated as a factor partly determining the outcome of therapy but she fails to come to terms with the crux of Howe's findings – that clients on the whole had no way of mapping or understanding the therapeutic process in which they were involved.

Walrond-Skinner's acceptance of the main findings of the study is understandable because she is well known in the family therapy movement for her willingness to raise ethical and political issues that therapists elect to ignore (as we shall see in Chapter 4). However, we are personally somewhat dubious about her conclusion. Experiential, contextual and dynamic models of family therapy may well avoid the pitfalls of the more technological approaches but we have little knowledge of what consumers of such approaches actually experience, because such models have, if anything, been less well researched than other models. However, we believe that Howe's results are very important and we will now summarize his findings in detail because they are controversial and have not been given the attention they really deserve.

Howe's study – a summary of his method and main findings

Details of the team studied by Howe   Therapy was undertaken by a six-person team (three women, three men) – four from an area social services team, two from an adolescent unit. Regular consultancy was provided by a visiting consultant psychiatrist. The team had worked together for three years but had 2–8 years of post-qualification experience as social workers.

Style of therapy	A mixture of brief systemic, structural and strategic family therapy. Therapist supervised via ear-bug; the team viewed sessions through closed-circuit TV. Clients were offered a maximum of six sessions, 1–3 weeks apart.
Families' backgrounds	Families offered therapy had severe problems with adolescent children, many of whom were on the brink of going into care.
Families' pathways to therapy	12 out of 32 had contacted Social Services before. 22 out of 32 were referred by other professionals.
Families' attendance record at sessions	139 sessions were booked but only 85 were kept; an attendance rate of 61 per cent.
Research interviews (undertaken after therapy had been completed – July 1985–July 1986)	Interviews were offered to 34 families in the study period; 32 accepted being interviewed: i.e. 21 out of 22 who accepted therapy and 11 out of 12 who rejected therapy. All family members from 29 of these 32 were interviewed so data was incomplete for only three families.

Main findings

Howe reports that the 21 families successfully engaged by therapists (and interviewed by him) could be divided into three categories:

1 *Relaxed and satisfied group* (3 families)
   These families remained in therapy, became engaged and felt that they could be helped. This group found the therapist friendly, valued his or her explanations, liked meeting as a family, and thought it appropriate to meet away from home. All three families felt helped by therapy but in one case the index client's behaviour got worse.
2 *The ambivalent group* (4 families)
   These families remained in therapy, were not engaged but still held on to the prospect of being helped. They felt that the therapist had them 'over a barrel', that they had to do it the therapist's way and that there was a clash of understanding between the family and the therapist. Typically they felt like guinea-pigs. None of these families felt helped by therapy.
3 *The early leavers* (14 families)
   These families withdrew early, were not engaged and did not have any prospect of being helped. According to Howe their unease about being in therapy hinged around 'machines, method and manner'. They disliked the video, the method (especially the supervisor who was connected to the therapist by a telephone) and the cold manner of the therapist which made them feel on trial. They also disliked the fact that their children were present

during the session. The room was experienced as uncomfortable and the supervisor as inquisitorial. All power was believed to lie with the supervisors who, though unseen themselves, were all-seeing.

Howe's conclusions concerning the engagement phase of therapy

Howe reports that families found that family therapy departed significantly from what they had expected, their usual experience of relating to an outside agent and their usual experience of relating to each other in the family.

> Clients will not follow, will not become engaged in emotional expeditions without discussion, rehearsal and reassurance. . . .
>
> All families felt that an introductory phase before therapy began was crucial so that they could cope with the transition from 'everyday ways of behaving' to 'extraordinary ways of behaving'. 'Relax me' was the prevailing message. Families wanted to be approached 'gently and sensitively, thoughtfully and slowly'. What was a familiar routine and taken-for-granted way of operating for the therapist is a unique and peculiar experience for the family.
>
> (Howe, 1989, pp. 58–59)

Howe's conclusions concerning users' understanding of the overall therapeutic process

According to Howe, families had a great need to understand two things – their problem and their experience of being in family therapy. The stance of the therapists, however, was to focus on behaviour rather than to develop an understanding. They believed that they should concentrate on changing the family behaviour and not worry about whether family members understood how the changes took place. So the situation was non-reflexive – the family was treated as the *object* not the subject of therapy. The rules for the family were therefore different from the rules for the therapists. Families could only make better sense of their situation if they behaved differently and could then reflect upon how the change had been achieved. The therapists could make sense of what was happening theoretically – they were informed by their intellectual effort and not just by the behavioural changes that occurred. So whereas the therapists could create new understandings, which could be matched with new experiences for them, this formula was not extended to the families, who were left adrift to struggle to understand what was happening to them. So, for therapists, theoretical understanding produced practice, but for clients practice alone was expected to produce understanding. Crucially, in a situation where *therapy failed to produce such behavioural change*, family members were left with neither a better understanding of their problems nor of their experience of therapy. The explanatory vacuum was filled by their assuming that they were being investigated and judged, manipulated and used, misled and maligned by a technique that defied understanding.

According to Howe, the majority of families did not feel that they were understood by their therapists on their own terms. There was a clash of understanding. Families were puzzled by lack of warmth and friendliness. Sessions were dominated by the therapists who were responsible for setting the agenda. Families felt they had no power to introduce discussions of issues that they (rather than the therapists) wanted to place on the agenda.

Howe's overarching conclusion is that systemic family therapy is unable to understand the significance of individual personal experience. It banishes the subjectivity of the user and prevents a genuine dialogue taking place between users and their therapists. Systemic family therapy is a one-sided encounter which involves users being disempowered by therapists who are themselves empowered by techniques and structures such as videotaping and supervision through an ear-bug, which are utilized unilaterally in order to enhance the power of the therapist.

Philippa Seligman's review of Howe's book does not address the crucial ethical and philosophical issues that lie at the heart of his critique. Our reading of his book is a sympathetic one because we share his preoccupations, if not necessarily his conclusions. The book's major strength is that it records users' impressions about being in therapy – it is, therefore, full of telling anecdotes which cannot easily be dismissed. For example, one family commented that their social worker was friendly and approachable when he called on a home visit, prior to beginning therapy with them. In the therapy room itself, he became transformed into a robot apparently controlled by his supervisor (in the adjacent room), who gave him instructions via an ear-bug.

Sigurd was in a similar position many years ago when setting up a family therapy clinic within a Social Services setting. A group of social workers interested in developing a family therapy approach within mainstream social work decided to meet together for a session a fortnight. A new video system was set up in place of a one-way screen together with an ear-bug system, and on the appointed afternoon the first family duly arrived. Sigurd had worked with 8-year-old Shane, his father and stepmother for some time in their home because of Shane's cruelty to animals and extremely disruptive behaviour at home and at school. Sigurd had enjoyed a good rapport with them all, and they had hesitantly agreed to come to the office to receive something that was intended to be better than what he had offered them at home. It was not long into the first session before Sigurd started talking to them according to a format and as if he had not met them before. They clearly felt awkward and Sigurd felt awkward as well, but he was desperate to break away from the previous homely, rather unfocused and what he thought was slightly 'collusive' style of home visiting. He was rapidly becoming one of the 'talking dummies' referred to by one of David Howe's respondents.

Having mistakenly adhered to a first-interview schedule, Sigurd realized by the end of the session that he was losing the family and that this was also likely to be the last interview. The stepmother left a message the following week saying that the situation had improved and they would not need to come again. A month later Sigurd discovered that Shane was in a children's home.

In this case, office-based family sessions could have played an important part in the overall package offered to the family, but a user-friendly perspective would have taken account of such matters as timing, issues of transition from home- to office-based interviewing, style of interview, and attention to blame-inducing procedures. It would also have challenged my need to have 'clinic cases' in order to inaugurate the Family Therapy Clinic.

David Howe's book is partisan – he abhors systemic approaches and his research data undoubtedly supports his idea that such approaches run the risk of being dehumanizing. However, we interpret his results more optimistically than he does because we believe that family therapists can learn from them. The crucial lesson for us is that therapy that is not custom-built to meet users' needs as they see them is likely to fail. The families studied by Howe had acting-out teenagers who were on the brink of going into care. Such families often have major problems to do with unemployment, alcoholism, illness and trans-generational patterns of abuse.

Whether a therapy package of only six sessions can possibly be of help is a very open question. Some families can respond if there is a careful clarification of realistic goals but other families, if given an opportunity, will want to work on a longer-term basis because they see their needs as different. Forcing such families to accept a six-session contract because that is the only one on offer is clearly user-unfriendly and fails to address a point that we will discuss in a later chapter – families differ in terms of their needs and their style of problem-solving. Offering them a short contract may be to force them to accept an offer that may not suit them. This is particularly true of families in which trust is a major issue.

So our understanding of the significance of Howe's work (as we hope to have demonstrated) is different from that of both the reviewers that we have cited. However, before moving on from Howe's work it is important to attempt to set his work against the background of other research into the value of family therapy. Howe's findings are uncomfortable for the family therapy movement but there are other findings which are equally problematic. For example, it is crucial to the movement to ask the straightforward question, how effective is family therapy?

EFFICACY AND FAMILY THERAPY

Alan Gurman, David Kniskern and William Pinsof (1986), in a much cited chapter in the *Handbook of Psychotherapy and Behavior Change*, edited by Garfield and Bergin, have argued that outcome studies generally support the idea that family therapy is efficacious. However, if we examine their findings about the efficacy of the major models of family therapy, then we discover an interesting paradox. Table 1, collating findings for no fewer than 15 models of therapy, is reproduced from that book chapter (with slight alterations to the footnotes made by us). The ratings recorded in each column signify the following: 3 means effectiveness is established; 2 effectiveness is probable; 1 effectiveness is uncertain; 0 effectiveness is untested.

Table 1 Overall estimates of the effectiveness of various marital and family therapies for specific disorders and problems

Type of therapy	Adult disorders				Psycho-somatic disorders	Child/adolescent disorders			Marital problems	
	Schizo-phrenia	Substance abuse	Affective disorders	Anxiety disorders		Juvenile delinquency	Conduct disorders	Mixed disorders	Marital discord	Divorce adjustment
Behavioral	2[a]	2[b]	1	3[c]	0	3[d]	3[d]	0	3	1[e]
Bowen FST	0	0	0	0	0	0	0	0	0	0
Contextual[j]	0	0	0	0	0	0	0	0	0	0
Functional[k]	0	0	0	0	0	2	0	0	0	0
Humanistic[f]	0	0	0	0	0	0	0	0	0	0
McMaster PCSTF	0	0	0	0	1	1	1	1	1	0
Milan Systemic	0	0	0	0	0	1	1	1	1	0
MRI Interactional	0	0	0	0	0	0	1	1	1	0
Multigenerational: other[g]	0	0	0	0	0	0	0	0	1	0
Psychoeducational	3	0	1	0	0	0	0	0	0	0
Psychodynamic-Eclectic	0	2[h]	0	0	1	0	1	1	2	1
Strategic	1	2[i]	0	0	1	0	0	0	0	0
Structural	0	2[i]	0	0	2	0	0	0	0	0
Symbolic-Experiential[l]	0	0	0	0	0	0	0	0	0	0
Triadic[m]	0	0	0	0	0	0	0	1	0	0

Note: 3 = effectiveness established; 2 = effectiveness probable; 1 = effectiveness uncertain; 0 = effectiveness untested

a = Behavioral Family Management
b = Alcohol abuse
c = Spouse-assisted exposure therapy
d = Parent Management Training
e = Divorce mediation
f = Satir
g = Based on Framo and Williamson
h = Conjoint couples groups for alcoholism
i = Integrative Structural/Strategic Therapy (Stanton)
j = Boszormenyi-Nagy
k = Barton and Alexander
l = Whitaker
m = Zuk

A close examination of this table reveals some interesting, if not worrying, findings. First, most models are not supported by any empirical findings. Second, if we use the criterion of 'effectiveness established' (rating 3), then only two models (the behavioural and the psychoeducational) stand up to examination – all the others fail to produce convincing results. This finding is discomfiting but it is worth noting that experiential, humanistic and psychodynamic models are least supported by this table (a finding that is at variance with Sue Walrond-Skinner's argument). Admittedly the research summarized here is outcome research rather than surveys of consumer satisfaction but we nevertheless believe that it is true to say that major theorists like Bowen, Boszormenyi-Nagy, Satir and Whitaker have shown remarkably little interest either in validating their results or recording what their users experience when they are at the receiving end of therapy.

As Andy has argued elsewhere (Treacher, 1983; Pilgrim and Treacher, 1992), there is little evidence demonstrating that the day-to-day practice of psychotherapy is directly influenced by outcome research findings. We can find no evidence that supports the idea that therapists are attracted to particular models of psychotherapy because there is convincing scientific evidence supporting the efficacy of the model. The attraction of the model is at a personal and not a rational-scientific level. As an illustration of this point, it is worth briefly reviewing a recent paper of Alan Carr (1991), who has effectively filled a gap in Gurman, Kniskern and Pinsof's table by reviewing Milan-style Family Therapy (MFT) published after the earlier review. The popularity of MFT increased strongly during the 1980s, particularly in Europe, but as Carr has recorded, the evidence supporting the model is no more convincing than for other forms of therapy. The majority of the studies surveyed by Carr were published between 1989 and 1991, that is, long after the model began to have a significant impact on the family therapy movement. Admittedly Carr does cite two earlier studies by Ian Bennun (1986, 1988) but it is ironic that Bennun himself has apparently abandoned using the Milan approach. Particularly in relation to schizophrenic users, he is now an advocate of the family management approach (see Bennun, 1993, for an exploration of his current approach).

Carr's study collated 10 studies which met unstated 'minimal methodological requirements'. Four were comparative outcome studies, two were process studies, one a single group outcome study, two were consumer surveys and the tenth was a clinical audit of a series of patients. In fact, as Carr himself points out (and a colleague of ours, Eddy Street (1994), has also noted), the 10 studies are impossible to interpret meaningfully because there was no quality control of therapy, that is, there was no attempt to define operationally what was meant by MFT. Since MFT is a continually evolving method of working, with distinctive differences between the model adopted in the late 1970s and that of the late 1980s, we are not left any the wiser about what features of MFT are crucial in producing positive therapeutic outcome.

From our point of view it is also interesting to note that the only study we can find (Meeda Mashal, Ronald Feldman and John Sigal, 1989) that asked users to express their views about how they felt about being in MFT therapy recorded an almost 50 per cent dissatisfaction rate. Parents in particular tended to dislike the team behind the screen and for fathers the long delay between sessions and overall length of treatment was disliked. Interestingly, 62 per cent of families sought further therapy from non-MFT practitioners. (See Chapter 9 for a further discussion of this important study.)

We should hasten to add that Milan-style therapists should not be singled out for criticism on this score. As therapists we are all in the same boat – what is required of us is the honesty to discuss openly how and why we are attracted to the model we use. Too often we retreat behind a scientific smoke-screen that obscures the fact that we are clearly not neutral and impartial professionals who are solely motivated by the desire to satisfy the needs of our users. We have feet of clay and are just as subject to career pressures as other professionals. In later chapters we will explore our own understanding of how and why we came to choose the model of family therapy (structural family therapy) that we are comfortable with and how our ideas have developed, not least because of users' views. However, in order to conclude this chapter we will explore another facet of the family therapy movement which is a cause for concern.

DISSEMINATING FAMILY THERAPY KNOWLEDGE

Through examining Gurman, Kniskern and Pinsof's work we have been able to establish that therapists' enthusiasm for different models of family therapy within the movement is not based upon scientific studies of efficacy. If efficacy were the main criterion for the success of a model, then it is clearly the behavioural model that should have pride of place, and yet this model has received relatively little professional attention within family therapy circles, especially in Britain. What, then, decides whether a given model has an impact or not? Unfortunately, as we have already pointed out, we know of no empirical studies that help us answer this question but an American anthropologist, Athena McLean (1986), has written an interesting and challenging exploration of how family therapy knowledge is constructed. She focuses in particular on the significance of family therapy demonstration workshops, and stresses – quite correctly in our opinion – that they have played a disproportionate role in influencing the development of the family therapy movement. McLean was employed as a researcher for about 12 years in three different psychiatric institutions. She was encouraged to attend workshops as part of her job and she used her experience of attending one of them as the main springboard for developing her critique. She describes the format of the workshop as follows:

> The demonstration workshop . . . was a two-day presentation – a 'dialogue' between two internationally known family systems therapists, both psychiatrists. . . . During the morning of the first day, one of the therapists treated one family. In the afternoon the second therapist treated . . . [another] . . .

family. On the second day, they exchanged families although at points both therapists appeared together with each of the families. The therapy sessions were videotaped and viewed by an audience of several hundred people. During breaks in the sessions the therapists 'dialogued' about the families' problems, discussing their differing approaches to treating the families. Occasionally the audience was given the opportunity to join the discussion. Then the therapist would re-enter the room and resume treatment, and afterwards the dialogue would continue.

(McLean, 1986, p. 109)

McLean reports that the two families used in the demonstration had been recruited from the institute that organized the workshop. They were already in treatment with another clinician but the 'demonstration' therapists were singularly uninterested either in previous work or in following their progress after the workshop ended. The invitation of the workshop, as McLean argues, was to behave like gurus who 'could convey their ability to treat the families virtually blind'. After the workshop it was the regular clinicians who would have to continue the treatment.

As McLean argues in precise detail, the families were, in fact, conned into participating in the workshop. They were indeed informed of the special chance on offer to receive family therapy from two internationally recognized experts but they were, of course, not told that they were being involved in the workshop. They signed the standard release form which permits video recordings of therapy to be used in the future for professional and training purposes but, as McLean comments, '[they] were not told, however, that for all practical purposes their therapy sessions were being observed "live" by several hundred people' (p. 109).

What happened in practice was that the session was indeed recorded but it was then replayed to the audience after a two- or three-minute delay. This ploy protected the institute legally but in practice it created a near-tragic situation as McLean points out:

[At] breaks (in the workshop) and at the end of each session the therapist left the room and discussed the 'case' with the audience while the family were still in the clinic, unaware that they were currently being 'studied' by a large audience who had purchased the opportunity to observe them. This fact was almost revealed to one of the families when several persons from the audience swarmed into a rest room discussing the morning 'case', only to discover some of the members of that family there!

(MacLean, 1986, p. 109)

But, as McLean reports, it was not just the structure of the workshop that was disturbing from an ethical point of view. Some of the therapeutic tactics adopted by one of the therapists were equally questionable:

On the second day one of the . . . [family therapists] . . . upon reviewing the situation of one family, observed the powerful position of control that the mother enjoyed in the family. He blithely declared that if the son were to be saved from becoming schizophrenic, the mother would have to 'go crazy', as would the father eventually. He then proceeded to conduct therapy with the family in a way that successfully provoked a hysterical outburst from the mother. This irate woman was understandably reacting to the demeaning manner in which she was being treated. She cried profusely, insistently demanding an explanation from the therapist for his behaviour towards her. He responded smugly '*I am* the doctor; I don't *have* to explain myself', only intensifying her rage as he promptly walked out with the other therapist who was present. . . . Their exit was accompanied by support throughout the audience, as evidenced by vigorous applause.

(McLean, 1989, p. 109)

McLean's account is fascinating to us because her example is an illustration of how an apparently well-meaning and committed therapist can behave in a staggeringly user-unfriendly way. Chapters 3 and 4 of our book will attempt to probe some historical developments within the family therapy movement which provide an explanation of how this contradiction could arise. McLean undertakes a similar task in her paper but her initial interpretation of the significance of the workshop is undoubtedly worth recording because it helps us to gain an insight into one of the ways family therapy knowledge is propagated.

McLean's first point concerns the peculiar role of charismatic figures in the family therapy movement:

It ought to be noted, for example, that within the field of family therapy, therapists as well known as the two in the 'dialogue' frequently carry a mystique and are regarded as charismatic [2].

Footnote 2 (not cited here), in fact, leads the reader to the following personal experience related by McLean herself:

I became well aware of this phenomenon (of adulation for charismatic figures) . . . during a break at another demonstration workshop where a young woman approached the renowned female therapist who was conducting it and asked "May I touch you? I have always looked forward to the day when I might be able to touch you".

We would argue that McLean has succeeded in highlighting an important pheno-menon within the family therapy movement which must be a cause for concern. The development of the movement has been disproportionately shaped by the influence of charismatic leaders performing (literally) as showmen (term used advisedly) at important conferences and workshops. Not surprisingly, clinicians are predominantly influenced by fellow practitioners who offer them pragmatic solutions to the problems that they face in day-to-day practice. They are usually not paid to undertake research and any time they spend consuming research (reading journals, attending research conferences, etc.) usually creates further problems for them because of their necessity to be constantly 'processing' users. Many private practitioners suffer from this pressure most acutely because any time not spent with users is a luxury since no fee can be charged.

It is perhaps not surprising that the influence of guru-style workshops is powerful. Typically, apparently highly effective – even charismatic – interventions are demonstrated by skilful practitioners who are excellent showmen. Failures are typically not shared and there is usually little attention paid to research findings. Many of the presenters of such workshops actually earn their living from their presentations so there is often a built-in marketing factor which militates against presenters being objective about their own successes and failures. Only good news about successes is communicated because to talk of failure is risky. People might be put off attending and defect to other presenters who claim more success.

There are, of course, honourable exceptions to the trend that we have just described. Some presenters are very ethical and will present their failures as well as their successes but family therapy has, in our opinion, suffered from its popularity. There is too little long-term painstaking research undertaken so that most clinical models are not tried and tested and refined over a long period of time. For us the work of Gerald Patterson (with families that have delinquent children) and Chris Dare (with families with anorexic children) are particularly good examples of long-term action research projects which provide us with a different model for developing family therapy. Both projects have been concerned with developing user-friendly, teamwork approaches which do not rely on the skills of charismatic therapists. Such approaches are painstaking and rely upon producing small but significant changes in the behaviour of family members – unfortunately they do not involve the type of within-session drama that makes for good video viewing at conferences. So it is perhaps not surprising that despite being supported by consistent research findings, neither approach has received the attention in family therapy circles that it deserves.

We believe this is an issue of fashionableness. Family therapy, as we have already begun to demonstrate, is a curiously ungrounded way of undertaking therapy. When historians come to write a critical history of the movement we are sure that they will remark upon its curious evolution. To us the movement seems to be all head and no feet. That is to say, it is prone to epistemological flights of fancy at the cost of grounding itself in painstaking and consistent research – a theme which we will return to again and again in the course of this book. Currently family therapy seems to be subject to a wave of therapies based upon ideas derived from second-order cybernetics. No doubt there are some important developments taking place because of the impact of these ideas but we are struck by the fact that there is, yet again, a crucial 'research gap' demonstrated by these approaches. Enthusiasm for the epistemological innovations that flow from these approaches is strangely bracketed with a lack of interest in how users experience them. In other words, therapeutic innovations seem once more to be driven by the preoccupations of therapists and not by a central concern for the development of services which are sensitive to, and respectful of, users' experiences of being in therapy.

It is possible to argue that we have overstated our case concerning family therapy workshops and the impact of fashionable ideas in family therapy. Indeed the impact of family therapy gurus does seem to be on the wane particularly as family therapy courses are becoming more firmly established in this country following the example of the USA, where there are hundreds of well-established courses. However, it is an open question whether courses actually train trainees to be capable of scrutinizing the basis of the models of family therapy that are taught. Courses are often monolithic and induct trainees into working within a single model. The structure of the course does not usually allow them to challenge the ethics of the model to which they are exposed. Professional bodies such as the Association for Family Therapy and the American Association of Marital and Family Therapy, have laid down guidelines for accrediting courses which do attempt to build in safeguards which inhibit this process, but they fail to address the vulnerability of trainees whose chances of graduating from a given course are so dependent on the say-so of their trainers.

DOES FAMILY THERAPY HAVE A FUTURE?

We are comforted by the knowledge that we are not alone in having second thoughts about how family therapy practice has evolved. Perhaps the most celebrated figure in the family therapy movement who has been prepared to explore her second and third thoughts about therapy is Lynn Hoffman. Ironically her classic book *Foundations of Family Therapy: A Conceptual Framework for Systems Change* (1981) was often cited as one of the most definitive summaries of systems theorizing and yet Hoffman has abandoned most of the ideas contained in the book (see Chapter 11 for further discussion of this point). Hoffman's change of direction is striking in a movement beset by competing schools that are often very effective at advertising the certainty that their way of undertaking therapy is best or briefest or both.

Since professions are typically inwardly directed and self-seeking there is usually little discussion within a given profession of the significance of the historical changes that occur within a profession. Mordecai Kaffman's (1987) paper published in the *Journal of Family Therapy* is an interesting example of such a discussion – it touches on important issues but in our opinion does not really dig deep enough. The observations shared are intriguing, as the following quotation reveals, but the reader may be left somewhat bemused about what conclusions to draw.

Kaffman argues that psychotherapy movements typically have a four-stage life cycle:

> Each of the first three stages spans about a decade. In the first, pioneering stage the initiator or small group of 'founding fathers' (*sic*) of the new method of therapy seek to gain a certain Lebensraum for their idea by publications, workshops and other ways of presenting the rationale behind the new

technique and its advantages over other approaches. The pioneers of the new method describe, in writing or on video, the clinical work they did with a small number of patients, all of them exhibiting significant improvement in their condition thanks to the new therapeutic procedure. In the second phase the circle of adherents . . . widens, as the pioneers are joined by trainees and others, and so does the stream of reported therapeutic successes. Omnipotence marks the third stage, particularly among the disciples of the original founders who report an ever-growing number of successful outcomes. By this time, many people in the profession are convinced that the new therapy model may be used successfully so widely that there is hardly a clinical problem beyond its reach. In the fourth period, some 30 years after the therapeutic model was first presented, a certain 'sobering up' occurs – something like a gradual return from an euphoric 'trip' back to a more balanced view of reality. At this stage, the first self-critical comments begin to appear, dealing with the constraints and limitations of what has changed from an experiential novelty to a recognized orthodoxy. One by one, therapists begin to report disillusionment and even failure. It is precisely at this stage – some 35 years after the appearance of the first paper in praise of psychoanalysis – that Freud published his recapitulation of the failures and weaknesses of psychoanalysis as a therapeutic technique in his courageous article 'Analysis terminable and interminable'. In similar fashion, exactly 35 years after a number of pioneers took the initial steps to introduce conjoint family therapy as a new method of treatment, a book entitled *Failures in Family Therapy* (Coleman, 1985), the first of its kind, made its appearance.

(Kaffman, 1987, p. 308)

Kaffman's statement is, we think, overly schematic – it is a pity from our point of view that he did not try to explore both the history of psychoanalysis and family therapy in more detail – but nevertheless we think his approach is valuable in understanding some of the changes that have occurred in family therapy. We think he puts too much stress on the magical number (35 years) and he singularly overlooks the fact that the psychoanalytic movement has a strong penchant for suppressing dissident accounts (e.g. the failure to publish Sandor Ferenczi's diary for 50 years, an issue we explore in detail in Chapter 3).

The strength of his approach is that it opens up the question of whether psychotherapy movements create situations in which they learn from the users they work with. Kaffman gives us a typically professional (top-down) explanation for the changes that occurred but the reality that he overlooks is that it is extremely painful for therapists when they fail to help the users with whom they are working. Therapists find all sorts of ways of insulating themselves from the fact that they have failed but truly reflective practitioners, who have the honesty to face the fact that they have on occasion failed their users, can learn a great deal from examining these failures. For example, Jenny Jenkins *et al.* have warned against terming families 'resistant', and have brought back the term 'counter-transference' to explain how easily therapists can become inflexible because of their own concerns. They continue:

> When we succeed in helping families change for the better we are keen to take the credit. When we fail we may well be right in deeming the family resistant, but we should add the rider that *we* were unable to help the family overcome its anxieties.
>
> (Jenkins *et al.*, 1982, p. 309)

Kaffman's analysis is useful because it helps us to have some sense of our own relationship to the life cycle of family therapy. We would argue that we are contributing to the fourth period – the 'sobering up' period.

CONCLUSION

This chapter, by reviewing quite disparate facets of contemporary family therapy, has attempted to set the scene for the rest of the book. We have intentionally started by looking at the dark side of the development of the family therapy movement. We firmly believe that family therapy has an important role in helping a wide range of users. However, we would insist that considerable changes need to be made if family therapy is to live up to its potential. In our opinion family therapy has been too strongly influenced by practitioners who are fascinated by versions of systems theory that are anti-humanistic. Within first-order cybernetics, users are rendered invisible since they are no longer primarily construed as being human. They become 'subsystems', inanimate parts of larger systems which can be dealt with as dispassionately as a car mechanic deals with an engine that fails to function correctly. Within second-order frameworks, users are apparently more visible but we would still argue that although the therapist in these models is invited to co-construct therapy with users, the *methods* utilized are never negotiated. For example, the systematic use of interventive inter-viewing techniques may appear to be user-friendly but the therapist within this model still calls the shots – there is no attempt to custom-build therapy in the true sense of the phrase.

In Chapter 3 we take one step back before exploring the issues raised by the present chapter. This step back is necessary, we believe, because family therapists are adept at ignoring issues that are important in the wider psycho-therapy movement. In this chapter we have explored several criticisms of family therapy but we have held on to the idea that an ethically sound, user-friendly form of family therapy is possible and essential. However, there are important and influential critics who have insisted that all forms of psychotherapy are intrin-sically damaging. In our next chapter we explore the crucial work of Jeffrey Masson, who has recently challenged the psychotherapy movement in very fundamental ways. We have found his criticisms so important that it has proved impossible for us to write our book without attempting to refute them.

Chapter 3

Coming to terms with Jeffrey Masson

Andy Treacher

INTRODUCTION

In Chapter 2 we explored David Howe's research which appears at first viewing to be so damaging to family therapy. Howe attacks therapies based upon systems theory but is willing to acknowledge that other forms of psychotherapy, based on humanistic concepts, are valid in helping users. In this chapter we will explore other critics of psychotherapy who take a much more radical stance. Interestingly, these critics, who have taken it upon themselves to criticize psychotherapy on behalf of users, tend to demonstrate a curious lack of interest in empirical studies that have revealed that users can have both bad *and good* experiences of psychotherapy. In reviewing their work we do not want to blunt their criticisms but at the same time we do want to utilize their ideas, if possible, to change the way that we conceptualize the role of the therapist in helping users to change the way that they grapple with the problems of living that prompt them to seek help in the first place.

In the 1970s it was Ivan Illich who led an onslaught on medicine and the caring professions in general. He insisted that caring professions, like all professions, are self-seeking cabals which tend to place their own needs before the needs of their users. His books, such as *The Limits of Medicine: Medical Nemesis – the Expropriation of Health* (1975) and *Disabling Professions* (Illich and colleagues, 1977), will always be uncomfortable reading for anybody in the caring professions but as paid professionals who provide a service we not unexpectedly cannot agree with his radical dismissal of all professionals as disabling. If we did agree fully with him, then we would have to resign in order to avoid accusations of blatant hypocrisy. However, Illich's critique raises issues for us that are important in writing this book. We passionately believe that family therapy can be helpful to families, but at the same time we are fully aware that therapy can be dangerous because it runs the risk of depoliticizing (an ugly term for an ugly process) issues that require political intervention.

Illich, writing in his usual grandiose style, draws attention to this issue in the following passage taken from *Disabling Professions*:

> One way to close an age is to give it a name that sticks. I propose that we name the mid-twentieth century, The Age of Disabling Professions, an age when

people had 'problems', experts had 'solutions' and scientists measured impon-
derables such as 'abilities' and 'needs'. This age is now at an end, just as the
age of energy splurges has ended. The illusions that made both ages possible
are increasingly visible to common sense. But no public choice has yet been
made. Social acceptance of the illusion of professional omniscience and
omnipotence may result either in compulsory political creeds (with their
accompanying versions of a new fascism) or in yet another historical emer-
gence of neo-Promethean but essentially ephemeral follies. Informed choice
requires that we examine the specific role of the professions in determining
who got what from whom and why, in this age.

(Illich, 1977, pp. 11–12)

Many researchers, commentators and users have, of course, written copiously
about 'who got what from whom and why' both before and after Illich issued his
invitation. Ideally, we should attempt to review this literature extensively, but the
scope of our book prevents us from doing so. However, whether we like it or not,
we feel that we do have to come to terms with Jeffrey Masson's book *Against
Therapy* (1990), which has thrown down the gauntlet to all psychotherapists.

It may at first sight seem rather curious that we should have chosen to pay so
much attention to Masson's work, which concentrates so heavily on psychoanalysis. However, we are sympathetic to the American family therapist Deborah
Luepnitz's (1988) view that one of the major weaknesses of family therapy is its
failure to come to terms with its history. Masson, in examining crucial historical
and ethical issues concerning psychoanalysis, opens up a whole range of issues
for discussion which are normally ignored by family therapists. Many leading
theorists have unfortunately created a climate of opinion within the family
therapy movement that stresses the discontinuity between the movement and
other psychotherapy traditions. Masson's work reminds us that there are striking
continuities that we ignore at our peril.

MASSON'S CHALLENGE TO PSYCHOTHERAPY

Curiously, Masson makes no mention of Illich and yet his book is written from a
very similar standpoint. Masson's challenge to psychotherapy is at times devastating. His critique of psychoanalysis is particularly savage – thanks to his
training as an analyst, he speaks with an insider's knowledge of the type of abuse
that can be perpetrated by therapists working within this tradition. He also
develops some penetrating criticisms of other schools of therapy, including
Rogerian client-centred therapy, family therapy and Ericksonian hypnotherapy.
In fact, Masson is prepared to criticize all forms of psychotherapy and to scru-
tinize the reputations of leading psychotherapists and family therapists. Freud,
Jung, Perls, Rogers, Erickson, Minuchin and Haley are amongst others whose
work is probed and analysed, but one of the most disturbing sections of the book
concerns the work of the American psychiatrist John Rosen, whose methods,
according to Masson, influenced many people (including Haley) in the 1950s and

1960s. Rosen's psychotherapeutic methods included vicious ways of confronting clients. The beating up of clients was justified as part of his method (so-called 'direct analysis') and some clients even died mysterious deaths while in his care. Rosen's methods also involved sexually abusing clients. Rosen and his staff regularly participated in the kidnapping of clients who were then subsequently held illegally in several psychiatric units to which he had access.

Perhaps the most frightening aspect of the whole gruesome tale is that Rosen (who eventually achieved an international reputation as an innovative therapist) was not denounced by anybody from his own profession. It was the bravery of a few of his ex-patients which finally led to his being charged with 67 violations of the Pennsylvania Medical Practices Act and 33 violations of the rules and regulations of the Medical Board. Infuriatingly, Rosen was never tried for these violations. By handing in his licence voluntarily, he escaped any further action being taken against him, so he has never been properly brought to book for any of the crimes he committed. Masson reports that the parents of an ex-patient did sue him successfully but the case was settled out of court for $100,000 and it was Rosen's insurance company that settled the bill so Rosen was not even out of pocket.

Masson uses an American example to help build his case against psychotherapy, but we should hasten to add that he could also have used examples from Britain. The use of pin-down in Staffordshire children's homes and the notorious regime of Beck in children's homes in Leicestershire are recent examples of British therapists abusing their power in frightening ways.

Masson's own comments about the significance of Rosen are undoubtedly controversial, because he refuses to accept that Rosen's behaviour was an isolated phenomenon.

> The events that took place tell us a great deal about psychotherapy in the United States. To learn about what John Rosen did to his patients may make the reader feel that Rosen belongs to a nightmare world of cruelty and gross excesses. I do not believe this is true. John Rosen is one of many, many therapists *who harm their patients under the guise of their greater wisdom*. He merely had the misfortune of being caught. There is nothing unusual about what he did to his patients. In many other disguises this kind of treatment goes undetected in thousands of psychiatric institutions throughout the United States. Indeed, far worse things happen on a daily basis. John Rosen is really only a tip of the iceberg. But he is symbolic because he was so praised by his colleagues when his star was ascending, and, perhaps even more telling for our purposes, once his crimes were exposed for the world to see, those same colleagues became strangely reluctant to speak about them. I am aware of only a handful of psychiatrists who are willing to publicly denounce what John Rosen stands for though privately, of course, most psychiatrists fulminate as loudly as anyone about these abuses. This solidarity tells us even more about psychotherapy than does exposure of a single case of abuse.
>
> (Masson 1990, p. 166. Emphasis added by SR and AT)

Some critics of Masson will attempt to dismiss his arguments by insisting that he confabulates institutional care with psychotherapeutic care. They will make a great play of the fact that the two men he exposes most prominently (John Rosen and his disciple Albert Honig) exploited their patients most blatantly in in-patient settings. It is undoubtedly true that in-patients are more vulnerable to abuse (because of their lack of concurrent contact with family and friends) but Rosen did not just work in secluded institutional settings. He shared his work (and demonstrated his abusiveness) with colleagues in the prestigious Department of Psychiatry at Temple University Medical School. Incredibly, one of Rosen's colleagues, Morris Brody, published a book in 1959 (*Observations on Direct Analysis: The Therapeutic Techniques of Dr John N. Rosen*) which actually records his observations of Rosen physically abusing and sexually harassing a young woman patient (see Masson, 1990, pp. 193–194 (footnote) for a brief summary of Brody's report). Brody was convinced that Rosen was an inspired healer so how could he have possibly been abusive?

Masson has a clear answer to this question. In a key passage in the book he argues that

> abuse of one form or another is built into the very fabric of psychotherapy in that power corrupts, that psychiatric power corrupts just as political power does, and that the greater the power (and a psychiatrist's power is greater indeed), the greater the propensity for corruption. Even more than politicians, therapists, by the very nature of their profession, are protected from usual forms of scrutiny. Psychotherapy is a self-policing profession. The psycho-therapeutic relationship is a privileged one, protected by a tradition of secrecy (usually called 'confidentiality'). Psychotherapists almost always encourage their patients not to speak about what happens during a session. To do so is branded a form of acting out. Talking (and, by extension, talking about the faults of the therapist) outside the session about the session is considered to dilute the force of the therapy. It is a diversion of energy, so goes the rationalization, but one that, conveniently, insulates the patient from the community of family and friends. The very fact of investing in therapy, both financially and emotionally, means that one is bound to attempt to protect it from criticism. . . . The ways that a therapist can harm a patient are as varied as they are in any intimate relationship. A person can be harmed financially (paying more money than is comfortable, or, if rich, being exploited for financial information) emotionally, physically (e.g. becoming dependent on drugs), and sexually.
>
> (Masson, 1990, pp. 210–211)

This is a very powerful statement which causes us, as family therapists, immense heart-searchings. If Masson is right, then we would need to resign and we could not continue writing this book. Our position is to accept many aspects of Masson's argument but to balk at full agreement with him. We would unreservedly accept that psychotherapeutic relationships can be exploitative but this does not mean that they are necessarily so. Masson is curiously very dismissive of clients' views concerning psychotherapy. Although he does not argue the point in any detail, it is clear from reading his book that he assumes that clients are basically deluded if they do report that psychotherapy is beneficial to them. Masson is clearly in difficulties over this issue because elsewhere in the book he argues that the major problem with psychotherapists is that they assume that they have greater wisdom than their clients. But it is Masson's 'greater wisdom' that enables him to argue that clients' views can be ignored.

It is difficult for us to escape the recursive trap of arguing that our wisdom enables us to rebut Masson's position but we would nevertheless insist that clients' views about, and experiences of, psychotherapy *must* and can be respectfully considered if we are to arrive at any conclusions about its value. Masson's concentration on the abuses that psychotherapists have perpetrated blinds him to any assessment of the positive case for psychotherapy. Our policy is to use Masson's important criticisms to sharpen our case for developing family therapy as a user-friendly approach. *Against Therapy* is a very important book and we cannot do it adequate justice in this volume. However, there are two major issues raised by Masson that we feel impelled to explore.

At first these issues (both concerned with psychoanalysis) will seem to have only peripheral relevance to our task of developing a critique of family therapy but in developing our ideas it is important for us to be aware of the crucial role that psychoanalysis played in shaping the development of all other psychotherapy movements. We would argue that psychoanalysis was, in fact, built upon very shaky foundations. Freud's attitude to his patients, as Masson demonstrates, was always highly equivocal and at crucial points in his career he was clearly motivated by his own personal and professional needs rather than the needs of his patients.

Freud's ability genuinely to listen to his patients

One of Masson's undoubted strengths is his ability to confront the myths and shibboleths of the psychoanalytic movement. His evaluation of Freud's account of the analysis of Dora (Ida Bauer) is particularly important. Dora's analysis is rightly considered to be crucial to the development of psychoanalysis and yet Masson convincingly demonstrates that Freud's treatment of her is both oppressive and destructive. In fact, it is clear even from Freud's own highly distorted account of the therapy that he does her harm under the guise of his (alleged) greater wisdom. Dora's father took her to Freud to be cured of her alleged depression but he was blatantly acting in bad faith. Dora's main complaint was that she had been sexually harassed by a friend of her father, Herr K, whose wife had been seduced by her (Dora's) own father. She felt, accurately from all accounts, that her father was expecting her to give in to Herr K's wishes so that he would then tolerate his wife's affair with Dora's father.

Freud listened to Dora's account with interest and was sufficiently honest to accept many aspects of it, but he insisted that she was not expressing her true feelings to him. He was, of course, the expert and assumed that she had feelings at a level outside consciousness which were the source of her symptoms. According to Masson, Freud was at first sympathetic to her account, but his sexist prejudices and her ability to stand up for her own point of view meant that the therapy was doomed from the start.

Freud disapproved of Dora's emancipated educational interests but at a deeper level his framing of Dora's response to Herr K's abusive sexual advances is clearly, in itself, abusive. Freud insists that Dora is hysterical because she does not respond to Herr K with sexual excitement when he attempts to seduce her in his office. Since Dora was 14 at the time of this event, Freud places himself in the position of actually condoning a criminal act. It is, of course, no surprise that Freud should take such a stance. He met Dora in 1906 at a time when he had already abandoned his earlier seduction hypothesis, i.e. that hysteria in adulthood was caused by actual sexual abuse in childhood. Faced by bitter opposition to his theory, Freud changed his position dramatically – instead of emphasizing the importance of real events occurring in the child's family, he began to develop his Oedipal theory which instead focused on biologically determined intrapsychic processes.

Many feminist writers have pilloried Freud for his grand betrayal on this issue and Masson himself has sided with them. Indeed, his book *The Assault on Truth: Freud and Sexual Abuse* (1992, but first published 1984) is correctly famous for its exposé of Freud's volte-face, which was a crucial turning point in the evolution of psychotherapy. Masson is strikingly, and perhaps unnecessarily, unsympathetic to Freud and does not really attempt to assess the enormous dilemma that Freud faced. If he had stuck to his original seduction theory position, he would have run the risk of being ostracized and having his career ruined. Tragically it seems that Freud did not have the courage to face these possibilities – he already felt very isolated within Viennese psychiatric circles and he felt the pressure of being the sole breadwinner for a large family very acutely.

Ironically, Freud needed the sort of courage that Masson himself has shown. Of course, Masson has been pilloried for exposing Freud by the American psychoanalytic movement, but his work has also been more subtly devalued by other commentators. For example, it is interesting to note how Deborah Luepnitz dismisses the impact of his book in her own very well reviewed book *The Family Interpreted: Feminist Theory in Clinical Practice* (1988). In Luepnitz's case she seems, ironically, to be more interested in providing a Freudian interpretation of Freud's behaviour than in establishing that his volte-face had enormous implications for the care of users who had been abused.

We believe, unlike Luepnitz, that Masson's analysis of Freud's management of Dora is convincing. Freud blatantly refused to listen to Dora's account of her distress. He operated from the outrageous premise that Dora should be flattered by Herr K's advances and that the best solution was for Dora to marry him, after he had duly divorced his wife. Dora knew instinctively that Freud only pretended to have her interests at heart and was fortunately assertive enough to refuse to go back to therapy after participating in a number of desultory sessions which she clearly found most unhelpful.

It is salutary to record that Freud's total failure to help Dora did not stop him from presenting the case as a major example of his technique. How ironic! Freud uses Dora to develop his ideas, and help to gain his place in history, and yet his patient terminates therapy knowing that his approach had nothing to offer her. She is abused by a friend of her father, who pays Freud to persuade her that her reality is wrong and that his (Freud's) is right. Dora senses that her father wants to offer her as a sacrifice to Herr K so that he himself can continue his affair with Herr K's wife. Freud goes one better through thinking that the ideal 'scientific' solution for Dora is to marry Herr K.

As Masson correctly comments, there is a staggering crudeness and clumsiness in Freud's attempts to force Dora to accept his interpretations. But the issue that is raised by Masson's critique of Freud's 'therapy' with Dora is quite devastating. Did Freud actually like and respect his patients or did his professional and scientific needs tend effectively to blot out any humanitarian tendencies that he may have had? Once again, Masson's extraordinary book helps us answer this question because it contains important evidence of how Sandor Ferenczi, Freud's favourite disciple, secretly documented Freud's antagonism to his patients. This is the second major issue raised by Masson that we need to discuss.

Freud's underlying antagonism to his clients

Ferenczi appeared to be in close agreement with Freud and collaborated with him extensively, but it is clear from his secret diary, written in 1932 during the last year of his life, that he began to question psychoanalysis in a very profound way. Sadly, we cannot go into these issues very deeply (but reading Masson's book, if you have not already done so, is fortunately a way of solving this problem). Nevertheless, it is essential for us not to move on before we have discussed two major issues that Ferenczi confronted in a way that was, in the 1930s, unique. The first issue concerns the origins of sexual abuse – Masson summarizes Ferenczi's position very succinctly in the following passage:

> Freud had told Ferenczi, and the rest of the world, that when women reported such abuse in childhood they were merely imagining the events. They were, said Freud, the product of childhood fantasies. But Ferenczi gave back to fantasy its innocent meaning. What the child has, according to Ferenczi, is a fantasy of being loved in the nonsexual sense of the term. The father, however, responds by raping the daughter. And, as if this weren't bad enough, he then denies the event, and devises methods whereby the girl is made to believe it never took place ('you are crazy'; 'you dreamed it'; 'you cannot distinguish between a thought and an action'). He also can no longer provide the daughter with affection of any kind, and withdraws from her emotionally, thereby abandoning her and refusing her the help she originally came to the father for.
>
> (Masson, 1990, p. 121)

Clearly, Ferenczi's demand that Freud should return to his original seduction theory was too uncomfortable for the psychoanalytic movement to tolerate. But Ferenczi also had a crucial ability to understand how the analyst–patient relationship could recapitulate the dark side of parent–child relationships. Masson continues:

> He likened the transference, the feelings that the patient supposedly develops for the analyst on the basis of other feelings in the past, to the original play/ affection/needs of the child. *And just as the father took advantage of these needs, either misunderstanding them or ignoring their importance, so the analyst takes advantage of the transference. Therapy is, Ferenczi said, like rape.*
>
> (Masson, 1990, p. 121. Emphasis added by SR and AT)

As Masson comments, this is a powerful indictment of psychoanalysis but does it really stand up to scrutiny? Sadly, there is good evidence, as Masson demonstrates, that therapy can involve seduction and even rape. Masson succinctly reviews the evidence documenting such behaviours in another chapter of his book. He cites two surveys that record, first, that 5 to 13 per cent of physicians (including psychiatrists) engaged in some kind of erotic behaviour with their patients (Sheldon Kardener, Marielle Fuller and Ivan Mensh, 1973), and second, that 10.9 per cent of psychologists did likewise (Jean Holroyd and Annette Brodsky 1977). A more recent, very exhaustive survey by the Dutch researchers Aghassy and Noot (1990) has provided further evidence of abuse by psychotherapists. Unfortunately for English readers this important book remains untranslated but the authors report that 5 per cent of psychotherapists admitted that they had had sexual intercourse with their clients while 20 per cent (of the total sample of psychotherapists) felt that sexual relations between therapists and clients could be beneficial. Mary Armsworth's survey of incest survivors (1989) is also disturbing reading because she reports that 23 per cent of the women in her sample reported that a therapist with whom they had contact had also abused them sexually.

The extent of abuse of users by family therapists is not explored by Masson, but Gregory Brock and Jeanette Coufal (1989) report some disquieting findings from their survey of a sample of clinical members of the American Association for Marriage and Family Therapy (AAMFT). Their survey of 1,000 members of the AAMFT elicited 540 responses. In their short report they present data recording the degree of sexual involvement between therapists and clients one year and two years after therapy had been terminated.

Answers to the question – Have you become sexually involved with a former client? (Figures in percentages.)

		Never	Rarely	Sometimes	Often	Always
(i)	Within one year of termination?	92.5	6.2	0.7	0.2	0.4
(ii)	Within two years of termination?	84.2	12.0	3.2	0.2	0.4

(Brock and Coufal, 1989)

Brock and Coufal's comment on these findings is really extraordinary; to quote it in full:

> Effective January 1, 1989, AAMFT changed its code prohibiting sexual involvement between therapist and client within one year of termination – one year was raised to two. Over 90 per cent of the respondents reported adhering to the old code, 7.5 per cent did not. The new codes require nearly 16 per cent of us (*sic*) to alter our behavior.
>
> (Brock and Coufal, 1989)

This seems to us to be a very insensitive statement implying as it does that these statistics are not really problematic and that it is only because the AAMFT guideline has changed that therapists need to change their behaviour.

A recent edition of the American journal the *Family Therapy Networker* (November/December 1992) has highlighted the problem of sexual abuse much more sharply. Laura Markovitz's (1992) article 'Crossing the line' is particularly disturbing reading but, unlike Brock and Coufal, she is prepared to make clear that abuse is predominantly a male phenomenon. She quotes research indicating that 1 in 10 male therapists has had sexual contact with clients and at least 50 per cent of these men are repeat offenders. However, she also cites a study by Nanette Gartwell who found that 3.1 per cent of female psychiatrists admitted to sexual misconduct. The group with the worst record turns out to be male psychologists – a survey conducted in 1988 reported that 17 per cent of respondents admitted to having had sexual contact with a current or former client. Markovitz's comments about family therapists as abusers are worth quoting in some detail:

> Family therapists traditionally have not believed they are as vulnerable to sexual relationships with clients as their individually oriented colleagues. It was thought that the particular format of the family therapy sessions, with families seen together and the use of one-way mirrors and reflecting teams, made it more difficult both to enter into sexual relationships with clients, and even to develop the kind of counter-transference feelings psychoanalysts routinely described. But the structure and setting of family therapy sessions have changed. Today fewer clinicians use one-way mirrors and reflecting teams once their training ends, and may work in private practices seeing as many individuals as families.
>
> (Markovitz, 1992, p. 27)

Markovitz's point is a telling one. We naively used to think that family therapists, because they worked with families rather than individuals, were unlikely to be abusive of their clients. But this is clearly not so. A family therapist who is intent upon developing a sexual relationship with a client within a family unfortunately has the power to engineer individual sessions so that he (or she) can pursue his (or her) goal (as Markovitz points out).

We will return to this issue in Chapter 12 of our book but it is important not to lose the thread of Masson's (and Ferenczi's) argument. Clearly some psychoanalysts are actively abusive to their clients, but both Masson and Ferenczi see psychoanalysis as intrinsically both disempowering and destructive because there is an essential phoniness built into the relationship by the analyst. One of Ferenczi's observations brings this point out very clearly:

> Psychoanalysis entices patients into 'transference'. Naturally the patient interprets the (imagined) deep understanding of the analyst, his great interest in the fine details of the story of her life and her emotions, as a sign of deep personal interest, even tenderness. Since most patients have been emotionally shipwrecked and will cling to any straw they become blind and deaf to signs that could show them how little *personal* interest analysts have in their patients.
>
> (Ferenczi, cited by Masson, 1990, p. 122)

In fact, Ferenczi is at pains to argue that inevitably patients do unconsciously perceive the negative feelings that the analyst may have towards his patient. The powerfulness of the analyst means that the patient is extremely vulnerable to pathological input from the analyst:

> Analysis is an easy opportunity to carry out unconscious, purely selfish, unscrupulous, immoral even criminal acts and a chance to act out such behaviour guiltlessly (without feeling guilt); for example, a feeling of power over the numbers of helplessly worshipful patients who admire the analyst unreservedly; a feeling of sadistic pleasure in their suffering and their helplessness; no concern for how long the analysis lasts, in fact the tendency to prolong it for purely financial reasons; and this way, if the analyst wishes, the patient is made a lifelong taxpayer.
>
> (Ferenczi, cited by Masson, 1990, p. 122)

And, of course, leaving therapy becomes a very big problem because of the emotional dependency that has been induced by the therapist. Through the process of therapy the patient has become infantilized, and it is the therapist that emerges the stronger.

Ferenczi's rethinking of therapy

Ferenczi was enormously troubled by his reflections on psychotherapy but he did not abandon therapy as Masson has done. Instead, he began radically to rethink his position. If the analyst wielded too much power and was incapable of truly validating his patients by genuinely engaging with them, then the answer was to democratize the process by inviting the patient both to become more active in the sessions and to analyse the analyst. Masson demonstrates that it was a particular woman patient (RN) who prompted him to have these thoughts. RN was a long-term patient of Ferenczi who had come to feel that he might want to torture patients and that the only solution to this problem that she could rehearse was for her to analyse Ferenczi and hence rid him of his tendency to persecute. Ferenczi was able to admit that the patient was substantially correct in her assessment of his attitudes to her – he undoubtedly did find her unlikeable. At her prompting, he did experiment in undertaking a mutual analysis with her, although Masson reports that, tantalizingly, Ferenczi left no record of how it progressed.

The crucial issue raised by Ferenczi is whether therapy can be successful if the therapist finds the patient unlikeable. The textbook answer is, of course, that analysis can and will proceed in such circumstances, but Masson is profoundly sceptical about this:

> Is there any reason to believe that an initial dislike will change, with time, into affection? It may do so but there is no guarantee; and what if it does not? Ferenczi . . . said that many patients told him that they felt that love coming from the therapist could cure them, that if Ferenczi could simply be there, more or less silent, without any attempt to interpret, this would help them. Ferenczi found this was true, and wondered if this love acted as a salve for the wounds left by early traumas. But he also recognized that the feeling the patient had of being helped did not always last beyond the end of the session. He asked whether this is not because 'our imagination endows us with more love than we in fact possess'. After all, he pointed out, when the analytic hour is over, the therapist simply sends the patient away and ushers in the next.
>
> (Masson, 1990, p. 125)

The conveyor belt nature of therapy is a crucial problem because it draws attention to the gross imbalance in power that exists between the two participants in the encounter. The analyst, seeing a stream of patients on the hour throughout a busy day, cannot possibly experience the encounter in the same way as an individual patient who attends a session and then departs. Masson believes that this essential asymmetry in experience destroys the possibility of a genuine relationship being established. Ferenczi, faced by the same contradiction, apparently experimented with offering his patients as much time as they wanted and even toyed with the idea of having only one patient at a time. Masson, needless to say, points out the impossibility of such a proposal but at the same time records that Ferenczi, honest as ever, admitted that he himself was 'in need of the soothing effects of love as much as his patients were; he, too, needed to be somebody's "only patient"' (Masson, 1990, p. 125).

Ferenczi's ability to understand both his own needs and the needs of his patients led him inevitably to expose yet another core problem of the analytic method, as Masson clearly demonstrates:

> [Ferenczi argued that the] therapist cannot be an indifferent spectator to the suffering. If one is to take it completely seriously, then one must really enter the past with the patient, that is, really believe in the reality of the event. 'Freud would not permit me to do this', Ferenczi complained. He wrote that to remain on an intellectual plane, without allowing one's feelings to enter, is subtly to encourage the patient to feel that the event could not have taken place. The child who has been abused often attempts to protect herself against

the full realization of what was done by saying, according to Ferenczi, 'It cannot be true, that all of this happened to me; for surely if it had, somebody would have come to my assistance'. It is preferable for the child (and latterly, the patient and the analyst) to doubt the veracity of memory than to become aware of the world's coldness and badness.

(Masson, 1990, p. 126)

As we have already noted in following Masson's discussion of Dora, parents who abuse typically seek to suppress discussion of abuse, but Ferenczi (and Masson) are crucially aware of the role that traditional methods of analysis can play in contributing to the denial. One reason why the analyst may not be able to hear the patient may be because the analyst is so needy that the patient's needs cannot be satisfied. Ferenczi himself reported an example of this – he began a mutual analysis with a patient but she decided instead to visit a relative who would give her the love and tenderness she felt her analyst could not give her.

Far from being rebuffed by this, Ferenczi was sympathetic because, as Masson argues, he was fully aware of the inadequacy of what he could offer. It is clear from his diary that he did understand, at an emotional level, just how devastating the effects of early trauma could be. He also felt that only genuine love could heal the hurts inflicted by trauma:

Otherwise, the child remains in mute and proud suffering, and if there is not at least one human being to whom it can open up, the child is suspended in majestic solitude above the events whereas in the symptoms, such as nightmares etc., and in trance states, the suffering is carried out without leaving any trace of conviction [as to the reality of what happened].

(Ferenczi, cited by Masson, 1990, p. 127)

Ferenczi continued to experiment with mutual analysis and was rewarded by some of the feedback that he got from his patients – in particular he felt more honest and frank about the feelings that he experienced. According to Masson, these developments led him to challenge the central core of analysis:

Certain phases of mutual analysis represent the total giving up of all force and all authority, on both sides. They give the impression of two children of the same age, who had been terrified, and who tell each other about their experiences. Because they have the same fate they understand each other completely, and instinctively seek to comfort one another. The knowledge that each has experienced a similar fate permits the partner to appear totally harmless, a person to whom one can safely entrust oneself.

(Ferenczi, cited by Masson, 1990, p. 128)

So Ferenczi, in the last year of his life, was elaborating an intriguing relationship model for analysis. His therapy involved the two participants – patient and analyst – sharing in solidarity their experiences of their own traumas. As Masson comments:

Ferenczi . . . clearly had something quite different in mind [from classical analysis]. He was referring to two survivors comforting one another. That is not analysis. Analysis has never had anything comforting about it. In analysis there is no sense of solidarity, of two people who have come through some tragedy still alive, but wounded in similar ways. This comes closer to what we find today in groups of women survivors of sexual abuse, or self-help groups such as Alcoholics Anonymous and Al-Anon.

(Masson, 1990, pp. 128–129)

Ferenczi's account of being analysed by Freud

Ferenczi's awareness of the inadequacies of analysis was clearly very acute, but Masson has pointed out that there is a link between Ferenczi's sensitivity to the needs of his clients and his own experiences of being analysed by Freud. Historically, Freud was, of course, the first analyst and Ferenczi the first analysand so what did Ferenczi make of Freud? His secret diary reveals all. He felt that Freud had, indeed, treated him badly, largely because he showed callousness to his suffering. The importance of this issue is such that we once again quote at length from Masson's account of Ferenczi's position. Masson bases his argument on what he calls the 'single most remarkable passage' from the diary (dated 1 May 1932):

Why should the patient place himself blindly in the hands of the doctor? Isn't it possible, indeed probable, that a doctor who has not been well analyzed (after all, who is well analyzed?) will not cure the patient, but rather will use her or him to play out his own neurotic or psychotic needs? As proof and justification of this suspicion, I remember certain statements Freud made to me. Obviously, he was relying on my discretion. He said that patients are only riff-raff. The only things patients were good for is to help the analyst to make a living and to provide material for theory. It is clear we cannot help them. This is therapeutic nihilism. Nevertheless, we entice patients by concealing these doubts and by arousing their hopes of being cured. I think that in the beginning Freud really believed in analysis; he followed Breuer enthusiastically, involved himself passionately and selflessly in the therapy of neurotics. . . . However certain experiences must have first alarmed him and then left him disillusioned more or less the way Breuer was when his patient [Anna O] suffered a relapse and he found himself faced, as before an abyss, with the counter transference. In Freud's case the equivalent was the discovery of the mendacity of hysterical women. Since the time of this discovery Freud no longer likes sick people.

(Ferenczi, cited by Masson, 1990, pp. 129–130)

Ferenczi's comments are devastating enough at an observational level, but the most telling aspect of Ferenczi's account is his ability to draw out the crucial theoretical shifts that occurred in Freud's position:

Since he suffered this shock, this disappointment, Freud speaks much less about traumas, and the constitution begins to play the major role. This involves, obviously, a degree of fatalism. After a wave of enthusiasm for the psychological, Freud has returned to biology; he considers the psychological to be nothing more than the superstructure over the biological and for him the latter is far more real. He is still attached to analysis intellectually, but not emotionally. Further, his method of treatment as well as his theories result from an ever greater interest in order, character and the substitution of a better superego for a weaker one. In a word he has become a pedagogue. . . . He looms like a god above his poor patient, who has been degraded to the status of a child. We claim that the transference comes from the patient, unaware of the fact that the greater part of what one calls the transference is artificially provoked by this very behaviour.

(Ferenczi, cited by Masson, 1990, p. 130)

Masson, with his usual skill, takes the argument still further by pointing out how Freud's scientism damaged the therapeutic potential of analysis:

Ferenczi explains that once Freud no longer believed in the reality of these early, terrifying traumas, he posited an explanation for their having been fantasized, that is, strictly biological. They are, Freud argued, universal fantasies. They cannot, therefore, evoke in the therapist any degree of real compassion for real human suffering.

The therapist's only task is that of the educator, to explain to his patient that these apparent memories are nothing but biologically determined fantasies; they are mistakes in perception. Therapy, Freud maintained, does not require any deep emotional commitment, but merely a certain intellectual grasp of theory. In effect, said Ferenczi, Freud's heart was no longer in therapy, because he could no longer believe in the uniqueness and the reality of each separate human being's experience of suffering. He had universalized suffering thereby robbing it of its power to move us individually. Just as the educator believes that the young student who must be educated is hopelessly inferior when in fact the child is merely younger, so also the analyst believes the patient has simply misunderstood the world around him, as an adult often believes a child does. Ferenczi knew that Freud had lost something uniquely valuable; the greater tragedy is that, with its loss to Freud, it seems to have been lost to therapy in general. And the greatest tragedy is the suffering this caused so many people since.

(Masson, 1990, pp. 130–131)

FERENCZI'S WORK AS AN EARLY EXAMPLE OF USER-FRIENDLINESS

Masson's exploration of Ferenczi's writings is particularly valuable to us because it documents what is effectively one of the earliest attempts to rethink therapy along user-friendly lines. An obvious weakness of Masson's book is that he does not attempt to establish whether other psychotherapists also arrived at similar conclusions to Ferenczi. The psychoanalytic tradition is, of course, well known for its ability to suppress heretical voices, so it is perhaps no surprise to find that Ferenczi's diary was effectively suppressed for 53 years until the publication of a French edition in 1985.

Some of the passages from the diary cited by Masson are very evocative of other psychotherapists who have attempted to challenge the 'expert' stance that so many forms of psychotherapy uncritically adopt. For example, on 27 July 1932 Ferenczi wrote in his diary the following very interesting comment:

> We greet the patient in a friendly manner, make sure the transference will take, and while the patient lies there in misery, we sit comfortably in our armchair, quietly smoking a cigar. We make conventional and formal interpretations in a bored tone and occasionally we fall asleep. In the best of cases the analyst makes a colossal effort to overcome his yawning boredom and behave in a friendly and compassionate manner. *Were we to encourage our patients to real freedom (of expression), and to overcome their anxiety and embarrass-ment towards us, we would soon learn that patients at some level are actually aware of all our real feelings and thoughts.*
>
> (Ferenczi, cited by Masson, 1990, p. 117. Emphasis added by SR and AT)

Tragically, Ferenczi died within a few months of writing these words. If he had lived it is possible that he would have abandoned psychotherapy (as Masson did, albeit some 50 years later). However, we believe it is possible to utilize his ideas in developing new approaches to therapy. His sensitivity both to clients' experiences and to the fallibility of therapists is refreshing to read, but his attempts to address these questions were curtailed by his untimely death.

As the reader, you may well feel that Ferenczi's argument is only relevant to individual psychotherapy. You may argue that family therapists, because they work with families rather than individuals, do not have to struggle with the same issue of phoniness that preoccupied Ferenczi. We would disagree. As family therapists ourselves, we have continually to struggle with the issues that preoccupied Ferenczi. The questions that preoccupy us are essentially the same: How can we get to like family members whom we initially dislike? How can we prevent our work from becoming routine and meaningless (as if on a conveyor belt)? How can we be sure that our users construe us as benign and supportive? How can we be sure that our power is not being used in a destructive way? These are all questions that flow from our reading of Ferenczi's position. Some family therapists would dismiss these questions as unimportant but for us they are central.

REFLECTING ON MASSON'S ACCOUNT OF FERENCZI'S WORK

We have explored Masson's presentation of Ferenczi's diary in some depth because the dilemmas that Ferenczi tussled with are, as we have already pointed out, very similar to the dilemmas that confront us in our everyday practice. Masson's profound pessimism about therapy is understandable but we believe his position is destructively nihilistic. He ignores a number of crucial questions including the sixty-four thousand dollar one: what is to happen to people who are clearly in need of help with psychological problems that do not spontaneously go away but repeatedly dog their lives? Masson stressed the importance of self-help groups and by implication the value of users' movements, but we do not believe that either can, by themselves, solve all the problems that users face.

We genuinely believe (without, we hope, an element of professional self-seeking) that professional help can be caring and ethically sound. Indeed, the purpose of this book is to subject family therapy to a type of criticism that is similar to the type of criticism that Masson has applied to psychoanalysis.

Rosemary Woodhead, in her brief but useful paper reflecting on Masson's position, has neatly summarized the essential crudeness of that position. She points out that basically Masson's argument can be boiled down to six major statements:

1. 'The very idea of therapy is wrong' (p. 24).
2. 'The structure of therapy is such that no matter how kindly a person is, when that person becomes a therapist he or she is engaged in acts that are bound to diminish the dignity, autonomy, and freedom of the person who comes for help' (p. 24).
3. 'It is therapy itself that is at the core of the corruption' (p. 298).
4. 'The profession itself is corrupt' (p. 298).
5. 'Almost every therapy shows a lack of interest in the world (in social injustice)' (p. 285).
6. 'Psychotherapy is merely an extension of the views of the dominant society (*sic*)' (p. 298).

(Woodhead, 1993. Pagination refers to Masson, 1988,
Against, London: Collins)

What is curiously lacking in Masson's analysis is a fine-grained examination of what structural features of the psychotherapeutic relationship are destructive and corrupting. He does, of course, state that it is the difference in power between the client and the therapist that is crucial but he makes no attempt to establish whether this power differential can be addressed in any way. His is clearly a utopian position that tries to establish unworkable criteria for professional relationships. The logical conclusion of his argument is that all professional relationships are suspect so that as citizens we are left in a totally stranded position – we cannot approach any professional for help because we immediately enter a situation in which the professional wields more power.

When I go to my dentist I am very aware of being in his power because he knows so much more about teeth than I do, but my dentist is very user-friendly and negotiative and involves me in informed decision-making about what he would like to do with my teeth. Recently, he felt that one of my back teeth should come out because it was apparently causing persistent difficulties. He was 80 per cent sure that the tooth he selected was the culprit but I was not so sure because the pain was very diffuse. We agreed to leave it a few days until diagnosis could be surer. To cut a long story short, my sense that it was an adjacent tooth causing the trouble turned out to be right and it was this one that was extracted much to my relief. The pain had become more focused and I could identify where it was coming from. If I had followed his initial advice, the wrong tooth would have been extracted. Because we negotiated the next step in therapy rather than relying on his expert advice, the result was more successful.

Masson's blanket condemnation of professionals cannot encompass this type of example in which a lay person and the professional negotiated the next step in therapy. Of course, all professional relationships are fraught with difficulty, but Masson's argument is based upon a major logical fallacy. In effect, he says, I have found major examples of psychotherapy involving abuse, therefore all forms of psychotherapy and all psychotherapists are abusive. Our position is very clear on these issues: we believe, from our knowledge of research and clients' accounts of therapy, that it is justifiable to argue that the majority of clients find the experience of therapy mostly helpful. Masson's criticisms of what can go wrong are very valuable because they enable us to begin to construct a manifesto for an ethically sound, user-friendly family therapy. Indeed, we can begin to construct such a manifesto precisely by turning Masson's statements on their head. For example, when a person is in training to become a therapist he or she must be trained in such a way that ethical issues become the central core of the training. To be ethical, therapy must be concerned with increasing the dignity, autonomy and freedom of the person who comes for help. Once trained, therapists must be exposed to an auditing procedure that enables clients to give feed back to a third party about the therapy they have received. Agencies providing therapy must take steps to establish work procedures that enable clients to feed back in this way.

In this era of increasing emphasis on auditing it is not utopian to expect that such mechanisms can be set up and adequately financed. The one arena where such possibilities are very limited is, of course, private practice. We are personally critical of private practice precisely because it is private and hence almost beyond effective surveillance. No doubt, ethical practitioners, working together in a consortium, could find ways of auditing each other's practice, but we suspect that there would be little enthusiasm for doing so because of the cost of providing such a surveillance method.

One of the reasons for writing this book is to answer the types of criticisms that Masson articulates. We became interested in user-friendliness before we read Masson's important books, but his work has helped us to refine and sharpen our work in order to create what we hope is a convincing case for an ethically sound user-friendly form of family therapy. The next nine chapters of our book leave Masson to one side as we set out to explore our journey in developing user-friendliness. However, although we will not be returning explicitly to

Masson's critique, his ideas effectively create a benchmark against which user-friendliness can be judged. We hope that you, as a reader, will find the journey worthwhile, but we suspect that Masson would find our work pointless because his position, as Rosemary Woodhead has argued, is essentially impossible to refute empirically. His concept of therapy insists that the therapist, *ipso facto*, must be abusive because the therapist wields all the power in the relationship and the user (by definition) is powerless.

We would challenge his argument by saying that a consistently user-friendly approach to therapy, which focuses on empowering users, can be developed by therapists if they are willing to make major modifications to the way they work. However, psychotherapy is too serious a business to be left to psychotherapists. Auditing procedures need to be developed so that all psychotherapists have their work regularly reviewed. Of necessity, users and ex-users will be key players in ensuring that their auditing procedures are valid and are actually effective in monitoring the activity of psychotherapists. The development of an adequate auditing system will require state intervention because it is clear to us that professional bodies, by themselves, are too self-seeking to establish procedures that are capable of really exposing poor therapy and malpractice.

We have enough optimism to think that the family therapy movement can contribute to putting its own house in order, but we have no illusions that it will succeed if it is left to its own devices. We are thankful for the work of Masson and other critics who have challenged psychotherapy in general and family therapy in particular. The remaining chapters of our book document our attempts to develop an alternative user-friendly form of family therapy, but we would be the first to admit that our approach is still incomplete and would benefit from the sort of analysis that Masson has undertaken in relation to other psychotherapeutic approaches. We argue that the therapist, if she is genuinely reflective, can demonstrate, on the basis of accounts from her clients, that therapy is both benign and life-enhancing.

In the next two chapters Andy starts the exploration of user-friendliness by discussing a series of overlapping projects, undertaken between 1983 and 1988, which helped to develop the idea of user-friendliness – a term we first began to use in relation to family therapy from about the end of 1988 onwards.

Chapter 4

Steps towards a user-friendly approach

Andy Treacher

My progress towards developing a user-friendly family therapy model has been both slow and convoluted. I first became involved in the family therapy movement in 1976, the year that the Association for Family Therapy was formed. In the winter of that year, Brian Cade (who, at that time, was at the Family Institute in Cardiff) and Phil Kingston (a lecturer in Social Work at Bristol University) ran an evening course in family therapy at the somewhat inauspiciously named Institute for the Deaf in Bristol. The course was very inspiring and had a profound influence on me. I had just begun training part-time as a clinical psychologist because I was wanting to make a career change after being an academic psychologist for 10 years. The previous year I had started training in individual psychotherapy but my trainer had been very disappointing to me. The family therapy training course offered me a very tangible, structured way of working that was far more appealing to me. Six months later (in April 1977) I was able to take a six-month sabbatical from my job in Bristol in order to go to the Family Institute in Cardiff.

TRAINING AT THE FAMILY INSTITUTE, CARDIFF

The Family Institute was a mecca for family therapists since it was one of the few places where formal family therapy training took place. At the time I went to the Institute Brian Cade played an important role in training. His training methods were very rigorous and at that time he based his work on Jay Haley's approach. Haley's *Problem Solving Therapy* (1976) was the key text and there was a strong emphasis on strategic techniques. For the first three months I worked in a training clinic with five other students and all the usual technology – one-way screen, videotaping and a telephone link between the observation room and the therapy room. For the remaining three months I worked less closely supervised and was able to include more home visiting in my work.

This was an exciting time for me because my skills as a therapist developed very rapidly given Brian's energetic and skilful input. However, with hindsight I am amazed at what was missing from my training. Ethical and professional issues were never discussed in any depth because the focus was so exclusively on the techniques of therapy. Personal aspects of therapy were also almost entirely ignored. As a group of trainees we did share our genograms during one training session with Sue Walrond-Skinner but personal issues (in true Haley fashion) received scant attention. There was no real emphasis on exploring the person of the therapist and no interest in the way that the process of working with clients could impact on the therapist at a personal level.

What I did not know at the time was that there was a major disagreement between Sue Walrond-Skinner and Brian Cade about how therapists should be trained. Sue had trained at the Ackerman Institute in New York and firmly believed that personal aspects of therapy needed to be central to any training programme (Walrond-Skinner, 1979). Brian adopted the highly pragmatic stance of Haley and other therapists who were hostile to psychoanalytic ideas. Since these two training stances were irreconcilable, the Family Institute had decided a training programme which was essentially two-track – alternate groups of trainees were either involved in strategic-style training or the more person-centred approach.

During my stay at the Institute I was aware of underlying tensions in the staff group but I was not able to clarify the issues involved. With hindsight I regret that there was not an open discussion of these issues. The split between Sue and Brian reflected a split in the family therapy movement at the time. The subsequent history of training in this country seems to have involved a process whereby the personal aspects of therapy were increasingly ignored as more systemically pure models of therapy (including the original Milan approach) became increasingly fashionable.

The underlying philosophical stance of the training was essentially pragmatic but the underlying ethical stance was never examined in any detail. I did indeed read *Problem Solving Therapy* which, unlike so many texts of that period, did have a chapter on ethics, but my main interest in reading it was to gain information about how to do therapy, not to consider whether the approach had any ethical justification. Re-reading Haley's chapter on ethics now (1994) I am struck by the clarity with which Haley defends his position. But this clarity is combined with an alarming complacency which amounts almost to blindness. Haley is convinced that the expert family therapist will find a way to develop ethical practice. The flavour of his approach (and much of what I was taught at the Institute) can be gained by quoting from the end of his chapter on ethics:

> Many therapists feel that too much is expected of them if they must judge what is best in the variety of social situations [*sic*] and make decisions for their clientele. They also feel that accepting the responsibility for changing people and keeping their knowledge of what is happening to themselves takes the wisdom of Solomon. Many therapists, therefore, choose to share their views with the client and push the responsibility for change onto him. *Yet if the therapist is trained to be expert, he should be willing to take responsibility and he should know what should be done in many different situations. Often he will not know but that does not mean he should not.* When therapy is seen from a

social network point of view, the teachers of therapists clearly have more responsibility to do an effective job than they had when training therapists in the past.

(Haley, 1976, p. 221. Emphasis added by AT and SR)

In 1977, in the context of training with a Haley enthusiast, I found such writing appealing. The theme that the expert does, and should, know best was irresistible to me at the time. I had almost no clinical experience and was an extremely marginal member of a Department of Mental Health, mostly staffed by psychiatrists. Family therapy was undoubtedly good for me in terms of a future career, so I was all too prepared to turn a blind eye to wider issues concerning the therapist–client relationship. The *Zeitgeist* of much of training at the Family Institute encouraged this uncritical stance which is best summed up by the final paragraph of Haley's chapter. After disingenuously commenting that many ethical issues had not been touched on in the chapter, Haley makes the following entirely self-justifying series of comments:

One crucial issue is whether it is ethical to take an experimental approach to therapy, tampering with people's lives with untried methods. Is it not more proper to use tested methods even if they have failed? The many social situations that appear in therapy force sudden ethical dilemmas on the clinician. *With experience in the field, a therapist develops an ethical posture and learns to consider each situation on its merit. Practitioners who have done therapy for many years know what is ethical behaviour and what is not. They may rationalize and attempt to deceive themselves and others about their own conduct, but they know.*

(Haley, 1976, p. 221. Emphasis added by AT and SR)

This is an extraordinary passage which Masson would quote as clear proof that therapists are inherently dangerous, self-deluded people. He would no doubt argue that John Rosen could, without a blush, adopt Haley's position and use it to justify his Direct Psychoanalysis. In fact Haley's argument is invalid. There is no reason to believe that by merely 'doing' therapy a therapist gets to know what is ethical or not. (Haley's pragmatism obviously runs away with him at this point.) Indeed it would be possible to argue that the reverse is more likely to be true especially if a therapist is trained in the Haley tradition – being taught to believe that *his* (pronoun used advisedly) professional knowledge is superior to his clients' knowledge. It is highly likely that such a therapist will be impervious to feedback (to use the jargon) and therefore be insensitive to ethical issues as well.

The use of one-way screens by therapists is a nice example of this point. For years their use was apparently never a problem in family therapy because therapists never bothered to find out their clients' attitudes to them. In fact their use raises many ethical issues which will be studiously ignored by therapists whose 'professional' knowledge tells them that their use is essential and that any contrary views expressed by clients are a barometer of their resistance to change.

This is a topic to which we will return several times in this book but suffice it to say that the use of screens was never discussed from an ethical point of view during my training and I am ashamed to say that I became entirely absorbed by the family therapy culture of the time that insisted screens were an essential feature of effective therapy. Working without screens was decidedly second best and to be avoided wherever possible.

RE-EDITING THE CARDIFF EXPERIENCE – LEARNING FROM PAST MISTAKES

With the benefit of hindsight I can now see that my training at Cardiff was far more problematic than I had first thought. My six months in Cardiff changed my life fundamentally – my mid-career crisis was resolved because I was able eventually to escape a dead-end academic job teaching behavioural science to medical students. Thanks to Brian Cade's training I gained a great deal of confidence about working with families and a great deal of zest to develop my skills further, but the down side of the experience also has to be acknowledged. The pragmatism of the approach was also its Achilles' heel. As a trainee I should have also been exposed to the wider political and ethical issues that confront therapists. Looking back I have difficulty in believing I could have been so myopic. But on deeper reflection I do know why. My own personal crisis as an academic meant that becoming a therapist was a real lifeline for me. If I had been more critical and sceptical about the approach I would have run the risk of not solving the identity crisis that confronted me. I was a failed academic hoping that I could become an effective therapist – any thoughts that family therapy was also problematic as a career were, not unexpectedly, banished from my mind.

Brian Cade's training offered me exactly what I needed at the time but in absorbing his ideas so strongly I entirely overlooked what other things the Family Institute could offer me. This meant that I ignored the contribution that Sue Walrond-Skinner was making to the development of family therapy. Her important book *Family Therapy: The Treatment of Natural Systems* had been published in 1976. I read it at the time I was at Cardiff but I am amazed that I read it with such unseeing eyes. Re-reading it now (in 1994) is a very salutary experience because the book raises a whole series of ethical and other questions which are central to the development of a user-friendly approach. When I read the book in 1977 I effectively ignored all the parts of it that dealt with wider issues. As a would-be systems therapist I concentrated on the chapters dealing with systems theory and action techniques and disregarded everything else. Reading the book now I would tend to do the reverse, i.e. concentrating on the important discussion of the contribution that psychoanalytic ideas can make to the development of family therapy practice and theory. In particular I would read the last chapter 'Special Problems' with much more attention because it discusses such issues as the problems of power in therapy and the ideological stances adopted by family therapists.

Unfortunately there was a gap of about eight years before I was able to collaborate with Sue. Together with the philosopher David Watson, she was instrumental in convening a seminar group which eventually resulted in the publication of the book *Ethical Issues in Family Therapy* (Walrond-Skinner and Watson, 1987). I will discuss my contribution to this project later in this chapter but before doing so I need to explore my experiences of being a family therapist in Bristol following my return from my sabbatical in Cardiff.

FAMILY THERAPY IN BRISTOL 1977–1984

After completing my training in Cardiff in October 1977 I returned to Bristol and was lucky to be able to continue my career as a family therapist in an honorary capacity at Gloucester House, Southmead Hospital, while retaining my job as an academic at the University of Bristol. Gloucester House was a therapeutic day centre set up largely as a result of the initiative of Dr Donal Early and his team. Early was sympathetic to family therapy and had attended workshops organized by the Family Institute in Cardiff. He asked me to act as a co-ordinator of family therapy at Gloucester House – a role I was very happy to take on despite my lack of experience. Looking back, I blush to think I took on the job but in family therapy terms I was more experienced than my colleagues, because even two years of experience (and six months of training) meant that I had more knowledge than most of them who, nevertheless, were much more experienced in working with clients in other ways.

Life at Gloucester House was hectic: I participated in five family therapy clinics a week and during the next three years learnt a great deal about families who presented with a wide range of symptoms, including anorexia, depression, anxiety and schizophrenia. Some of our work was successful but we also failed miserably with some families – an issue that was largely ignored because the pressure of referral was always so great that families who dropped out or failed to change were scarcely noticed. Initially our approach was mainly pure Haley: information about the presenting symptoms was gained and the main 'work' of the session took place in the observation room devising strategic messages and homework tasks. However, my own style was beginning to change, largely because I had discovered the structural school of Salvador Minuchin and his colleagues at the Philadelphia Child Guidance Clinic.

THE INFLUENCE OF MINUCHIN'S STRUCTURAL APPROACH

Haley and Minuchin had in fact overlapped at the Clinic for about six years but stylistically they were quite different despite sharing many theoretical ideas. Minuchin had presented a workshop at the Everyman Theatre in Cardiff in February 1979 which I had attended. A friend of mine, Donna Smith, and I had been so impressed that we decided to sign up for a four-week practicum at the Clinic later in the year. We spent July in Philadelphia being bedazzled by the work going on there. The skill and enthusiam of our trainers (Marianne Walters, Salvador Minuchin, Bill Silver and Jamshed Moreno) was very impressive and we both became hooked on the structural style which, unlike the strategic model, allows therapists to be much more active and involved in the sessions that they hold with families. Minuchin's emphasis on joining was much greater than Haley's but I was particularly intrigued by the emphasis on enactment (and role play) which invited families actually to make changes during sessions. Haley's emphasis on information-gathering and directive-giving was, to me at least, a much colder style that kept the family at a distance. To me, Minuchin's approach seemed more honest and direct – directives and homework tasks were utilized and the back-up team played a significant role in devising these but nevertheless there was a strong invitation for the therapist to be available to the family in ways that the Haley model did not encourage.

With the benefit of hindsight I can now see the down side of Minuchin's approach more clearly. At the time I trained in Philadelphia (1979) there was little or no discussion of feminist issues within family therapy. Marianne Walters, with other colleagues, had just formed the Women's Therapy Forum but there was little trace of feminist thinking in the work that I saw at Philadelphia. Minuchin's approach was appealing to me because, to my eyes, he modelled the benign use of the personal power of the therapist to create change. Minuchin's performances on tape were warm, affectionate, challenging and even provocative. Through my eyes he seemed to create a benign mood in his sessions which enabled his clients to risk making changes which they would otherwise have avoided.

As a therapist who was struggling to create a style of doing therapy that was comfortable and suited me personally, I found Minuchin a revelation. His enthusiasm for actually getting people to interact with each other in new ways within sessions appealed to my interest in psychodrama. Haley's method, which relied so heavily on questioning – while being very valuable especially when exploring the nature of the problems that users presented – seemed too cold and the repetitive use of directives and strategic messages ran the risk of dehumanizing therapy, turning it into a complex game of move and counter-move.

I returned from the month-long practicum determined to build on my new experiences but on reflection I can now see that my acceptance of the structural approach was too uncritical. Minuchin has been taken to task most effectively from a feminist perspective by Deborah Luepnitz, whose chapter on structural family therapy in her book *The Family Interpreted* (1988) is essential reading, in my opinion, for anybody who wants to come to terms both with the strengths and weaknesses of the approach. We will return to these criticisms in a later chapter but it is important for me to acknowledge that my enthusiasm for the structural approach had both positive and negative consequences. I think I did gain a great deal of confidence with families because of my experiences in Philadelphia. I came to trust my own hunches and feelings about families much more and I felt much more able to take risks with families – for example, saying the 'unsayable' things that I was feeling in a session. (Later when I witnessed examples of Carl

Whitaker working I saw further possibilities with this approach.) The negative side of my experience resulted from being too willing to overlook the ethical difficulties that the model failed to address. Somewhat hypocritically (as I now feel) I concentrated on the strategic model and not the ethical issues that it posed.

COMING TO TERMS WITH STRATEGIC APPROACHES

My feelings of uneasiness about strategic work took a long time to surface and it was not until 1983–1984 that I really began to articulate my thoughts in any clear way. Part of the stimulus for doing so was re-reading Haley's book *Uncommon Therapy – The Psychiatric Techniques of Milton H. Erickson MD* (1973). My initial enthusiasm for the book, which I first read when I was training, became clouded by actually seeing Erickson performing on videotape. For reasons I cannot fully understand I found his approach very unsettling – I disliked his paternalistic style and I also disliked the way many therapists elevated him to guru status. Interestingly, my misgivings about him were confirmed (but 10 years later) when I read Masson's exposure of the dangers of his way of working with clients. What disquieted me about Erickson was the very powerful way in which he took responsibility for changing his clients' behaviour. I have never been attracted to hypnotherapy as a way of working with clients because I have always worried about the ethics of using trance states to change behaviour. Clients may well give permission for their therapists to utilize trance states but the potential for abuse is enormous (as Masson, 1990, illustrates). The passivity of the client and the powerfulness of the therapist within such a model has always created problems for me because such a power relationship recapitulates, in my mind, all the most questionable features of the doctor–patient relationship which had been the focus of research that I undertook with my colleague Geoff Baruch in the 1970s (see Baruch and Treacher, 1978, for a full discussion of the way that psychiatrists can get caught up in processes that effectively undermine the agency of their patients).

Haley's adaptations of Erickson's work were challenging, and to many people very exciting, but I began to become increasingly unhappy with utilizing paradoxical or defiance-based interventions. During this same period (early 1980s) Mara Selvini Palazzoli's work became more fashionable in Britain and I attended workshops both by her and Luigi Boscolo and Gianfranco Cecchin. However, despite buying *Paradox and Counterparadox* (Palazzoli *et al.*, 1978) I was curiously unable to bring myself to read it for a long time. The work failed to inspire me in a way that Minuchin's had done.

I suppose it could be argued that my lack of enthusiasm for the Milan approach is a case of sour grapes because of my prior commitment to the structural approach. But I don't think so. The approach then advocated by the Milan group had many features which have troubled many therapists, not just me. What the model offered, as Michael Whan (1983) has argued, was a very powerful approach which would have an appeal to therapists who felt powerless. As I have already acknowledged earlier in this chapter, training in family therapy certainly solved my own problems of feeling powerless – I felt that many people who adopted the Milan approach did so for the same reason. I would not deny that they also felt the approach was helpful to their clients but part of the disquieting heritage of family therapy is the tendency to paper over any discussion of personal motivation. Family therapists are allegedly scientist practitioners and hence their work is to be construed within the domain of scientific knowledge and not within other domains, such as the sociology of professions or ethics (see Drane, 1982, for further discussion of this point).

THE AFT PLENARY PROJECT

In 1984 I was asked by the National Committee of the Association for Family Therapy to give the plenary address at the annual conference at York. The stimulus of preparing the address coincided with a major change in my life. After teaching behavioural science to medical students at the University of Bristol for 15 years (1969–1984), I was burnt out and wanting to concentrate exclusively on clinical work. Fortunately I was able to get a job as a clinical psychologist at Chippenham and Bath. Launching myself into a full-time clinical career was very challenging for me, so I think it was quite natural that I wanted to take stock of where I was in relation to family therapy and being a family therapist.

Fortunately the transition to the job was fairly gradual because I had already been working as a consultant with Donna Smith and her colleagues at Chippenham Child and Family Guidance Clinic. My work at Chippenham was very stimulating and I felt I was beginning to create a new level of rapport with the families I was working with. This level of rapport was noticeably different from the level I had achieved at Gloucester House. Possibly I was, by then, more experienced but I also think that working with child-focused problems opened up possibilities of working together which I could not create in adult-focused settings. My own children were then in their teens and I felt quite confident about working with families which had children either of approximately the same age or younger. Sharing my own experiences of parenting my children with the parents I worked with helped to create an easy working relationship which could not be created so easily with parents whose children were adults.

It was experiences like these that made it difficult for me to empathize with the approach of the Milan group in particular. Admittedly they initially worked mainly with users presenting with anorexia (Palazzoli, 1974) or schizophrenia (Palazzoli et al., 1978), which I rarely worked with, but I do not think the differences could be explained away just on that basis. (Minuchin, after all, had utilized his structural model successfully with anorexics and I had already absorbed his approach partly by reading the book *Psychosomatic Families* (Minuchin et al., 1978) and partly through the training I had received in Philadelphia.) When I did summon up the energy to read *Paradox and Counterparadox* I was put off most, I think, by the monolithic nature of the approach. The claim to have found a new model of therapy for families in schizophrenic transaction was challenging but it was the certainty with which this claim was put forward that worried me. To be frank, I read the book with great scepticism and this scepticism became deeper when I discovered, much to my surprise, that the pure systems approach was utilized monolithically by the group with all the families they worked with, and not just with families in schizophrenic transaction. I have always been puzzled by this: if we accept that families in schizophrenic transaction have unique ways of communicating and therefore require a special approach from a therapeutic point of view, why should other families also fit the model? I suppose Milan enthusiasts would argue that the therapeutic method they developed in relation to families in schizophrenic transaction was such a fundamental step forward that it revolutionized the way of working with all families. Needless to say, I am not convinced by this argument.

With the benefit of hindsight I think it is fair to say that my almost instinctive distrust of the claims of this approach were well founded and it is no surprise to me that Palazzoli and her group, which now includes her son Matteo, have abandoned a great deal of their 1978 approach; Boscolo and Cecchin have also abandoned many aspects of the original approach. As we will argue in a later chapter, many of the developments that have taken place since the original Milan group split up can be understood in user-friendly terms. In particular, the original 'pure systems' approach has been eroded and the significance of the relationship between the clients and the therapists has been given much more prominence – paralleling developments in other schools of therapy.

Some of my misgivings about the Milan approach and strategic approaches in general were brought together in my plenary address at York which was published two years later (Treacher, 1986). My plenary address was actually called 'Invisible patients, invisible families – a critique of some technological trends in family therapy'. In writing the paper I drew upon some of my earlier research work that had been published under the title *Psychiatry Observed* (Baruch and Treacher, 1978). As I have already mentioned, this research had been important to me because it had helped me understand how psychiatry had been able to achieve a position of professional dominance in relation to other caring professions. In the paper I explored my feelings about how family therapy was in danger of following a similar path to psychiatry but at a more personal level I was also concerned in estimating what effects becoming a family therapist had had on my own personal development. Reflecting on this development I commented:

> I think it was Laing who was first responsible for splitting the word 'therapist' into two words – 'the rapist' – and I used to treat this as a mere party trick, but I am becoming increasingly aware that there is a facet of the role (the wielding of real interpersonal power) that influences me quite profoundly. I do not think I am alone in being seduced or attracted by this power, although it is a difficult point to establish because I do not think therapists are inclined to examine their own motivation too frankly.

> (Treacher, 1986, p. 285)

This passage from my earlier paper summarized my misgivings at that time fairly accurately. In the remainder of the paper I went on to explore many different aspects of these issues but the main dimension that I want to comment on here is the issue of professional power and the way it can be used to render users invisible. One of the reasons I was particularly sensitive to this issue was because of a recent interesting experience I had at a conference organized by the Clinical Division of the British Psychological Society. The purpose of the conference had been to explore the role of clinical psychologists in providing services for children. One of the speakers reported a consumer-based research study of a Child Development Centre which he had helped to set up. Parents had been interviewed in depth by researchers from the Department of Social Work at the University of Warwick. The criticisms they made of the unit were found to be totally at odds with the views of the staff that ran the unit. This disparity was very striking, but what brought the whole issue alive for me was the fact that two parents (who had participated in a similar survey) had been asked along to address the conference. The wry comments about what it was like to meet a clinical psychologist and have their child tested or treated by the psychologist were quite startling.

As a family therapist attending the conference, I was ashamed to admit to myself that I had no idea what would have happened if I had brought some of 'my' ex-users to the conference and asked them to share their experiences of coming to see me. These painful thoughts led me to ask the more general question: why had users in general become so invisible as far as the family therapy movement was concerned? At a theoretical level I could no doubt understand why, but how was it possible that my own practice was so insensitive to users' views? Terry Johnson (1972) has pointed out in his important book *Professions and Power* that a profession, in seeking to establish itself in competition with other competing occupational groups, instinctively tries to limit consumer choice (and hence consumer control) in relation to its activities. The profession eventually controls who shall call themselves a 'doctor' or 'psychologist' and hence seeks to invalidate any other worker who tries to make claims about having expertise in the disputed area of competence. The professional group becomes more and more homogeneous as it lays down stricter training criteria, adopts stricter standards for selecting its members and attacks other occupational groupings as 'charlatans' or 'incompetents'.

It seemed to me (in 1984) that family therapy was beginning to be ensnared in this process of increased professionalization but curiously this increased professionalization seemed to go hand in glove with decreased interest in the views and attitudes of users. The parallel with professionalization in medicine seemed alarmingly close to me. David Armstrong's work, which I had included in a previous book *The Problem of Medical Knowledge* (Wright and Treacher, 1982), was particularly relevant to this issue. I had worked on this book between 1978 and 1981 with an old friend of mine, the sociologist Peter Wright. We shared a mutual interest in attempting to understand how the development of medical knowledge was influenced by social and historical factors, which traditional accounts of medicine ignore in presenting the development of medicine as a non-problematic and natural evolution from ignorance and obscurantism to secure knowledge based on science. To initiate the project we had held a seminar at the 1979 York Conference of Medical Sociology Group of the British Sociological Association. The success of the seminar encouraged us to launch the book project. David Armstrong's important chapter documented an interesting sociological phenomenon which permeated late nineteenth- and early twentieth-century Western medicine. Patients as sentient beings disappeared – instead they became objects for manipulation as medicine became increasingly scientific in the latter half of the nineteenth century. It was only in the 1930s and 1940s that doctors were grudgingly forced once again to pay attention to the patient – literally the sufferer – who has the illness and is therefore inseparable from it. The distressing heritage of a 'personless' medicine is still alive and well, despite the evident necessity for a sophisticated medicine that adopts a truly holistic view of illness. But it was ironic for me to find that many family therapists had similarly constructed (through the mechanistic theories they had adopted) a personless family which was similarly so reified that it could be treated as an object lacking subjectivity.

As we will explore in more detail in a later chapter, so-called first-order systems theorizing, while apparently offering a more holistic view of many types of interactional phenomena, has many weaknesses including its tendency to ignore the role of individuals (and the role of individual consciousness) in determining behaviour. As a way of theorizing it is, in a curious way, custom-built to mislead theorists by helping them render users invisible. In the second half of the nineteenth century, medical discoveries, particularly within the disciplines of bacteriology and surgery, resulted in medical practitioners constricting their 'gaze' to the physical aspects of their patients. The patient's body fluids, organs and cells became the focus of attention – holistic approaches that attempted to understand the patient as a sufferer who lived in a complex social and physical environment were banished from medicine.

Systems theory seems at first sight to avoid this problem of constricting the practitioner's 'gaze' but because individual consciousness cannot be encompassed by such theorizing the individual is rendered invisible. Individuals become parts of a sub-system, or sub-systems themselves (to use the jargon), but their voices are not heard because they are merely parts of the system. What they may be heard to say by the practitioner is treated as an epiphenomenon – more 'information' which allows the expert practitioner to understand how the system 'works'.

The full extent of this process of not 'hearing' users was not entirely clear to me in 1984 when I wrote my paper but, as I will demonstrate later in this chapter, the most doctrinaire systemic theorists (notably the original Milan group) took the systemic position so seriously that they did (demonstrably) end up actively denying the significance of the felt experience of their users. In 1984 I was also clearer about the flip side of rendering users invisible – the invisibility of the user is curiously mirrored by the invisibility of the expert that utilizes systems ideas. A major weakness of systems theorizing in its original formulations was its lack of self-reflexivity – the theorizing pays no attention to the theorist who theorizes – a hallmark of the scientism that was endemic to the approach.

This lack of self-reflexivity – the unwillingness to explore the relationship between theory and theorist is paralleled at a practical everyday level by an unwillingness to examine the relationship between therapist and user within systems theory. The power differential between the two was not considered a legitimate subject for discussion just as power differentials between members of a family (particularly husband and wife) were studiously ignored, as feminist writers have pointed out (see Rachel Hare-Mustin, 1978; Virginia Goldner, 1985; and Kate Osborne, 1982, for further discussion of this point). In my plenary paper I concentrated my attention mostly on the power differential between therapist and user because, in my opinion, this topic had been most neglected by family therapists. I utilized an important article by Barofsky (1978) to open up the issue.

THE POLITICS OF THE THERAPIST–USER RELATIONSHIP

My primary concern was to establish how relationships between doctors and patients could be restructured to enable patients to break out of the 'normal', passive-dependent roles in which they are cast and to begin to develop forms of self-care. Given this framework, Barofsky's discussion therefore raised many issues which are relevant to psychotherapeutic relationships. At the centre of this discussion is his basic assumption that all therapy is political:

> At the core of the phenomenology of all patients is a sense of loss: a sense of losing personal control over oneself in order to become part of a system that is to restore health, but by unfamiliar methods. This loss of power seems to be the key event that justifies looking at the health care process as a political process.
>
> (Barofsky, 1978)

I suspect that many therapists, particularly those who are sympathetic to strategic frameworks, would be untroubled by what Barofsky says here. They would say 'just so – what such patients need is my expertise to solve their problems'. Indeed such therapists might well wish that their patients would adopt the traditional passive-dependent sick role (as outlined by Parsons, 1951).

Any family therapy approach which seeks to break from the tradition of reinstating 'the clinical paradigm' (to use Mary Tushen's useful term; Tushen, 1977) must confront this issue of loss of power and seek ways to ensure that therapy does not also contribute to disempowerment. This means that the issue of expertise and expertness moves to centre stage – knowledge is one form of power and it is the way in which different professionals use power that is indicative of their underlying approach to users. Michael Whan in his important paper 'Tricks of the trade: questionable theory and practice in family therapy', which I have mentioned already in this chapter, explored this issue, focusing in particular on one of the much quoted papers published by the Milan group in 1980:

Expertise implies directiveness by virtue of its supposed ownership of knowledge and the techniques for applying it. The promise of expertise is that by the application of 'human relations technology' a solution to many difficulties in human relations can be found. The trappings of such certain knowledge and techniques are often the positivist and methodological ones of scientific rationalism. . . . A paper indicative of this approach within the context of family therapy speaks of casting off 'the stereotypes that endow the therapist with those intangible personal qualities of "intimation", "charisma", "concern"' (Selvini-Palazzoli *et al.* 1980). These 'conceptually unclarified stereotypes' are to be replaced by 'precise methodologies'. Throughout this paper a scientific vocabulary is used to describe the activity and reflective mode of the therapists. Terms like 'hypothesis' 'verification', 'observation' and 'experimentation' as well as more technical concepts such as 'negentropy' give a flavour of the scientifically prestigious 'experimental' method. It is science therefore that authorises the activity of this therapeutic approach. What remains problematic here is the nature of the therapist's subjectivity and person. For the attempt to cast off 'intangible personal qualities' can be understood as a call to depersonalization and for the therapist to adopt a stance indicative of the experimental method of natural science. What is not questioned is whether this positivist version of science is applicable to the realm of experience of the human sciences. And what is at stake is whether the authors in their prescriptions of a methodological formalism are not inculcating a technocratic vision of the human being!

(Whan, 1983)

I have quoted Whan at some length because he does in fact explore many of the major misgivings that I have about the strategic schools. But Whan makes a further extremely telling point that helps explain the seductive quality of the type of systems thinking that strategic therapists adopt:

The reason for . . . [the] influence [of these ideas] may have to do with the situation in social work described by David Howe (1980) who writes: 'Uncomfortable in the face of the denseness of the real world and its resistance to control and manipulation, social workers have been seduced . . . into looking in vain for a style of knowledge which offers to embrace social reality and promise control over it'. Systems and cybernetic theory are modernity's versions of a long tradition in thought that seeks to construct an overall theoretical system. However, this predilection for systematizing the realms of individual and social being, compromises both the idea of the person and his inner experience and the moral principle of respect for persons as well.

(Whan, 1983)

I found this a shattering point when I first read it while preparing my own paper. I think I have always hankered after an all-embracing explanatory system (perhaps this is a vestige of my enforced Christian upbringing) and part of me heavily resisted Whan's argument nevertheless. I felt that his assessment of systems theory thinking was largely correct. But this argument resonated strongly with my own thoughts and feelings about my own powerlessness as a professional. Family therapy (as I have already commented earlier in this chapter) provided me with a ready-made vehicle for solving my own problem of being professionally powerless. The only ethical way forward for me was to develop a form of practice which addressed this issue by saying: is it possible to develop a form of therapy which benefits *users* first and foremost (and therapists serendipitously)?

To develop therapy in this direction necessarily involved insisting that only a highly self-reflexive theory of therapy could be the vehicle for future progress. Whan himself made a similar point very eloquently by using a quotation from Kierkegaard, who had previously explored the relationship between a thinker and her system of thought in the following way:

> A thinker erects an immense building, a system, a system which embraces the whole of existence and world history etc. – and if we contemplate his personal life, we discover to our astonishment this terrible and ludicrous fact that he himself personally does not live in this immense high-vaulted palace, but in a barn alongside of it or in a dog kennel, or at the most in the porter's lodge. If one were to take the liberty of calling his attention to this by a single word, he would be offended. For he has no fear of being under a delusion, if only he can get the system completed by means of a delusion.
>
> (Kierkegaard, 1974; cited by Whan, 1983)

Whan used this quotation from Kierkegaard to insist that we need to be extremely cautious in our attempts to build theories of human behaviour. I too would accept this argument, although I would prefer to draw out a rather different lesson from Kierkegaard. It seems to me that the demand for self-reflexivity (to include ourselves in our own theorizing) is of paramount importance if we are to avoid the trap of positivism and scientism that is implicit in so many family therapy frameworks.

It is this failure which worries me most about any form of strategic work, or, to use Sue Walrond-Skinner's words, 'As outsiders [critics like Whan] . . . seem to have grasped, the problem with which we are confronted . . . [is over-emphasizing] . . . pragmatics at the expense of aesthetics, or control to the detriment of participation' (Walrond-Skinner, 1984). Ironically this double error leads inexorably to therapists not just failing to look inwards – to examine themselves, their own morals, politics and personal motivation in becoming therapists – but it also leads to a failure to look outwards. The actual help provided for a family cannot be divorced from interventions involving the family's cultural and political context. Or, to cite Bateson himself, as Walrond-Skinner does, 'the ecological ideas implicit in our plans are more important than the plans themselves, and it would be foolish to sacrifice these ideas on the altar of pragmatism' (Bateson, 1972, p. 505).

It is easy for a non-practitioner and theoretician such as Bateson to make statements like this. As practitioners we have little choice but to continue our day-to-day practice; the crucial issue is whether we can prevent our practice from becoming conservative and pragmatic and merely recapitulating many of the features of psychiatric practice which I found so easy to criticize. If we settle for this easy option, then we condemn ourselves to impotence – to being an optional (luxury) extra at the periphery of the main development of services. Bill Jordan, in his plenary to an AFT national conference (1981), had forcibly argued that family therapy was already developing in this direction in this country, and I felt that the more we developed strategic and pragmatic methods of intervention the more we would disappear into the woodwork and lose the battle to change the way that agencies actually function.

To illustrate this latter point, I cited an article by Sebastian Kraemer, whose work was a good illustration of the pragmatism that dominated strategic thinking at that time:

> One of the most tenacious ideas in therapy is that the client has to learn something consciously. Strategic or systemic therapy has this in common with behavioural learning theory, that conscious reflection is not required for change to occur. Those who try to understand how it works tend to puzzle over the absence of any attempts to explain to the clients why they have the problems they have. This puzzle arises because they assume wrongly that families and networks have the same capacity for thought as an individual. I do not believe that this is so. People say 'the family wants to . . .' or 'the family thinks that . . .' as if it had a mind of its own. This is a misleading shorthand, however, since families are not flexible and skilful and cannot really think at all. What they do is to organise, and they are organised for various extremely important activities.
>
> It is really only the human individual that can achieve the pinnacle of evolution which is independent thought. The relatively primitive processes of human groups work more automatically, and have the same inevitability as physiological and evolutionary events; they just happen. Sometimes it is useful to think of a family group as if it were an animal, just carrying on the way animals do. When, for whatever reason, it cannot carry on in the ordinary way, help is required to remove the block. Just as an untamed animal is not grateful or co-operative when a human tries to rescue it from a trap, or take a thorn from its paw, so the family is not organised to receive 'therapy' which is so obviously artificial and embarrassing compared to the regular gatherings of social life. The sooner these meetings are over, and the sooner forgotten, the better.
>
> (Kraemer, 1983, p. 9)

There are very many facets of this quotation which could be disputed. For example, Kraemer seems totally unaware of the major debates in behaviour therapy about the role of cognitive factors or that some of the most successful behaviour therapy techniques rely on directly developing clients' ability not only consciously to manipulate their own ideas, but fundamentally to change their methods of thinking and fantasizing (Murray and Jacobson, 1978; Mahoney, 1978). But the crucial issue by far is the claim that families do not think. Of course he stacks his argument in his own favour by pointing out that phrases like 'the family wants to' or 'the family thinks' are strictly nonsense. For statements like this to make any sense we would have to postulate the existence of a group mind or a collective unconscious. Such concepts have been postulated, but they are usually rejected because of their metaphysical connotations. But that does not mean the argument is over. David Reiss's work on family construct systems (Reiss, 1980), coupled with the Kellyian-inspired work of Harry Procter (1984) and Rudi Dallos (1991) enables us to understand these issues at a much more sophisticated level.

George Kelly's famous dictum that 'all men are scientists' (Kelly, 1955) is one of the most liberating ideas that I have ever come across. (It is so powerful for me that I could even forgive him the chauvinism contained in the statement.) Above all else it invites us *not* to treat family members as objects to be manipulated by superior beings (scientists/therapists) who think differently. Kraemer does concede that individuals are sophisticated thinkers but I would challenge his proposition that they lose that quality when operating within their families. If I think about whether Kraemer is right about this as I sit alone at my desk writing this chapter and then go upstairs to talk to my wife, do I suddenly lose the use of my neocortex? Do we as a couple not have an ability to talk about what he says and establish whether we think he's right or wrong?

These are clearly questions which cause Kraemer great difficulty but, nevertheless, Kraemer is, I believe, essentially correct in stressing that there are powerful processes in families which make for conformity and the burying of different ways of thinking about issues that confront the family. But to base a therapeutic approach on these facets of family behaviour is to overlook the other side of the coin. There are equally important processes that create differences within families. Family members also participate in other groups (peer groups, work groups) and social situations which impact on them very significantly, so their thoughts and behaviour are obviously not solely determined by intrafamilial processes. The use of the metaphor of the ensnared animal (like most biological metaphors applied to human behaviour) clearly does not do justice to the complexity of family life but it does empower the therapist to be crudely behaviourist in attempting to change the family's behaviour.

Family members (because of their age, gender, position in the birth order, and so on) have different thoughts and feelings about being members of the family. Traditional systems theorists ignored such differences because too many of their ideas were drawn from the examination of 'non-sentient' systems. It is the ability to be self-reflexive that, above all else, causes difficulty for such systems theorizing. But the impact of such ideas on any notions of user-friendliness also needs to be directly estimated. Clearly, if a therapist believes that families are wild (and threatening) like caged animals, then any notion of being user-friendly is utopian. The best strategy for the therapist is to keep the family at a distance and utilize intervention techniques that do not rely on the family's co-operation and do not rely on empowering the family. And, of course, ethical issues can be ignored, because a human being faced by a threatening animal is justified in using whatever means he or she thinks necessary to ensure safety.

The value of coming to terms with the strategic position of Kraemer is, I hope, obvious from my discussion. Many of the ideas that are central to user-friendliness emerged from challenging the underlying assumptions of such extreme positions as Kraemer's. His use of the animal metaphor was particularly challenging: clearly, user-friendly approaches need to develop alternative metaphors which stress the co-operative possibilities of encounters between families and therapists.

NETWORKING – THE FORGOTTEN TRADITION WITHIN FAMILY THERAPY

The remainder of my plenary paper moved away from analysing the negative contribution of strategic approaches and explored approaches within family therapy that attempted to empower clients by utilizing methods that did not accept the constraints of the clinical paradigm which dominated so much of contemporary family therapy. The methods I explored mainly involved networking – an approach which (as its name implies) seeks to involve a family's wider network in solving the problems that the family may be experiencing. Ross Speck and Carolyn Attneave's book *Family Networks* (1974) is an inspiring source for such work. The approach, if utilized correctly, can stimulate a network to solve problems that an individual family cannot possibly solve.

Networking is, I believe, the most fundamental answer to the problem of disempowerment which is associated with any form of therapy that relies heavily on professionals playing the central role in achieving change. However, since most professional agencies are geared to delivering their service on the basis of individual practitioners working with clients, it requires a radical intervention to establish a networking approach. Family therapists do manage to establish teams in order to undertake their work, and many agencies do have multidisciplinary ways of working, but the type of team involved in networking is radically different, because the team's method of functioning involves breaking out of the confines of the clinical paradigm in order to engage in a whole range of activities which cannot be neatly encompassed in conventional professional–client relationships.

CONCLUSION

I have explored the content of my plenary address in detail because it did eventually (and belatedly) make a significant contribution to re-orientating my therapeutic work. My therapeutic style was shifting away from the authoritarian style of my initial training. My approach to 'my' users was, I think, much more co-operative and I was less concerned to be the 'expert' who was adept at 'fixing' their problems. I found the climate in the child guidance setting in Chippenham where I worked much more conducive to such an approach and I was delighted that a couple (Helen and Graham White) with whom I had worked had felt able to accept my invitation to come to York with me to participate in my plenary presentation. They gave a user's-eye view of being in therapy which hopefully balanced my rather grandiose desire to probe the theoretical implications of adopting a more user-centred approach.

The lessons I learned in writing the plenary address were not immediately obvious to me at the time because I was so caught up in making a transition from being an academic (and part-time clinician) to being a full-time clinician. However, at least two of the strands that were to contribute to the later development of a coherent user-friendly position were already in place. These strands can be summarized as follows:

1 The systems theories I had encountered shared a common weakness because they stressed the all-pervading role of the family system in determining behaviour and they inevitably neglected the role of individual consciousness. Family members became invisible and their individuality was ignored – they became interchangeable parts of the family system.
2 The metaphors and language utilized by systems theorists in understanding families prompted and confirmed the antagonistic stance adopted by therapists. Since families were seen as powerful systems resistant to change, therapists were empowered to be endlessly inventive and instrumental in getting them to change. Interventions were judged pragmatically in terms of whether or not they succeeded in achieving change. Ethical issues were therefore largely ignored.

Obviously a genuinely user-friendly approach to therapy would need to challenge both these technocratic tendencies within family therapy. In the next chapter I will explore three further projects which helped to clarify and develop user-friendliness. However, it is important to stress that my own therapeutic practice post-1984 remained relatively traditional and uninfluenced by developments on the theoretical front. The reason for this hinges around my failure really to draw out the lessons of the plenary paper for my own practice (a flagrant example of divorcing practice from theory).

Chapter 5

Further steps towards a user-friendly approach

Andy Treacher

Before discussing the next important step in developing user-friendliness (the Swindon Project), it is important to mention another project which, while not contributing directly to developing ideas about user friendliness, did focus on an important related issue that had been largely ignored by the family therapy literature, particularly in Britain. This project, undertaken by the Bristol-based Family Therapy Co-operative (to which both Sigurd and I belonged), was concerned with writing a book about how family therapy could be developed in different agencies. Eleven members of the Co-operative contributed chapters to a book, *Using Family Therapy*, which was eventually published in 1984. We wrote about our experiences of developing family therapy in a very varied spectrum of settings including child guidance clinics, social service departments, mental hospitals and general practitioner practices (Treacher and Carpenter, 1984).

The book had many strengths but unfortunately its main preoccupations were professional ones. A 'user's-eye view' of the development of services was entirely absent – it was a very 'top-down' book, preoccupied with how agencies can develop family therapy services. User-friendliness was not on its agenda, but in concentrating on how agencies could develop family therapy, it inadvertently raised the important (but unanswered) question: How can family therapy services be custom-built to suit the users that come to different agencies? This general issue will re-emerge in later chapters of this book but fortunately the Swindon Project was able to clarify how custom-building can be achieved in a specific setting.

THE SWINDON PROJECT

In September 1984, a year after being involved in the *Using Family Therapy* book project (1981–1983), I changed jobs in order to work as a clinical psychologist and family therapist in Bath Health District. After being in post a few months, I was asked by Pam Pimpernell (a probation officer working in Swindon) to supervise her clinical training at the Child and Family Guidance Clinic in Chippenham, where I was working. Pam had been able to take a short sabbatical fellowship at the Department of Social Work in Bristol. We shared a common interest in methods which enabled clinics and other centres undertaking family therapy to become more open to the needs of their potential users. For some time I had been interested in the problem of convening reluctant families but Pam's interest in probation users led us to explore a wider literature. One crucial discovery was a chapter by Raymond Lorion (1978) in Garfield and Bergin's influential *Handbook of Psychotherapy and Behavior Change*. Lorion's chapter summarized an impressive range of papers concerned with developing psycho-therapy techniques which would be helpful to disadvantaged users. Lorion's approach involved looking at two different literatures – one concerned with therapist and one concerned with patient (for us, user) preparation. Unsurpris-ingly, his extensive review clearly demonstrates that if psychotherapists are trained to be more sensitive to the cultural background and values of their clients, they then succeed in engaging their clients much more reliably. Obviously family therapists need similarly to pay careful attention to their engagement tactics but it is equally important for therapists to pay close attention to the reverse side of the coin. Therapists have attitudes towards their clients but what about users' attitudes towards psychotherapy and family therapy in particular?

As Lorion clearly suggests, there is no reason for therapists to be pessimistic about making their work more accessible to users from a wide range of different social and ethnic backgrounds. For example, as Lorion pointed out very clearly in his chapter, American surveys showed that social class attitude differences in relation to psychotherapy changed markedly between the 1950s and the 1970s so that psychotherapy was much more widely accepted. Possibly family therapy can be construed as more threatening than individual psychotherapy, but given this basic shift in attitudes, there is good reason to assume that a policy of carefully explaining the process and progress of family therapy can be effective in over-coming clients' reluctance to engage in family therapy.

Some of the studies reviewed by Lorion were very thought-provoking and helped us to imagine how family therapists could build on such work. For example, early studies by Albronda, Dean and Starkweather (1964) and Baum and Felzer (1964) demonstrated that a pre-treatment informational interview carried out by social workers was useful in formulating specific treatment goals, answering questions about the psychotherapeutic process, and defining therapist and user roles. Following this interview, there was a significant increase in the proportion of users who both attended their first formal psychotherapy interview and remained in treatment. Orne and Wender (1968) introduced a similar type of interview for users who were about to begin psychoanalytically oriented psycho-therapy. However, it is an important series of studies by Hoehn-Saric *et al.* (1964) at the Phipps Psychiatric Clinic that has contributed most to the development of user-preparation techniques. Hoehn-Saric developed a Role Induction Interview (RII) which was specifically designed to help users understand their role in psychotherapy. Prepared users did indeed behave differently in therapy but they also reported greater change as a result of treatment than did controls – a finding confirmed independently by 'blind' interviewers who saw the clients after treat-ment had finished. Strikingly, Nash *et al.* (1965) report that utilizing the RII with clients increases their perceived attractiveness for therapists. But an equally interesting finding (Stone *et al.*, 1966) reveals that the impact of the RII can be enhanced if a significant other from the user's network (e.g. wife, friend, parent) participates in the RII and then subsequently supports the ongoing therapy. Crucially the positive use of the RII has been validated in replication studies by Schonfield *et al.* (1969) and Sloane *et al.* (1970).

An interesting variant of the RII approach reported by Lorion has been developed by Warren and Rice (1972) who utilized a user 'preparation' technique *during* the course of treatment. The appeal of this approach to use is very strong since it avoids the fixed 'one-off' procedure involved in the RII; it also makes a link to the 'anti-stuckness' techniques which have been explored in previous work (Carpenter and Treacher, 1989).

Warren and Rice assigned clients randomly to either therapy plus 'stabilizating' (*sic*) sessions (designed to encourage discussion of transference issues) or therapy plus 'stabilizating' and 'structuring' (socialization) sessions. Comparing results for prepared versus unprepared clients, it was clear that the former clearly benefited in terms of measures of treatment duration, involvement in the therapeutic process and symptom improvement. The structuring sessions were also shown to be crucial to the maintenance of the therapeutic alliance.

Interestingly, Lorion reports that Strupp and Bloxom (1973) have used the RII interview (plus an RII type of film) in preparing clients for group treatment. One hundred and twenty-two disadvantaged clients were assigned either to group treatment, or to group treatment plus the RII, or group treatment plus the film. Prepared clients benefited from the therapy more markedly than unprepared clients but it was noticeable that the two induction procedures produced different results – the RII imparted specific information about treatment roles while the film maximized the client's motivation to begin and engage in treatment.

Lorion ended his review of user-preparation techniques with a quite definitive statement about good practice. Given the usually desultory concluding statements that emerge from reviews of psychotherapy research, it is refreshing to be able to quote something as affirmative as this:

> Given the consistency of reported findings, it appears that some form of pretreatment preparation should be made available to disadvantaged patients. The evidence for the positive impact of preparatory procedures is too overwhelming to ignore. All potential patients cannot and should not be expected to be equally sophisticated about the nature of mental health treatment. Most can, however, be expected to gain therapeutically valuable insights into the treatment process if they are given an opportunity to learn about therapy prior to or early in its inception. Thus, a relatively simple modification of the standard intake to allow for the *provision* instead of the *collection* of information promises to increase significantly the availability and potential impact of psychotherapy for the disadvantaged.
>
> (Lorion, 1978)

This quotation is significant because it accurately expresses Lorion's rather technique-orientated approach. Notions of empowerment and user-friendliness are not really integral to his approach since he is mainly interested in the technicalities of improving the information flow from therapist to user. However, it was ideas emanating from Lorion's work, together with the seminal work of Teismann (1980) on convening strategies, that helped prompt Pam to undertake her project in Swindon.

The families that Pam was attempting to help within a probation setting were understandably reluctant to work with her. The reasons underlying their reluctance were complex but usually the parents involved directed their anger and blame at the offender for what he or she had done. They felt that the offender should take responsibility (and hence the punishment) for his or her actions, on his or her own and without involving them in any way. Coupled with this would be fear and anxiety about all the police and court involvement in their lives and a lot of stress associated with painfully long periods of time waiting for the final disposal of the case. At the same time parents would acknowledge that their sense of failure was symbolized by the court appearances and acquisition of a conviction which conferred a 'failed label' on them as parents. Such a label is hard to shake off and becomes, all too easily, the property of the local community, friends and relatives, who know what has happened to the offender.

The families Pam worked with had usually had considerable contact with probation and other helping agencies, but often the outcome had been bad. It was no surprise to Pam to realize that the amount of previous contact that had been experienced by the families was in direct proportion to the reluctance that she encountered when she attempted to engage them. It was often a case of 'here we go again – here's another interfering social worker with whom we have to seem to co-operate to ensure a good outcome in court'. At the same time the families were preparing themselves for yet another exasperating round of days at the police station and in the courts. The families were generally very disadvantaged, had experienced long-term poverty and lived in areas with poor amenities. Typically, marital and step-family problems were also very prominent. As a probation officer, Pam necessarily had to be offence-orientated, but she needed to be sensitive to the fact that, for many families, there would be a plethora of problems and offending was just one part of what was often painful and chaotic family life.

In trying to join with these families it seemed vital to demonstrate to them that she could understand their feelings of anger and despair, and to open up the possibility that contact with a professional like herself could be fruitful and not just another burden. Following Lorion's lead, she therefore decided to develop a project which would involve making a special videotape which could then be used to introduce family therapy as a commonsensical and worthwhile way of solving problems.

To this end, Pam used part of her study leave to make a videotape called *So Convince Me*. She was able to employ professional film-makers and did not have to concern herself with the technicalities of producing the video. The video begins with a series of brief vignettes that demonstrate some of the main concerns and fears that are experienced by offenders and their families. However, the main story-line running through the tape is a recapitulation of work that Pam undertook with a single-parent family (a mother and two sons). The youngest son was a persistent joyrider who was the subject of a probation order. With his mother and elder brother, he also participated in family therapy sessions which were briefly summarized by role-played segments of the tape. (For further details of the tape, see Pimpernell and Treacher, 1990.)

Unfortunately, because of time and work pressures, Pam was not able to set up a controlled study during the time that the videotape was used for recruiting purposes (June 1985–June 1987). However, she was able to use the videotape with a small number of families selected from her caseload. A videotape showing was offered to each family as part of her initial contact – usually the second session and before the court appearance had taken place. Since some families possessed video machines themselves, it was also possible to leave a copy of a tape with them so that they could view it by themselves. Pam's preference was to view the tape with the family since she could then get immediate feedback and make sure that any queries could be answered immediately.

The response of the families to the videotape was very interesting. They either became more enthusiastic customers for family therapy or they decided to find their own solutions to the problems they faced. Within a user-friendly framework, either outcome is to be welcomed, because the tape seems to have contributed to the empowerment of clients to take active decisions to deal with the problems confronting them. Obviously the project is open to a number of criticisms – for example, were the results just to be dismissed as a Hawthorne effect? Equally, would routine use of videotape just become a bureaucratic procedure that sorted users into sheep and goats – the compliant and the resistant? To settle such questions, a major research study would have to be undertaken. Unfortunately, neither Pam nor myself was able even to think of such a project since both of us changed jobs in 1987. However, it is clear from the response that we have had to demonstrating the tape that the approach does have potential in a wide range of settings.

THE BRISTOL ETHICS PROJECT

While Pam's project was still being completed, I was also involved in another, much more wide-ranging project which also helped to develop my thinking about user-friendliness. Sue Walrond-Skinner and David Watson, a philosopher, using funds donated by the Sir Halley Stewart Trust, were able to convene a series of seminars in Bristol which brought together a group of philosophers, researchers and practitioners who were interested in exploring the ethical basis of family therapy.

Participating in the seminars was very stimulating and I was able to contribute a chapter to the book that was prompted by them (Walrond-Skinner and Watson, 1987). The title I chose, 'Family therapists are potentially damaging to families and their wider networks. Discuss', was designed to be critical in its tone because I was concentrating my attention on what I thought were ethically very dubious practices adopted by strategic family therapists. My chapter was quite wide-ranging but the most important part of it concentrated on developing a theme of invisibility first explored by me in my plenary address at the 1984 AFT Conference. In this paper I concentrated not on the invisibility of users but on the invisibility of strategic therapists who tended to concern themselves with the technicalities of their approach. The central plank of my argument was based on the very honest and thoughtful work of the American therapist David Calof, who had been invited to submit a case study to the ongoing series of case studies that are published in each edition of the *Family Therapy Networker*.

The case history Calof presented was first written in 1977 but was not published at that time. The report describes an extremely successful piece of strategic work undertaken with a husband and wife whose marriage was at the point of breakdown. On his own admission, Calof insists that the therapy was an extended ego trip:

> At the time I saw this couple I was a young, lay-hypnotherapist swept away with the idea of hypnosis as the great panacea. I placed great emphasis on disguised, tricky varieties of techniques while hoping never to be caught by my clients in the act of attempting to change them. I sometimes saw clients as consciously stupid and not to be trusted except unconsciously. Consequently in the case report . . . I was primarily interested in portraying my rather flamboyant, grandiose, and manipulative technique, *while the client's behaviour and resources remain as background.*
>
> (Calof, 1984, pp. 52–53. Emphasis added by AT)

It is extremely rare for therapists to write so frankly about their work so we must be grateful to Calof for his bravery in breaking the usually accepted professional norm that is involved when therapists write up their case studies. But Calof was by no means involved in a piece of public breast-beating. His purpose was far more serious than that, since he sought to link his change in therapeutic style to changes in his own life, as the following further quotation reveals:

> Milton Erickson was unquestionably the model for the kind of therapist I wanted to be. I was attempting to imitate and emulate Erickson . . . trying to disregard myself in favour of a persona of seeming invincibility and invulnerability. At various times Dr Erickson had, like my father, terrified, confused, frustrated and nourished me. He had powerfully elicited my love, envy and respect. Certainly it is no coincidence that following Dr Erickson's death, I began taking steps to rejoin my family and to end a decade-long chilly stand-off with my father.
>
> (Calof, 1984, p. 53)

Calof's presentation reads almost like one of the fables so beloved of his mentor Erickson: 'Once upon a time there was a young man who wished to apprentice himself to a magician, but being an apprentice magician had its pitfalls. . . .' I should hasten to add, however, that my purpose is not to demean Calof in any way. Indeed my intention is the reverse of this. He raises many crucial issues here – one that always fascinated me concerns the reason why some therapists are almost instinctively drawn to adopting paradoxical or defiance-based interventions, while other therapists are drawn towards using more direct methods. Calof gives us a clue to possible answers in the next two paragraphs of his article in which he points out which crucial aspects of the case he actually neglected in favour of his passion for technique:

> It is clear to me now that [back in 1977] . . . I regarded the couple's relations with their families of origin and parenting issues as largely irrelevant. Transgenerational and systems issues, patterns and themes were reduced in the report to mere problems with in-laws, mere differences in parenting styles, communication gaps and the like. The main focus was on the therapist's technique.
>
> I am less interested in technique today. In fact I now view any need I may have to perform or use tricky technique as more my own need than something required by the clinical situation. While I am proud of this case as an early example of my work, I wouldn't be satisfied with it today because of the authoritarian, therapist-centred, manipulative style.
>
> (Calof, 1984, p. 53)

The importance of Calof's work in developing a user-friendly approach may not be immediately obvious but it did help to develop the line of thought that I had begun to develop in my AFT plenary paper. Therapists who allow themselves to get caught up in theories that are not self-reflexive run the risk of overlooking the crucial fact that users and therapists meet in therapy as fellow human beings. Therapists (whether they like it or not) are incapable of delivering 'pure' therapeutic interventions mimicking types of medical intervention (like surgery) which are relatively free of interpersonal processes. The person of the therapist is something which cannot be expunged from our attempts to understand therapeutic processes. Indeed, as Calof so clearly demonstrates, there are crucial links between a therapist's personhood (to use a rather ugly term) and the therapy that he or she practises. Calof, in reflecting on his evolution as a therapist, makes clear that his earlier work was problematic because it was driven too much by his own immature and narcissistic needs and was concerned too little with other more important issues, including the crucial question of whether the approach was ethically defensible.

I would argue that the life cycle of the family therapy movement in many ways parallels Calof's life cycle as a family therapist. Most of the early pioneers paid scant attention to ethical issues in their enthusiasm to develop a new paradigm. The only notable exception was Ivan Boszormenyi-Nagy (Boszormenyi-Nagy and David Ulrich, 1981), whose lonely voice has raised ethical issues within the family therapy movement while other schools of family therapy have turned their attention to technical and scientific issues which are much more central to the process of building lucrative careers and recruiting acolytes.

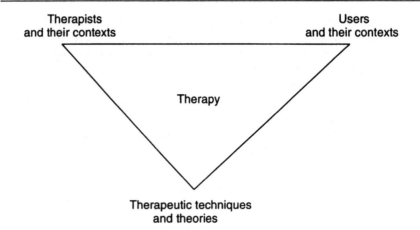

Figure 1 The triangular 'phenomenon' of therapy

The value of Calof's work to me was many-faceted. It helped me to be clearer about my lack of enthusiasm for strategic family therapy but it also helped me to understand that developing a user-friendly approach would necessarily need to involve a broad examination of the role of the therapist in contributing to the complex triangular 'phenomenon' which constitutes therapy. This can best be summarized by the diagram shown as Figure 1.

My training, and involvement in the family therapy movement for eight or nine years, had resulted in my concentrating too much on just one of these three components of therapy – therapeutic techniques and the theories that backed them up. Calof, like many other theorists, insists that the therapist, and his or her life experience, must be drawn into the discussions. But encouraging therapists to be self-reflexive and to address their own experiences also facilitates a process which makes users' experiences much more vital and significant. It, of course, encourages the idea that therapy is much more of an encounter between human beings striving to create meaningful ways of overcoming challenging dilemmas and far less about technically fixing 'problems' that users allegedly bring to therapy.

I would guess that you as a reader may be puzzled by the point that I have just made. Surely, you may argue, family therapists have paid attention to users. For example, the notion of the family life cycle is a crucial concept in family therapy, and indeed it was Jay Haley in his book on Milton Erickson who helped to popularize the concept (Haley, 1973). There is, no doubt, some truth in this point but, with the benefit of hindsight, I think it is possible to argue that many therapists, particularly those like Haley who were most strongly influenced by systemic ideas, paid only lip service to the notion of the family life cycle. The *experiential* importance of the cycle was largely ignored and there was a strong tendency to reify the concept, treating it as a normative process. The danger inherent in using the term '*family* life cycle' was largely ignored – and yet male and female experiences of participating in the so-called family life cycle may be saliently different. Fortunately many of the weaknesses in the original formulation of the concept have been corrected by the feminist-informed work of Betty Carter and Monica McGoldrick (1980) but the heritage of the original formulation lives on, particularly within strategic models. Crudely put, Haley's original position can be boiled down to a kind of credo – families with problems typically get stuck at transition points in their life cycles. The therapist's role is to intervene in order to get them unstuck.

This is too narrow a view in my opinion – Calof and many other theorists who are genuinely sensitive to family and individual life cycle issues encourage us to hold up a mirror and ask questions like, 'And what of you? Forget you're a therapist for the moment and tell us where you are – what life experiences are you struggling with?' 'And what are you avoiding in therapy? Are you encouraging, for example, the husband in this family you are working with to reconnect with his father even though you are more cut off from your own father than he is?'

It is important to add that many other family therapists – particularly transgenerational theorists, including, of course, Murray Bowen (1972) – have always insisted that these issues are crucial. My own training initially led me away from such theorists but Calof's work was particularly helpful in re-awakening my interest in transgenerational issues. Unfortunately, despite good intentions to the contrary, I was not able to absorb Boszormenyi-Nagy's work. I bought his book *Invisible Loyalties* (Boszormenyi-Nagy and Spark, 1983) but, like many other people with whom I have compared notes, I found the book very difficult to read. It was the work of Norman and Betty Paul (Paul and Paul, 1986) and Stuart Lieberman (1979) that was most influential in changing my ideas, but paradoxically the work of Mara Selvini Palazzoli was equally influential albeit in a negative sense (see below).

The preparation of my plenary address and my participation in the ethics project had helped me to make a conceptual shift towards a more user-centred way of thinking about therapy but my practice still lagged behind the theoretical developments I was making. Unfortunately the Swindon Project did not make a very tangible impact on my work because the type of users that I worked with were much more willing to attend sessions, so I never felt the necessity to make a tape like *So Convince Me*. I take a different view of this issue now because I would argue that important ethical issues are involved. If we are really concerned to be user-friendly, then we need to find ways of genuinely informing users about how we work. Most family therapists rely upon inducting users into the process of family therapy, but this approach has its pitfalls because family members have little conception of what the therapy will entail and have to take too much on trust.

COMING TO TERMS WITH THE MILAN APPROACH

During the winter of 1986 I attempted to write a wide-ranging critique of the Milan approach. As a therapist who was mainly structural in orientation, I was unsettled by the popularity of the model which was so different from my own. I felt I could not just ignore the model and concentrate on my own methods because I had a nagging feeling that the Milan approach was leading the family therapy movement in a direction that I felt was dangerous. The paper I produced was over-ambitious and much too rambling to be published in journal article form. However, the publication of my 1984 AFT plenary paper very belatedly (in late 1986) prompted a response from Jürgen Hargens, the editor of the German family therapy journal *Zeitschrift für Systemische Therapie*. He invited me to write a short paper critiquing the Milan approach. He asked for only 2,000 words, so it was difficult to do justice to the task in the space allowed. (Ironically the publication of my article in the German journal (Treacher, 1987) in turn prompted Bryan Lask, the editor of the *British Journal of Family Therapy*, to ask for permission to publish it in English (Treacher 1988a). In order to write the paper I decided to focus my attention primarily on Palazzoli *et al.*'s key book *Paradox and Counterparadox*. Given my heightened sensitivity to ethical issues, it was intriguing to read this much-cited book which I had resisted reading for far too long. I felt a little like the boy in the Emperor's clothes folk tale because what I discovered was really very disquieting to me. I already knew that Palazzoli's understanding of 'the schizophrenic transaction' (to use her term) was based on the hypothesis that family members are caught up in a unique systemic process which must be the key focus for intervention by therapists. If schizophrenic transactions can be disrupted, then the family system will no longer be maintained homeostatically and it becomes possible for change to occur.

This model obviously stressed the significance of systemic processes, but I was not aware that Palazzoli was extremely dismissive of family members' felt experiences. This issue is best explored by quoting directly from the book:

> It has often been stated by students of the family in schizophrenic transaction that the parents in these families have fragile personalities, that they cling to their partner in the constant fear of abandonment as well as true intimacy. Our own experience with these families has made us understand that such a belief, which initially we had shared, had seriously held back our work and led us to commit errors. . . .
>
> This erroneous belief led us to consider the feelings shown in the session as a 'reality'. . . . We had . . . been conditioned by the linguistic model, according to which the predicate we link to the subject becomes an inherent quality of that subject *while, in effect, it is no more than a function of the relationship.* For example, if a patient appeared to be sad, we concluded he was sad and we went so far as to try to understand why he was sad.
>
> (Palazzoli *et al.*, 1978, p. 26. Emphasis added by AT)

The 'scientific' reason why they were able to proceed in this way without any ethical or philosophical questioning is explained in the following passage:

> In order to bracket [*sic*] the sentiments, in the sense of intrapsychic reality, we had to force ourselves to systematically substitute the verb *to seem* for the verb

to be. Thus, if Mr Bianchi *seemed* sad during a session we had to make an effort to avoid thinking that he was sad (this being undecidable) and therefore not to be interested in finding out why.

(Palazzoli *et al.*, 1978, p. 27)

I find it very difficult to accept this sort of statement, since it contains a type of scientistic arrogance that really distresses me. What upsets me most is Palazzoli's message that her clients' felt experience is unreal – after all, family members are only participating in the systemic game which brings them to therapy. What they say can therefore either be dismissed as meaningless or reinterpreted at will by the therapist who (to use Masson's phrase) has superior wisdom.

Clearly the original Milan approach incorporates ideas which are the antithesis of user-friendliness – thoughts and feelings are construed as epiphenomena. Family members are caught up in endless games, so they must be approached by therapists who are armed with techniques which enable them to escape entanglement or enmeshment in the family game. The use of positive connotation and the maintenance of neutrality through the use of circular questioning are the key tactics that the therapist utilizes in her struggle to avoid being influenced by the family. Neutrality is one of the most controversial concepts in the psychotherapy literature and yet its discussion in Palazzoli's paper is ironically so brief (barely half a page) that there is space here to reproduce it verbatim. In my 1987 paper I did not have enough space to pay much attention to the concept because I concentrated most of my criticism on the issue of users' felt experience of being in therapy. However, in order to make a link to the remainder of this book it is essential to focus directly on the concept because it is an almost direct negation of user-friendliness. (Positive connotation is also problematic, so I will add some comments about it later in this chapter.)

Let me start my discussion by quoting Palazzoli *et al.* in full:

By neutrality of the therapist we mean a specific pragmatic effect that his other total behaviour during the session exerts on the family (and not his intrapsychic disposition). We shall try to explain exactly what this pragmatic effect is by describing a hypothetical situation. Let us imagine that when one of our team members has terminated his interview with the family and has gone to discuss the information he has gathered with the rest of the team, an interviewer approaches the family and asks the various members their impressions of the therapist. If the session has proceeded according to the systemic epistemology, the various members of the family will have plenty to say about the personality of the therapist (his possession or lack of intelligence, human warmth, agreeability, style, etc.). However, if they are asked to state whom he had supported or sided with or what judgement he had made concerning one or another individual or his respective behaviour or of the entire family, they should remain puzzled and uncertain.

In fact, as long as the therapist invites one member to comment upon the relationship of two other members, he appears *at that time* to be allied to that person. However, this alliance shifts the moment he asks another family member and yet another to do the same. The end result of the successive alliances is that the therapist is allied with everyone and no one at the same time.

Furthermore, the more the therapist assimilates the systemic epistemology, the more interested he is in provoking feedback and collecting information and the less apt to make moral judgement of any kind. The declaration of any judgement, whether it be of approval or of disapproval, implicitly and inevitably allies him with one of the individuals or groups within the family. At the same time, we try to observe and neutralize as early as possible any attempt towards coalition, seduction, or privileged relationships with the therapist made by any member or subgroup of the family.

In fact, it is our belief that the therapist can be effective only to the extent that he is able to obtain and maintain a different level (*metalevel*) from that of the family.

(Palazzoli *et al.*, 1980, p. 11)

We have quoted Palazzoli *et al.* in full because it enables us to communicate the flavour of the approach. In fact, the definition of neutrality is curiously vague and does not strictly make sense. Perhaps this is a result of mistranslation but the phrase 'his other total behaviour' is a contradiction in terms. If I delete the word 'other', then the phrase does make sense, but I can really only grasp the meaning of the term because Palazzoli offers us a concrete (if hypothetical) example. What intrigues me about the concept is its curious linearity. I can accept that by relentlessly using circular questioning, the therapist does attempt to keep herself equidistant from individual family members and can attempt to remain allied with all family members, but it is curious that Palazzoli does not bother to take a user's-eye view and attempt to understand what users would be thinking and feeling as they experience a therapist who floats away from them directly they make an attempt to engage her in conversation in culturally accepted ways.

Through my eyes, Palazzoli *et al.*'s presentation of neutrality is yet another example of a family therapist creating user invisibility. Users' feelings and thoughts are seen as irrelevant but the invisibility involved here also hinges around a refusal to examine gender and power differences which permeate family life. It is perhaps Virginia Goldner who has understood this crucial flaw in systems-based theorizing most clearly. In a crucial passage in her important paper she says the following:

By ignoring the complex interpenetration between the structure of family relations and the world of work, family therapists tacitly endorse the nineteenth-century fiction that the family is a domestic retreat from the market place economy. The dichotomization of these social domains is a mystification and distortion that masks a fundamental organizing principle of contemporary family life. The division of labour (both affective and instrumental) and the distribution of power in families are structured not only to generational hierarchies but also around gendered spheres of influence that derive their legitimacy precisely because of the creation of public/private dichotomy. To rely on a theory that neither confronts, nor even acknowledges, this reality is to operate in the realm of illusion.

(Goldner, 1985, pp. 43–44)

This quotation is, I think, powerful enough to burst the bubble of the original Milan model's alleged neutrality but Goldner drives home her point by stressing how systems theory evolved in a period of extreme political backwardness:

This illusory picture of family life is clearly a legacy of the early, formative years in the history of our field. The post war families who formed the clinical basis for family systems theory represented both a culmination and an intensification of the doctrine of separate spheres. They were more nuclear, more socially isolated, and more gender-dichotomized than any in previous history.

(Goldner, 1985, p. 44)

It is not surprising that the American theoreticians who developed family systems theory should reflect the prevailing sexism of their times. Neither is it surprising that the Milan group (all psychiatrists) should take over the ideas of these early pioneers and uncritically develop them into a 'pure' theoretical position which fails to understand that the modern nuclear family contains one of the most divisive splits in the whole fabric of society, i.e. men versus women, women versus men.

Palazzoli's concept of therapist neutrality can retain credibility only if it is part of a theoretical package that assumes (to use the jargon) that families are systems whose sub-systems are relatively undifferentiated. With a family whose members are in general agreement about most things it is possible to imagine that a skilled therapist (with ongoing help from a back-up team) could maintain a position of relative neutrality (in the sense of equidistance) from all family members. But how is it possible if there are major schisms in the family or major power differences, or family members have had manifestly different life experiences, particularly, for example, in relation to being badly treated by helping agencies?

Palazzoli, as we have seen in the quotation I have cited, uses a hypothetical example in order to provide some flesh for the notion of neutrality. Let me pick an equally hypothetical example to illustrate the concept's difficulty. Supposing the family being interviewed has the following characteristics:

– The father is violent and brutal, a marine whose professional life as a sergeant involves him in ordering men and women around within a very hierarchical structure.
– 'His' (possessive adjective used advisedly) wife is isolated from next of kin and from friends because of moves necessitated by the husband's career; her own father was equally violent and brutal and sexually abused her; she feels powerless and has discovered that helping agencies she has contacted before do not help her because they have never been able to cope with her husband who has always sabotaged any help.

– The children (both girls, aged 7 and 10) also feel powerless because of physical abuse by their father and lack of support from their mother, who is too depressed and needy to help them.

How is a therapist whose main therapeutic approach is based on a concept of neutrality and the asking of circular questions able to work with such a family? What questions could the therapist ask which would themselves help to maintain neutrality and avoid offending any of the family members? Would a male or a female therapist be better able to maintain neutrality if they were to work with this family? I have never been able to gain satisfactory answers to these sorts of questions but in attempting to understand the then existing Milan approach I became more and more convinced that a user-friendly approach was necessary. I found the Milan approach quite alien to my value system and, just as importantly, totally alien to the way in which I felt I achieved success with the users I worked with. As I was working in child guidance settings, it was predominantly through developing a strong therapeutic alliance with parents that I think I achieved success. In practice, I was attempting to modify the paternalistic structural formula of Minuchin (i.e. that the therapist should parent the parent(s) so that they are able to parent the children) into a different one – build a careful alliance with the parent(s) and they will then feel empowered to help their children. My approach stressed the need to build carefully an alliance with the parents – if and when they felt safe and supported, they would be able both to change their own attitudes and behaviour and to help their child (children) change theirs.

The original Milan group's methodical (some would say relentless) use of circular questioning raises many questions about reciprocity between users and therapists. Circular questioning was designed to create neutrality but (at least through the eyes of a structural family therapist) it was a hazardous technique because it did not, of course, allow the therapist to create a strong joining relationship with any family member. Family members naturally interact with their therapist using their normal everyday communication patterns. What they receive back from their therapist is a stream of questions. (Little wonder, then, that drop-out is a major problem within this model, as Fisher, Anderson and Jones (1981) have pointed out.) A user-friendly approach can accept that circular questioning has its place as a possible tool to be utilized some of the time by a therapist, but its perpetual use is clearly alienating and process-wise continually establishes and re-establishes a non-egalitarian relationship between the users and their therapist.

It is also important to add some brief comments about the use of positive connotation and paradoxical injunctions. In my 1988 paper I pointed out that positive connotation is logically linked to the concept of neutrality. Indeed the use of positive connotation and circular questions are designed to maintain neutrality. However, it is very important, I think, to examine the ethical status of these linked concepts. As I said in my original paper:

I personally side with Anderson (1986) who has pointed out the strange paradox that positive connotation may be merely a thin veneer that covers a very demeaning and critical approach to families. Anderson points out that Palazzoli has an alarming habit of referring to families as being 'conniving', of families using 'foul means' and 'subtle cunning', 'brazen lies', 'relentless revenge', 'treachery', 'manipulation', 'seduction', 'ambiguous promises' and 'ambiguous betrayals' (Palazzoli, 1986).

Anderson is surprised by this way of framing family behaviour but I am not at all surprised because, as I have stressed, the Milan group has a misanthropic view of humankind that is built into their theory. After all, they believe that it is the family game that has to be addressed in therapy. Family members are not really individuals, to be approached as human beings, they are mere participants in the 'game'. Why worry, therefore, about what language you use to discuss their behaviour? And remember, positive connotation is a systemically dictated tactic, not a generic Rogerian-like stance taken up by the therapist for humanistic reasons.

(Treacher, 1988a, p. 6)

My ideas about the difficulties in using positive connotation prompted an interesting reply from Sebastian Kraemer, which has caused me partially to rethink my original criticism of positive connotation. I find his comments so interesting and important that it is worth quoting them more or less in full:

Most therapists, when they first 'use' this technique, think they can just say that black is white and that any bad thing is all for the best hoping to shock the family into miraculous change. This is the unacceptable and omnipotent force of family therapy and a terrible abuse of a good idea.

I wonder if I was mistaken in taking positive connotation to heart. I found only one paper that even mentions its effect on the therapist's attitude. Karl Tomm's important series of papers on therapist activity (e.g. 1988) does not quite get to this point. What I am referring to is the profound transformation that occurs in me before I am able to positively connote a person with any sincerity. This is how it works. What is often thought of as a simultaneous process (e.g. of co-evolution) is actually a series of linear sequences starting somewhere in the identified patient. Stimulated by the pressure to do something about the problem the therapist offers a new view of it to the patient and others involved. The positive reframing of my perception of clients precedes change in their perceptions of each other, and positive connotation is a particularly powerful new view because it reaches unexpected depths, particularly the secret love and loyalty that family members in conflict still have for each other.

If it had not been for the impact of Milan therapy, I doubt that I would have taken the trouble in my clinical work to practise positively connoting people who annoyed or upset me, so that it became a discipline, not of pretending to approve of something I did not like, but of actually coming to see what was good in it. In any consultation you will meet someone who irritates you, even provoking contempt. It is just these individuals who need to be reached, and I suspect that clumsy attempts to do so with positive connotation are what Anderson and Treacher are referring to.

I say that I might have been mistaken because I took a technique and used it for a purpose for which it was not designed. Positive connotation was introduced to prevent paradoxical injunctions from blaming members or sub-systems of the family in therapy (Palazzoli *et al.*, 1978; ch.7). For the original Milan team, it began almost as an incidental discovery, but for me (and I think for them, too) it was a breakthrough, helping me to join my clinical scapegoat, the one who I imagined was really causing the trouble. I would not under-estimate this problem. Nice words like neutrality will do nothing for you in the heat of the moment, when anger rises up at the outrageousness of one family member's treatment of another, and I am distressed by the absence in the literature of any discussion (in anything I have read) of these daily difficulties which our trainees have to deal with and master painfully and slowly. No, positive connotation is not just any kind of patronizing whitewash, nor is it simply the Rogerian unconditional positive regard (although they are related). It is more a desperate clutching at straws to rescue yourself from behaving badly and punishing a client for being wrong. As Minuchin has shown so powerfully (although positive connotation is not in his vocabulary), after you have made this kind of contact it is possible, and often necessary, to 'have a go' at the individual in question, but then the challenge is based on some kind of affection and not on scorn.

The grossest misunderstanding of positive connotation has been that it approves of actions which are obviously offensive. Properly and ethically applied, it is a discipline that forces you to find the better, and often heroic, motives behind bad behaviour and attitudes. The behaviour is not approved of nor justified but the person is. This is a necessary condition of therapeutic change.

(Kraemer, 1988, pp. 413–414)

Kraemer's comments are very valuable because they deal crucially with the experience of positively connoting users' actions and behaviour. I think that he is essentially right in saying that the process of positively connoting helps the therapist to maintain a stance of unconditional positive regard towards the users but if I am frank with myself I need to say that my irritation with much of the original Milan group's work hinges around its apparent ignorance of other tradi-tions in psychotherapy. For example, I would insist that family therapists must be prepared to connect to other important psychotherapy traditions. We need to debate, for example, a crucial question: What is the difference between neutrality and unconditional positive regard? For me the essential difference lies in the difference of philosophical stance, with Roger's humanism clashing funda-mentally with Milan misanthropy.

Kraemer's comments were useful to me when I first read them because they enabled me to see that positive connotation could be reconstrued. Within a humanistic framework, positive connotation, *if used selectively, rather than monolithically*, could be very valuable because, as Kraemer argues, it challenges the therapist to find ways to avoid being critical of family members and their actions. If positive connotation is seen as a useful joining approach that a therapist can utilize when it seems appropriate therapeutically, then it can become a useful facet of a therapist's work with a family. Clearly positive connotation then becomes more akin to the reframing approach of strategic therapists. Both have similar pitfalls but if used selectively both can help family members reconstrue both their own behaviour and the behaviour of others.

Kraemer's comments were very valuable to me but, as I have already stressed, I cannot resist pointing out that he still provides us with a 'therapist's-eye view' of positive connotation. For me there is still a crucial unanswered question: What is the felt experience of users who are at the receiving end of positive connotation (or paradoxical injunction, for that matter)? In my 1988 paper, for polemical reasons, I asked the question, 'Is there any real difference from the client's point of view, between receiving ECT and receiving a paradoxical injunction from a Milan-style therapist?'

So far I have not received a satisfactory answer to this question, but equally important questions can be asked about positive connotation. How, for example, do users feel when they have an aspect of their behaviour positively connoted and yet they themselves feel extremely guilty about the behaviour in question? Obviously there is a real possibility of the therapist's input being construed as invasive and condescending and yet it may have a positive side too, since it may prompt reconstruing by the user. Only careful research, involving the interviewing of ex-users, will resolve these issues, but five years ago (as now) there was no research that helps us to begin to resolve such questions.

My criticisms of the original Milan approach were, I think, well justified. As we will report in a later chapter, the group's work evolved very rapidly from the early 1980s onwards so that it has been genuinely difficult to keep up with their progress (see Chapter 11 for a discussion of the so-called 'post-Milan' developments). However, the theoretical work I undertook in trying to understand and critique the work of the original Milan group was valuable in sharpening my understanding of how I wanted to develop my work. Curiously, their stress on neutrality and positive connotation prompted me to turn their approach on its head – I began to explore what could be achieved by being less distant from the users I worked with. The structure of my clinical practice also prompted me to develop along these lines.

My job involved working in two places: Chippenham Child and Family Guidance Clinic and the Department of Child and Family Psychiatry at the Royal United Hospital, Bath. The former setting had an excellent custom-built family therapy suite, while the latter had a poorly equipped one, which was very uncomfortable and bothersome to use because of poor soundproofing, no fixed camera, and a screen that was too small and placed so high up in one of the walls of the therapy room that it was difficult to view families through it. In Chippenham I worked as part of a very well organized team; in Bath I worked either solo or with a single regular co-therapist, Nuala Sheehan. Over a two-year period I discovered that I became increasingly uncomfortable with my work in Chippenham. The crucial difference between the two settings revolved around the greater intimacy in Bath. I (or we) rarely used the screen or videotaping. Stylistically I was different too – using much more self-disclosure in the Bath setting which was much more intimate (basically a large hut, free-standing in the hospital grounds). The team working in Chippenham certainly had its strengths, and I worked with very talented and committed colleagues, but I found that teamworking itself (particularly the phoning-in of messages from the back-up team) often disrupted the flow of therapy and unsettled both me and the users I worked with.

Working in these very different settings helped me to be much more aware that the structure of therapy itself has a major influence on both users' and therapists' experiences of therapy – a point that is perhaps almost too obvious to make, but so many of the major theoreticians of family therapy seem to have worked in highly structured settings in which teamworking is *de rigueur*. Practice and theory seem often to be so interwoven that the experience of working in other ways seems to have been totally ignored. And yet it is perhaps only in other settings – home visiting or just meeting with a family within the four walls of a traditional interview room – that families feel safe and contained enough to contribute to therapy in ways that are precluded by therapists using the technological paraphernalia of 'kosher' family therapy.

There are, of course, other ways in which teamworking strongly influences the way that therapy unfolds. Unsurprisingly, the very context of a family therapy suite (and the teamworking associated with it) creates a pressure that therapy should be undertaken to a timetable dictated by the team and not by the needs of individual family members. The interleaving of individual sessions (in response to the needs of individual family members) can create big difficulties because it is often inappropriate for this individual work to be team-supervised. For example, a user wanting to disclose very traumatic experiences is not going to be encouraged to do so if a team is listening in to and viewing the therapist at work.

Contrasting my experiences at Bath and at Chippenham was important – it helped me to loosen up my ideas about what was user-friendly practice and what was not. But at the same time I was also developing another aspect of user-friendliness. This was partly prompted by being commissioned by Eddy Street and Windy Dryden to write a chapter on family therapy for a book that they were editing. The chapter I wrote (Treacher, 1988b) forced me to put my own family therapy work really under the microscope for the first time, but in doing so I was able to explore how far my practice had developed away from the style that I had originally been taught in Cardiff in 1977. In writing the chapter I was very aware of being influenced by a paper written by Peter Hudson, who had worked at the Family Institute in Cardiff for several years. His seminal article 'Different strokes for different folks: a comparative examination of behavioural, structural and paradoxical methods in family therapy' (Hudson, 1980) was very thought-provoking.

Hudson's paper was no doubt prompted by his experiences at the Institute, which had earned itself a reputation as a centre for propagating Milan ideas. In his paper Peter argues that since families can differ markedly, it is important for therapists to change style in order to offer an approach that suits them rather than the therapist. His notion of custom-building therapy was an increasingly attractive idea for me – as I worked with more and more families, I became increasingly aware of how different families could be. Some could respond easily and directly to well thought-out advice while others were clearly locked in stuck processes which required therapists to be far more creative and flexible in their efforts to help the family change. My chapter ended up exploring what was effectively an integrated, three-tier model which attempted to incorporate ideas from structural, strategic and transgenerational frameworks. Since I had also absorbed ideas from brief therapists (through attending workshops led by Lynn Segal) and had always had a profound respect for the work of George Kelly (Kelly, 1955), I also incorporated ideas from brief therapy and personal construct theory. I argued that an integrated approach offered more to families than either monolithic, one-theory approaches or Hudson's (1980) version of custom-building which advocated selecting a model of therapy to suit the style of the family that was in therapy.

A truly integrated approach allows a therapist more freedom than this, as the methods adopted by the therapist can change as therapy unfolds – addressing the process phenomenon that a family (or individual family members) may require a different approach at different stages in therapy. Writing this chapter could have made a clearer contribution to my developing a coherent user-friendly approach. However, a clear emphasis on user-friendliness was still missing from my work because I had been so heavily inducted into a top-down, therapist-driven way of understanding therapy.

CONCLUSION

Ideally the theoretical work I had undertaken both in relation to the Milan group and writing the book chapter should have prompted me to undertake an action research project in order to develop user-friendly ideas. However, at that time I was employed as the head of the Child Clinical Specialism in Bath Health District. In practice (since I had no staff) I was the only psychologist working with children in the whole health district, so research was the least of my priorities. However, it did prove possible for me to help set up a project in Western Wiltshire, as we explain in the next chapter.

Chapter 6

Learning from users

Sigurd Reimers and Carolyn White

The first phase of our Western Wiltshire user survey got underway because of a happy set of circumstances. In October 1986, Carolyn started a sandwich-year work experience placement with Andy in the Department of Child and Family Psychiatry at the Royal United Hospital in Bath, as part of a social studies degree at Bath University. Her contact with Andy came about primarily because she was interested in learning family therapy skills, but since she was also interested in undertaking a project as part of her degree the idea of a consumer study developed organically through her contact with Andy and Sigurd.

Sigurd had recently been appointed social work team leader with Western Wiltshire Child and Family Guidance and was working at both the Chippenham and Trowbridge Child and Family Guidance Centres. Together with a number of colleagues at both centres, he had for some time been interested in users' experiences of family therapy – in particular some of the more controversial and technical aspects of therapy like the use of the one-way screen and video.

Quite naturally the initial meetings between the teams and the would-be researcher concentrated on familiar research issues. What were to be the overall aims of the study? How long would it take? What were the advantages and disadvantages of interviewing rather than using a postal questionnaire? How were the users going to be contacted? How would confidentiality be preserved?

Another interesting question also emerged concerning the interviewer. What were the advantages and disadvantages of having a researcher who was not a member of either of the therapeutic teams? How would team members feel about users talking to a complete stranger about their experience of therapy? Would they feel less threatened because they would not run the risk of having their work 'judged' by a close colleague who was a team member? Would they feel more vulnerable because someone who did not know the team and who was not a family therapist might have a different, less relevant set of priorities from which to interpret users' experiences?

On balance, the teams felt that having a researcher who was an outsider but knew something about their work was a positive factor. However, it should be stressed that the relationship between the researcher and the teams whose users are researched is a very important one. For example, David Howe's attitude to the team he researched was, in our view, a disrespectful one, and we do not gain the impression that he had any real desire to feed his results back to the team in such a way that they could readily modify their methods of working. Fortunately the relationship between the Western Wiltshire teams and the researcher helped to ensure that the research findings did not create a rift between the researcher and the researched. Clearly teams can only utilize research of this type if they feel that the researcher is genuinely interested in both the team and the users who are interviewed. Feedback from users may at times be painful to hear, but can be used to change practice in a productive way if there is a fundamental relationship of trust between researcher and team.

In order to preserve confidentiality it was agreed that Carolyn would not have access to users' files and would only be provided with the minimum of information which would allow her to contact the users. In order to help users to be as frank as possible in giving their views, results were collected in such a way that individual respondents could not be identified by Sigurd and the other team members.

The main aim of the study was to explore users' experiences of therapy – in particular we were interested in finding out which aspects of the service had been positive (and perhaps contributed to users staying in therapy) and which aspects had been negative (and perhaps contributed to their leaving therapy). These factors were incorporated into the interview schedule along with other issues which the team wanted explored. The full interview schedule therefore covered a large number of areas and has 36 questions (see Appendix 1). Since it is impossible to present the results for all 36 questions (and many of these were not relevant to the development of user-friendly ideas), we have only selected the results from questions that explored the following six areas:

1 Users' expectations of help at the time of referral.
2 Users' feelings before going to the first interview.
3 Users' experience of the interviews, particularly how helpful or unhelpful they had been.
4 Users' experiences of the one-way screen and the video.
5 Users' perceptions of the therapist.
6 Issues relating to gender match and mismatch between users and therapists.

The study started with a pilot study using eight unstructured interviews. These allowed us to look both at the issues which we wanted to address and the issues that were important for the users. The pilot interviews were successful in allowing us to design a more focused interview schedule which could be used in later tape-recorded interviews.

In order to gain a fairly representative sample, every fifth family was selected by Sigurd from a chronological list of closures during a 3–6 month period immediately preceding the study. He then wrote to families asking for their help with the study, explaining confidentiality and asking permission for Carolyn to contact them directly to arrange an interview time. As it turned out, some families had moved away, others declined to be interviewed or were not at home when Carolyn called. Nineteen of the respondents were women and three were men, including one young man who had been referred (and was therefore the identified client). These statistics clearly highlight a limitation of the study. The gender imbalance was caused partly by the fact that most of the interviews had to be carried out during the day, and partly by the fact that women were more willing than men to participate in the study. The imbalance may reflect the degree of willingness with which many men engage in therapy as well. As a reader you will therefore have to bear in mind that what you will hear in the next sections of the book will mainly be the views of women. Men's views will, unfortunately, be neglected – a weakness which we will attempt to correct in Chapters 8 and 9, by reviewing studies that have examined both men and women's attitudes to therapy. Actual names have been changed, as have a number of other identifying features.

WHAT THE USERS TOLD US

The question numbers are those used in the interview schedule (see Appendix 1).

Q.4 In what ways were you expecting to be helped?

   14 users expected to be given practical advice and guidance.
   6 users expected to talk about their problems.
   2 users expressed no particular expectations.

It is interesting to note that a clear majority were expecting expert advice, and yet their therapists, like most family therapists, tended to treat advice-giving with great caution. This discrepancy between the users' expectations and the theoretical orientation of the therapist is obviously an important issue that needs debating, and we shall return to it later in this chapter. It is intriguing to illustrate how some users dealt with this discrepancy. Mrs Atwell's opinions were very interesting and we will quote her at length because she demonstrated how some users adapted to the method which was offered them:

> I didn't know quite what to expect. . . . I think I thought I'd go in and they would say to me, if you do this, that and the other, then the problem would be solved. And I must admit that when I came away the first time I did think, oh dear! what was the point of all that? . . . it wasn't until we had been going along for quite a few sessions that I realized what benefit I was achieving from it . . . it's just talking, talking it through with someone totally impartial who won't decide about you or put you down or whatever. And you make the answers in your own mind – you solve the problem, that's the point, and that was why after the first session I thought, well, what was all that about? It didn't really make sense to me, then . . . suddenly you come up with the answers yourself then, which is what they want you to do. They can't say to you, we want you to do this, you come to that conclusion yourself . . . eventually.

It is natural to expect that people who had never received therapeutic help before would have a mixture of expectations. Mrs Unwin was quite open about her confusion:

> I don't think we had any expectations. In fact, quite the opposite, because we had been through so many professionals in the year . . . but I think that we were both hoping that there would be some sort of miracle worker with a solution.

Not all the users were expecting to receive practical help. Mrs Kane-Smith had felt very isolated when she had asked for help:

> I was expecting to be helped just by having someone understand . . . not criticize.

It was interesting for us to learn that users came with conflicting expectations, despite their reporting that no one had told them what to expect. Although some people may be more aware, and articulate their views more clearly, than others, we must assume that all users will have some ideas in their minds – perhaps based on past experiences of receiving advice – about what may happen when they turn up for the first session. These ideas provide a useful focus for discussion during the first session and help set the scene for a more collaborative way of working, and prompted us to think of new questions which could be incorporated into the first interview.

Q.2 Before you went, can you remember what your feelings were about going?

5 users felt generally positive about going.
13 users felt generally negative about going.
4 users expressed mixed feelings.

Positive feelings tended to be expressed in a matter-of-fact way:

> I felt very open-minded . . . it was a problem that needed resolving and I was happy to, sort of, you know, use any help available.

> I was quite confident to go, you know, and to listen.

> Relief and interest really. I actually looked forward to going. I was interested in going along . . . relieved to have somebody to go to for help.

These statements suggest a feeling about problems which does not include notions of personal blame, but rather one of problems as occurring 'out there'. We did, however, notice that the majority of users had quite complex concerns about therapy before the first meeting. For some, like Mrs Cartwright, not knowing what was going to happen caused some anxiety:

> I was a bit dubious about going, because I didn't know the arrangements, what the situation would be. Whether I'd be on my own, whether there'd be lots of parents. I didn't have any information before I went.

Others, like Mrs Thomas, had a clearer picture in their minds:

> Very sceptical . . . well I had a fair idea you'd just sit and talk.

Those who approached the first session with mixed feelings are represented by the views of Mrs Kingston:

> I was very anxious. But at the same time I was glad something was happening.

Mrs Holloway said something similar:

> I was pleased in one way and nervous in another because my family . . . that's my mother . . . was very sort of against it. She felt that I shouldn't deal with people like that . . . the old fashioned attitude which made me feel a bit half and half.

The views of the older generation about seeking help outside the family were referred to by other mothers, and some, like Mrs Sinclair, had to deal with their own dilemma of whether to live with their problem or seek professional help:

> I think how I felt, if I just talked to somebody that was out of the family . . . I used to, well I still do now, talk to my Mum, 'cos she went through the same experience as I am with Kevin, with me. But she said I wasn't so bad as Kevin. And apparently Kevin's got my father's temper: so it's in the family do you know what I mean?

Mr Sinclair was also present during the interview but said nothing about his feelings about going to the Centre.

As we have seen, moving the discussion about problems from the private world to the public world was a source of relief for some people. For others it carried a feeling of discomfort, as Mrs Jackson said:

> The only thing that did bother me was that we'd be down as a problem, you know. I didn't like to think that, but then that's probably a bit silly.

Although we can see that a wide variety of concerns were expressed, the most common ones centred on fear of the unknown and the feeling of being a failure.

Q.7 Can you say which aspects of going to the Centre were the most valuable?

Q.8 Can you say which aspects of going to the Centre were the least valuable?

With these questions we were wanting to move on from the expectations of therapy and some of the hopes and fears and to explore the actual experiences of the therapy itself.

Mrs Cartwright was one whose original worries had been somewhat allayed:

> It was very friendly. They had toys and that for the children to play with . . . they put you at your ease and that, so it was all right . . . I thought, gosh it's going to be all hospitalized, clinicized, you know . . . but it wasn't, it was very nice.

In fact, nearly half the respondents had found that their original feelings about going to the Centre had changed – and mostly for the better. Mrs Atwell was one who had felt relieved once she had been to her first session:

> I went originally with a problem with Lucy, but in actual fact it helped me really, and I suppose through helping me then I could cope with the children better . . . so apprehension turned to . . . I looked forward to going, I needed to go really. It was nice to be able to go.

It does seem that those parents who felt most helped were those who either had originally felt that they were failures or who wanted to improve their communication at home. Family therapy, with its traditional emphasis on positive reframing, on seeking strengths and on improved communication, appears to have helped those parents who were willing to accept that their 'problem' was not just their child but also involved wider issues related to family life. There is, however, a delicate balance between looking at family issues and feeling to blame for problems surrounding the child. The balance seems to have been right for Mrs Atwell:

> I was normal, that was the point. That was what I didn't think I was. And the children were normal and that was worth a lot at the time to know that.

Another mother, Mrs Holloway, had had a similar experience:

> Get out of the house . . . they gave me permission, something I didn't think I was entitled to do.

Some felt helped by having to communicate openly with other family members during the sessions, like Mrs Unwin:

> Partly because my husband is not the most communicative of people and when he was . . . actually being there and forced to participate helped me to realize a bit how he felt.

An aspect of therapy which is perhaps related to communication in the minds of some users seems to be to get unsaid things into the open. This was certainly important for Mrs Walton, and probably others who appreciated an opportunity to talk:

> They helped a lot . . . I'm sure that going there helped because I don't think I'd ever have said the things I did if I hadn't said them there . . . there wouldn't have been the opportunity to say them at home.

Mrs Mullen was more detailed in her comments:

> . . . helping me to communicate with my husband. I had to look at him and I was quite embarrassed then, but that was quite helpful because that learned us to talk, to communicate, you know.

Mrs Mullen was referring to the use of enactment, a technique used regularly by a team which largely based its work on a structural approach. Not all users appreciated the use of enactment, and some of them may have been parents who, throughout therapy, saw the problem as located in the child, or certainly outside themselves. Mrs Hanson said:

> I didn't get out of it what I needed . . . we needed somebody to give us advice on how to treat these problems, not for us to sit there and tell Paul what his problems were, 'cos he already knew.

Mr Shaw had approached therapy with optimism, but found that communication with his wife had deteriorated:

> It didn't accomplish anything. My wife didn't like the video . . . she felt in the wrong . . . so even though I found it interesting and agreed with what they suggested, we ended up biting against each other.

Mrs Pettit had also found enactment very hard, although she had understood the reason for it:

> I think the fact that you sometimes had to more or less act things out . . . was really hard to do . . . we'd never really discussed our child at home . . . and when we got there they asked us to discuss him, and of course we came to an absolute blank over this because I knew he didn't want to go . . . and it put a lot of tension there.

Discomfort about speaking openly sometimes extended beyond enactment to more generally talking about problems in each other's presence. Some parents seemed to feel 'protective' of their children, like Mr Wyatt:

> My daughter found it negative, hearing her mother discuss all her problems.

Mrs Collins also thought that having parents and children interviewed together was not helpful:

> I think he should have been seen on his own. I do feel that if a child like him, you know, had problems, that talking about them in front of the parents, he might just have come out with the one thing that could have helped solve it and still not be having the problems.

The dilemma for a whole-family approach can perhaps best be summed up by Mrs Kingston, who came to see the family sessions as something positive, having at first expected a more conventional individual approach:

> I didn't realize that we would be seen as a whole family together. For some reason I thought that perhaps it would be my husband and I chatting and then the child guidance person would talk to my child, but at the same time I can see that it was a positive thing for us to be interviewed as a whole family.

Q.21 In what ways, if any, did it seem helpful to use the one-way screen?

Q.22 In what ways, if any, did it seem unhelpful to use the one-way screen?

The one-way screen had been used with 11 out of the 22 families.

> 6 users said they had found it unhelpful
> 5 users said they had found it helpful.

Those who found it unhelpful did so for various reasons. We have already heard what Mrs Jackson said about being labelled as a problem. This extended to the meaning she attached to the use of the one-way screen:

> There were people behind the screen and I found that quite off-putting . . . because then I did feel very much as though I was or we were a problem . . . I can see its use in lots of cases, but I still didn't feel it was terribly necessary.

Mrs Jackson added that she would have preferred having the team in the room. So did a number of other parents, including Mrs Langford, who had felt very self-conscious about being a stepmother:

> I didn't like it just being a mirror. I'd have preferred it if people had been in the room. I could hear what was being said, why couldn't they say it to me? It caused a lot of friction . . . the sheet of glass – not being able to see people.

Mrs Mullen had told Carolyn that she had suffered from paranoid problems in the past, and the one-way screen had worried her:

> I was very nervous then and I kept . . . I was very self-conscious and I kept touching my hair and my face and I think I would have opened up a lot more, and with the telephone ringing occasionally. . . .

Others also reported feeling self-conscious about the way they sat, and shared Mrs Mullen's concern about the telephone ringing. We wonder whether this had been a particular problem for the mothers, who may have felt more responsible for the problems in the first place, and also seemed to attach particular importance to talking and to telling their story. Mrs Sinclair explained:

> They kept ringing through and cutting my concentration off, and then when the therapist got back to us, I had forgotten everything.

It seemed, then, that many of the concerns about the one-way screen centred on three main factors:

1 Being defined as a big problem.
2 Being scrutinized by unseen people.
3 Having one's concentration broken, and feeling put down by telephone calls from the team in the observation room. (At the time team members were not introduced to the families, but some users explained that this would have helped them.)

A number of people thought that the one-way screen was useful, some of them speaking with a touching sense of generosity, like Mrs Hanson:

> Well, I think the people there that are trying to help people like us, and people have got to learn, haven't they, like anything, and I think . . . I don't mind people learning off our mistakes or our misfortunes.

From some of the critical comments made, we might imagine that people would prefer having the team or supervisor in the the room with them. Yet John Sinclair, a teenager who had experienced the supervisor in the room during the first session, said he preferred the screen to live supervision:

> I didn't mind them being behind that glass window so much, 'cos you couldn't see them.

Mrs Pettit had found live supervision in the room quite confusing, despite explanations:

> . . . one person to be talking to you, but the other person to be writing it down and you didn't quite know who you were supposed to be talking to.

Discomfort with the screen had been clearly expressed by a number of users. It is worth noting, however, that most people had generally felt well cared for – the therapeutic alliance seems to have been good enough to help them stay in therapy. Mrs Langford, who, as we have already seen, was concerned about the screen, continued:

> Well, apart from that, I thought it was a very good place to go. I mean, they were all, each person we saw was completely different in how they dealt with us and yet I thought they were all very helpful and very good.

Let us give the last word to Mrs Holloway, who like a number of other users, had come to take the screen for granted:

> Sometimes you tend to look ahead and you see this screen and you know people were behind there because they used to telephone through . . . I suppose in the end I was so engrossed with what I was saying that I didn't really notice.

Q.16 In what ways, if any, did it seem helpful to use the video?

Q.17 In what ways, if any, did it seem unhelpful to use the video?

The video had been used with 14 out of the 22 families.

> 12 felt that they had been clear about why it had been used.
> 10 had been happy about the explanation they had been given.
> 6 had become used to the video or forgotten about it.

5 thought that it had only been of use to the therapist, but a further 5 thought that it had indirectly been of use to them because it helped the therapist do a better job.
4 described feeling nervous about the video throughout therapy.
3 thought the video had been entirely unhelpful.

Behind these figures lay a multitude of feelings, as we can imagine. Formal consent had been given in all cases. The therapist had given a written confirmation of confidentiality, but this obviously did not ensure that use of the video was meaningful to all the users. Some of the users' concerns were expressed quite briefly:

'No point in it', 'invasion of privacy', 'I was aware of it', 'I would like to have seen where it was.'

Other users clearly struggled to make some sense of the video, particularly if they had felt comfortable with other aspects of the therapy. Mrs Rodgers seemed to represent this point of view:

She [the therapist] liked to record it to play it back and maybe pick something up from that . . . you can't remember every word what you've said . . . but I felt a bit nervy – they watch everything you've said. I think I would have felt easier if they had never had it and I know my husband would have done.

Mrs Pettit had also made some negative connections between the use of the video and the team, in this case the live supervisor in the room:

It would be of no advantage to us because we weren't going to see the video anyway . . . it was only for their benefit and we couldn't see why they needed it, seeing as they had two people in the room . . . they would probably sit there and watch our reactions to the questions . . . and we didn't like that . . . neither of us liked them really in a way discussing us behind our backs. We prefer them to say while we were there.

Some, like Mrs Pettit, linked their negative experiences of the video with that of the one-way screen, although Mrs Pettit had found other aspects of the therapy extremely useful – like the therapist drawing a circularity diagram on the blackboard to explore how family members interacted:

Well, when we asked them that we didn't want it videoed, but anyway why do you video it, and they explained that they do it to get more information out of it . . . like my husband and I discussed it when we came home – they probably sit there and watch our reaction to questions [laughs], shock horror, you know.

The links people make in their minds are hard to predict, and they are also likely to change. Mrs Kingston said of the video:

Well, at the time I don't suppose I'd have given it any thought but looking back . . . that to have someone observing from the outside objectively rather than being involved subjectively in the conversation.

Mrs Kingston was a teacher, and had felt particularly anxious and guilty about feeling she had to bring one of her children to the Centre. One might have expected her to have been more concerned than most people about the video and the one-way screen. However, not only was she clear in her own mind that she could have refused to give consent; she was also one of the few users who had said that one of the crucial issues relating to the problem would probably not have come out if it had not been raised by one of the team members behind the screen.

Another person who was quite dispassionate about the use of the video was Mrs Wallace, who had been pleased at how the children had been involved through the use of drawings and play, and looked forward to the meetings:

> Well she [the therapist] just said it was for her, you know like, for her monitoring, for her notes and things like that. We said we didn't mind, so that was OK . . . well, I suppose it was to see what our facial reactions were to questions and things like that, I suppose, 'cos your face tells you a lot of things, you know.

No doubt it was thoughts about close observation that worried some users. This had to be contrasted with a touching sense of altruism demonstrated by those users who had in other respects had a good enough experience of the therapy. Mrs Kane-Smith had not experienced the video and said:

> I would have been quite happy for them to . . . [have used the video]. I'd hate it though . . . the more that people use these facilities, then I think you almost have a duty to give whatever feedback you can, because it's always going to improve the service and help other people. Maybe in a year's time I'll have another problem and the service will be that much better as a result.

From the diversity of responses given it was clearly going to be difficult to draw generalized conclusions which would guide our practice in the future, other than make the consent-giving exercise a more extended one. This might involve checking with users at various stages how the video and one-way screen were being experienced by them. However, as so often in this study, users came up with valuable ideas themselves. Let us look at Mrs Unwin's account, and her hints which were to be useful to us later:

> I think they said that they did it [use the video] to replay so that they could assess in the light of what they'd learnt, which is fair enough . . . I think it probably had a very valuable part to play. Obviously, it's as I said, it's slightly unnerving knowing that it's there, but more or less I think its benefits probably outweigh its disadvantages . . . I think to play to an anonymous camera is one thing, but to have someone sitting there – as you feel – in judgement on you is another . . . if we had met them, it would have been different . . . [I felt] curiosity, I would, I think I would like to have had it kept if for no other reason than we have played it back now and maybe he has improved [laughter].

Q.32 Was your therapist male or female? Would it have made any difference?

10 users thought that the sex of the therapist mattered.
7 users thought it did not matter.
3 users were unsure.

The appropriate gender for a particular family is a matter which has been regularly discussed in teams we have worked in. It is also a topic on which it is notoriously difficult to reach a conclusion, both in general and specifically in relation to individual cases. Most of the users interviewed were female, as were most of the therapists. By and large, users said that they were happy about the gender of the therapist, or that it did not matter. Responses were usually fairly brief:

I feel that females are more tuned in to the sleeping habits of a child than a man really.

Um, yeah, I preferred a female.

I think just some people you can relate better to than others, and it doesn't matter whether they are male or female.

He's always got along better with men at school and that . . . yes, choose a man, not for me, but for him.

I think a man was better for her [teenage daughter].

As yes/no answers it would be hard to draw any generalizations from these responses, although we suspect that gender is a matter with which most people are preoccupied, or are interested in, at various times, perhaps particularly when things go wrong. What was interesting for us was the few occasions when users expanded on this question. Mrs Kingston said:

I thought at first when I went in, oh you know, she's quite young, and I felt a bit like a granny being taught how to suck eggs, sort of thing, but she was so understanding, it was so amazing, so I think no. I think if it was an equally understanding male it wouldn't have made any difference.

A hint of interest or preoccupation may be found in Mrs Unwin's comments about the one-way screen:

I mean to have someone faceless that you don't know . . . I didn't even know what sex they were . . . didn't even know whether they were male or female or what.

There may have been a hint of feeling threatened in the last comment, and there certainly was in what Mrs Sinclair said:

I don't think I'd have been able to speak my mind to a man like I did to Mrs K . . . don't think I'd have said what I needed. He [husband] was glad it was a woman. Didn't think he could have talked to a man. If you'd been a man sat there . . . I'd be tied in a knot, I put chains on both doors when I'm on my own.

We will see in Chapter 13 how we have tried to build into our therapy questions relating to gender even if these have not been specifically raised by family members. It seems both from these research questions and from so many therapeutic interviews that issues of gender – and with them issues of power – are never far away, providing we are willing to raise our own and other people's interest in them.

We did not specifically ask about gender as an issue within the family relationships. However, looking back on the transcripts, we became interested in some of the incidental statements made which have – five years on – taken on a different meaning for us in the light of our subsequent experiences. These statements may give us some insight into the different experiences of therapy by women and men.

Some women clearly felt alone in their sense of failure, and protective towards their husbands as they recounted their experience of therapy, like Mrs Holloway:

> He came twice, I think, because it was really . . . though I feel they felt it was concerning him and they wanted him for his opinions. He was very nervous, he didn't like that kind of thing. I don't know honestly whether he was, really liked, I don't really know whether he liked it or not, but he did go . . . don't get me wrong . . . he's very interested in the children, but on the one hand it was difficult for him to take time . . . and I felt it was to do with me in the end . . . it was nothing to do with him.

Mrs Jackson seemed to be making a similar point:

> He actually works away, and we wasn't really . . . I mean he would have gone if he felt he had to go, but he . . . obviously I told him what went on.

Not all the women felt this way. As we saw earlier, some wives were quite insistent that their husbands should come and participate. One mother, Mrs Jackson, answered the question in a very reflective way, and did not claim that either she or her husband was necessarily right – just different:

> He didn't view the situation the same. He didn't see it in quite the way I did where Pauline was concerned. He thought Pauline was just going through a stage and he said this to the child guidance person at the end of the interview, that he wasn't worried. Part of her personality and it would work its way through as things do with a family. It was me who felt there was probably something more deep-rooted and that Pauline and I were clashing. . . . He still felt afterwards that it was probably a lot of my guilt feelings, but we did discuss it more afterwards in the light of what we'd been told and agreed that we would have the same sort of responses to Pauline for certain things. If she did something wrong then we would both try and respond in the same way and so on, so it was quite positive.

Some of the accounts bear a strong resemblance to the descriptions given by Marianne Walters *et al.* (1988) who have highlighted the strong sense of guilt and responsibility women often bring to family therapy. It also seems that there can be a difference between the expectations which men and women have of therapy itself. Ian Bennun (1989) found that women tend to seek understanding of the problem, whereas men tend to be more interested in direct advice. A sense of responsibility certainly appears to be present in Mrs Sinclair's description of the first session. Her son, John, was also present:

John: What I didn't like about it was when we first went with that lady. She had someone else in the room – a bloke.

Mrs S: She had a gentleman sat in the room and it put . . . our son retaliated to that so when we got out . . .

John: I just didn't like him being there.

Mrs S: It made him uneasy.

Q.30 Did you feel that your therapist understood how you felt about your problem?

    17 users felt that the therapist had understood.

    2 users felt that the therapist had not understood.

    3 users were undecided.

Listening and understanding (or trying to understand) are important skills in any user-friendly therapy, but understanding is not a static concept. Therapy often involves a change in understanding, both on the part of therapists and users. Many family therapists are rightly concerned about inadvertently creating a mismatch between themselves and users if an expert position is adopted. But, used supportively, such expertness can help those users for whom such a stance is part of their expectation of therapy. Mrs Holloway said:

Oh, yes, because I remember I kept getting told off for using words, in a nice way; things like I felt guilty and things like that and they kept telling me off. And I found that very hard to understand up to now.

The therapist had here 'understood' what Mrs Holloway had struggled to under-stand. We may wonder how far she had found this helpful, although talking to the researcher clearly meant a lot to her. Mrs Kingston seemed to have felt helped by her therapist's 'understanding' how she was feeling:

Yes, straightaway she turned round and said to me, 'You feel very guilty about Carol for some reason. Why?' and that sort of pulled me up with a start because I hadn't realized I did feel guilty. Although I talk about how I felt guilty now, I didn't realize that it was guilt that I was feeling at the time.

For others such seemingly instinctive understanding did not come about so easily. The gap between user and therapist may have been greater either because of the sheer exhaustion of the user or the apparent differences in life style between the two. Mrs Pettit is an example of the former:

In some ways, yes, I think she did; in other ways, I think she really didn't understand just how sort of tired and fed up I was feeling of having to get up every night. It was virtually like going back to having a small baby in the house again.

Mrs Cartwright was not too sure about how far her therapist could understand her:

Well, they seemed sympathetic, put it that way. I don't know if they had families. I know one wasn't married, so obviously she probably didn't have children.

Q.31 Did your therapist understand how you thought the problem could be helped?

8 users felt that the therapist had understood.
14 users were either undecided or felt that the therapist had not understood.

This question was asked on the assumption that many users have their own ideas about the way in which they want to be helped. We have already seen that a number of users had not received the type of help they had originally wanted, but had been pleased with what they had received instead. As Mrs Williams put it:

Well, I thought the problem would be helped by Pat [her husband] talking, but I think it was probably me. She certainly succeeded in making me feel much better in myself than I'd felt for a very long time. And how you are in yourself reflects in your children.

Mrs Langford had perceived something of a paradox in the question. She had also felt helped in the end:

Er, no, because I didn't know how it could be helped, so probably not. Well, she must have done because it did seem as though it helped in the end, so . . . I didn't go with a clear idea of how it could be helped, otherwise I don't feel as though I'd needed to go.

The users who felt helped may have been those who, as we have already seen, were able to make the adjustment to, and subsequently understand, the therapist's way of working. Some users even went so far as to take responsibility for the fact that they themselves had not helped the therapist understand. Mrs Thomas said:

Well, he never gave me any practical advice, you know, treat him this way or treat him that way. I expect if I'd asked him he would have.

Mrs Holloway also seemed to have felt that she had not explained adequately to the therapist what she had hoped for:

No, I don't know. Well, unless they did I don't know, but I don't know whether I was clear enough at the time . . . I don't think I'd just come out with it like I have now and said . . .

Indeed, Mrs Holloway's various statements have haunted us somewhat and reminded us of the fact that users may continue thinking about therapy even when it is over. So often, the process of researching probed old dilemmas, and several users commented on how good it had felt to talk about the therapy – and not least to have been able to be of help to someone in return, by answering questions.

THROUGH THE STAGES OF THERAPY

In this chapter we have looked at what strikes us as being some of the crucial questions about what it may mean to be a user of family therapy. We have tried as far as possible to let the user speak, although we have had to be selective with the quotations and have presumed to offer some cautious interpretations and connections. We hope that the excerpts we have included in the chapter will have brought alive the users' 'voices' but as the reader you may still be left with the feeling of having received a somewhat jumbled collection of disembodied quotations and very little context. We therefore want to conclude this chapter by following just one user through some of her responses to the questions posed. This may go some way to explain how diverse and full of apparent inconsistencies a user's experience of family therapy can be. But it will also illustrate how important a positive therapeutic alliance with users can be in helping them through the minefield of therapy and the mistakes which we can all make as therapists.

Mrs Partridge was talking about her stepson Michael (aged 17), her husband Bill, and Bill's first wife Linda:

The first time I went I think the most useful thing was that she [therapist] helped me to understand that I was managing . . . that we were just like any other family. It wasn't because we were a stepfamily. She said, no, we were just the same, like complete families . . .

She kept on doing these family trees, about two or three sessions, I can't remember, anyway I was completely on the outside and everyone else was part of it. . . .

We had to go with that mirror. He [Bill] didn't like the mirror, none of us liked it, and Michael especially didn't like it the way they kept on interrupting, you know, coming through on that phone. . . .

The second time we went they decided that I was too domineering and took too much upon myself, I think they said. I should try and take a back seat and let my husband do more. And I did, and it was surprising how much easier I found life after that. . . .

After we forgot one session she [therapist] phoned during tea, and he [Bill] made some excuse why we hadn't gone. But because she spoke to him directly, he wouldn't say, 'Oh, we're not coming again'. So we continued . . .

So what with that mirror and the family tree, I didn't think it was helpful. Anyway, Michael went to live with an aunt soon afterwards, and he's a different boy now. . . .

Apart from that I thought it was a very good place to go. I mean they were all completely different in how they dealt with us, and yet I thought they were all very helpful and very good.

In quoting Mrs Partridge's comments in some detail we are not wanting to imply that she was involved in a particularly good or bad piece of structural family therapy. We could, with hindsight, comment on ways of completing a genogram more sensitively; of being sympathetic to the particularly complex tasks of being a stepmother; of being aware of the gender issues around whose responsibility it is to bring people into therapy; and of using one-way screens more openly. However, what we want to highlight instead is a more over-arching issue. We believe that the somewhat ragged therapy experienced by Mrs Partridge ended on a relatively positive note because the therapist and the family were able to build a good enough therapeutic alliance. At a more general level, what excited us when Carolyn's results were shared with the teams was the possibility that our hit-or-miss methods of building alliances with users could be modified in meaningful ways so that therapists would become more sensitive to their users' experiences of (coming to and) being in therapy. In our next chapter, Sigurd explores how the teams were able to utilize Carolyn's research in order to achieve a more user-friendly approach to family therapy.

Chapter 7

Research and practice, practice and research

Sigurd Reimers

In the last chapter we saw how our project had provided us with important information about how a small sample of users had experienced the Child and Family Guidance Service in Western Wiltshire. In this chapter we will examine how the results of this study influenced the therapeutic practice of the teams involved. The impetus created by this initial work prompted two further studies to be undertaken in due course. The remaining part of the chapter will discuss the lessons that were learnt from both these studies. Users had reported to us many positive aspects of their experiences of therapy but there were five major areas which needed attention:

1 More than half of the respondents who had experienced the screen were unhappy about its use.
2 More than half of those who had experienced the video had been unhappy about its use despite having given consent to its use.
3 Many had felt uninformed about the service before coming to the first session.
4 Many parents had come expecting advice, and some had found that the therapist's emphasis on exploring relationships and on developing the family's own ideas did not match their expectations of therapy.
5 Some parents had found it uncomfortable being seen as a family, and would also have liked their child to have been seen alone, or to have seen the therapist by themselves without their child.

THE EFFECTS OF THE RESEARCH ON THE TEAMS

The effects of the findings on the teams involved were quite varied. Teams tend not to think as one person any more than families do. Also the extent to which family therapy was practised within the teams varied between team members, some of whom used a number of other methods as well as family therapy. There was, however, a dilemma which was shared by all of us. To what extent was there a need for any changes in our practice of family therapy? After all, although some concern had been expressed by many users about some specific details of family therapy, there was general satisfaction with the service overall. Nearly all the users had felt well cared for and understood by the therapist. The great majority of the parents would either return for further help if they needed to or would recommend the service to their friends. Most had found that either the problem itself had changed for the better or that their own sense of coping with the problem had improved.

What, then, was the case for making any changes in our practice? Is it ever possible to please everyone? Will users, who have mixed feelings about receiving help in the first place, tend to find something 'objective', like the one-way screen or the video, on to which they can project their concerns about therapy? If the outcome is good enough in most cases, perhaps the medicine sometimes needs to be uncomfortable? These questions might all be valid, but not unexpectedly the process of becoming more aware of how users think about the therapy made it more difficult to leave an existing practice entirely unchanged. Also, other teams were beginning to make discoveries similar to our own. Jackie Russell and M. Leyland (1986), for example, in their study of users' views of therapy, reported that a majority of families could accept the technology of family therapy but a minority were concerned about the use of the video. One of the respondents in their study had also pointed out that the major difficulty for families experiencing the one-way screen was that 'there is no eye contact with the observers, so it is difficult to know what reaction you are getting, and impossible to correct mis-understandings'. (See Chapter 9 for a further discussion of their findings.)

Russell and Leyland's work is significant because it actually focuses on a rare type of data – feedback about therapy from a user perspective. It is ironic, but true, that family therapy, which claims to base itself so firmly on the notion of feedback, has paid relatively little attention to feedback from users about their experiences of therapy (a point we will establish more clearly in Chapter 9). However, we have also noted in previous chapters that therapists tend not to be influenced by empirical research, and it is disappointing to have to record that even critical feedback from users easily goes unheeded. For example, Mitchell and Fowkes (1985), in their own study of the effects of research within general medicine, found that research feedback was negligible in changing clinical practice, mainly because researchers and practitioners inhabit two very different professional worlds which are rarely linked. Harlene Anderson and Harold Goolishian (1988), writing about family therapy, make this point succinctly: 'At the end we are reminded that we can think of no theory of psychotherapy that has ever been abandoned because of clear observational data and evidence.'

Fortunately the teams in Western Wiltshire were already concerned with providing an improved service as well as being aware of the risks involved in undertaking research. On the basis of the five areas of concern outlined above, team members decided both to make some clear changes in team practice and also to encourage each other to try out some new ideas in response to user feedback within a team culture which encouraged diversity as well as cohesion.

Changes in the use of the one-way screen

We were now more aware that many users found the one-way screen both impersonal and threatening. We decided that when we used the screen, we would introduce members of the back-up team to the family at the beginning of the first session. For a few families this seemed to be unnecessary, but the majority eagerly took up the idea of meeting team members face to face, albeit briefly. The therapists also began using the name of the person phoning through from the observation room, again to try and humanize what always risked being a mechanical way of working. So, for instance, a therapist might preface a comment with a remark like, 'Trevor has asked me to comment . . .', 'Clare wonders whether . . .' and so on. Simultaneously we were becoming ever more aware of the importance of the gender of the therapist within the therapeutic process. The naming of colleagues, especially in a mixed gender team, was a reminder to both therapist and family members that both men and women were present. (See Chapter 13 for a discussion on how gender issues can be brought alive within family therapy sessions.)

As we became less perfunctory and defensive about our use of the one-way screen, we noticed that many children were fascinated by the largely unseen team. They welcomed our offer of going behind the screen at the end of the session, and this seemed to give some parents 'permission' to satisfy their own curiosity about the team process. Alison O'Brien and Penny Louden (1985) have described some delightful uses of the 'magic mirror' (the one-way screen) in work with the families of young children.

Before Carolyn's study had been completed it was not unusual for us to have four or five colleagues behind the one-way screen. Apart from team members, students and other observers interested in how family therapy was conducted were often present. Once we started introducing families to team members, it became increasingly difficult for us to justify the presence of so many people. No doubt a few families felt flattered by the amount of attention they were receiving, but others expressed a polite concern at the fact that their problem should be considered so serious as to warrant such a large team. It seemed as if we risked confusing the idea of giving families the best with giving them the most. An unanticipated effect of introducing families to the team was, therefore, that we reduced the size of the therapeutic team to the point where it became more customary to have one, two or at most three people behind the one-way screen. Outside observers would now only be welcome when they had a specific interest in developing family therapy skills rather than participating in the 'tourism' of earlier days. More crucially for developing our practice, permission was now sought from the users specifically for observers or trainees to be present behind the screen.

The actual way we introduced the one-way screen to users did not change drastically. However, we did spend more time explaining the thinking behind its use, taking a pause to listen to any comments from family members, and then proceeding either with or without the screen. No doubt we will at times have come across as a little unsure of ourselves, but we generally preferred this risk to that of rushing through the consent-giving process in a perfunctory way which could, at this very early stage in therapy, easily be taken to reflect our general approach to therapy.

Live supervision/live consultation

This method of 'in-the-room' consultation (which avoids using a screen) had been used for many years, and had been well described by Donna Smith and Phil Kingston (1980). Donna had been my predecessor as social work team leader in Wiltshire and live supervision had been used widely by both teams at the time of the study. The decision about its use had tended to be made by the therapist, rather than in conjunction with family members, in line with the then current thinking about expert teams. Live supervision would be used in preference to the screen where a sense of proximity and immediacy – even of intimacy – was thought to be called for. It was also often used in instances where family members expressed unhappiness about the use of the screen, and it was particularly this last consideration which influenced us at this point. Live supervision came to be used more since, when asked, some family members said they preferred to see (and hear) the supervisor. We should, however, note from the survey that a few people had said that they preferred to have the supervisor less obtrusive, and out of sight behind the screen.

Changes in the use of the video

Most of our respondents had felt uncomfortable with the video. We now felt we had to justify more clearly to ourselves why we wanted to make recordings, particularly as we had very little time for reviewing the tapes anyway. We started using the video less than in the past. When we did use it, it tended to be when we anticipated meeting with large families, or when we were working with parti- cularly complex situations or on our own. Some members of the team abandoned its use completely.

The question of gaining consent, however, still remained an important issue. Jim Birch (1990) makes the point that seeking consent to the use of video recordings should be congruent with the type of therapy being used. He takes Gregory Bateson's point that communication has both a 'command' and a 'report' function. Birch claims that a therapy which is based on emphasizing empowerment rather than a power hierarchy must also work towards a consent- seeking approach which goes beyond what the user may experience as an 'illusion of choice'.

Over the years, most people (including ourselves) have become more familiar with the use of video cameras, and most homes in the United Kingdom now have a video recorder. We sense that the majority of users are therefore more accustomed to video recordings. We have, at the same time, noticed an opposite trend as well. Closed-circuit television cameras are used for surveillance of public places, and video recordings are used for evidence-taking, particularly in cases of suspected child abuse. Many users are aware of this, and we have had to bear this in mind when seeking consent.

The findings of the study created a new situation for us. If we were to be truly user-friendly, then all aspects of therapy needed to make sense to users as well as to ourselves. It was therefore important for us to ask permission to use the video in a more flexible and sensitive way, giving clearer explanations of why and how we wanted to use it. We were also prompted to discuss the use of video at various stages of the therapy in case people had changed their minds about its use but were afraid to say so. For my own part, I also found that I wanted to change my standard practice for seeking permission to release videos for training purposes. The engagement stage in therapy no longer seemed the best point to ask about this, and I now began to wait until nearer the end of therapy, when the family and I understood each other better. I would explain that there were certain passages on the tapes which I thought would be of use for the training of other professionals, and I would suggest to the families that they might like to see the episodes concerned before deciding whether to give consent. Some users take up this suggestion, and seem to feel more comfortable with the idea once they know that they really have the power to say no. Signing what amounts to a blank cheque at the beginning of therapy is problematic ethically because users feel at their most vulnerable and are therefore most likely to agree to training videos although they might prefer not to give permission.

Publicity about family therapy

As we have seen, many people in our study had been worried about coming to the first session and some had said that they would like to have been better informed about therapy beforehand. It seemed to us that one way to do this was through making an information leaflet – something which in post-Citizen's Charter and post-Children Act times may now seem obvious. A number of principles influenced the way we wrote the leaflet:

(a) It should be in plain English.
(b) It should recognize that family problems are a common and normal experience.
(c) It should make clear that therapy involves people talking to each other.
(d) It should point out that it can be helpful to involve the family as a resource in dealing with difficulties.
(e) It should explain how long a session lasts and that it may be useful to return for further sessions.
(f) It should make it clear that responsibility will not be taken away from the family.

An example of the first version of the leaflet can be found in Appendix 2. Unfortunately we did not involve users themselves in designing and testing the leaflet, so what we did was not a model for good practice. Clearly users can be very helpful in designing and writing such leaflets but it is important to keep updating the leaflets as agency policy and practices often change.

Advice-giving

A number of our respondents had said that they wished they could have had more direct advice about dealing with their children's difficulties. This is not surprising. We live in a society where we have come to expect technical solutions to everyday problems and a family life which 'should' not need to be problematic. At the same time as becoming more aware of the wishes of some users for advice, as therapists we were also being told by some referrers that some users found the whole idea of formal referrals, attending pre-set appointments and bringing the whole family to sessions too demanding. They wanted something more informal. We therefore decided to set up a 'walk-in' service in one of our centres, and advertised this widely in various agencies and other public places. One afternoon per week in term-time was set aside so that parents could come for a guaranteed half-hour consultation without either having to give a name and address or having to make an appointment.

Between 1987 and 1992 our experience of running the service produced interesting results. About half of those parents who used the service found one session to be enough, and the other half decided to refer themselves more formally and returned with their families for further work. The half-hour walk-in consultation required some quick thinking on the part of the team member on duty, and it lacked the benefit of planning or team support but it became an effective way of helping parents explore what help, if any, they might want before having to commit themselves to any therapeutic plan. Where direct advice was given in the sessions, it would often take a tentative form, the therapist perhaps pointing out that ideas which worked in some situations might not automatically work in all other situations.

Interview composition: together or apart?

As we have seen, a number of parents had assumed that we would be seeing their children on their own, perhaps in the belief that the problem was 'inside' the child and needed to be 'brought out' by an expert. Also, some parents felt uncomfortable about talking about problems in front of their children, and would have preferred to speak to the therapist on their own. Rather than make a whole-family session an absolute requirement we moved further towards a position which offered users a variety of choices. It also became more common to reach such decisions in consultation with family members. At first such consultations felt to some of us like abandoning our responsibility to know what was best for the families, or at times to be colluding with conflict-avoiding tactics on the part of family members. In due course a number of us developed a three-pronged approach to the issue by arranging for family, individual and parent appointments, where relevant, but this move became more established after the next user survey had been completed.

FROM PRACTICE TO QUESTIONS, FROM QUESTIONS TO PRACTICE: THE SECOND USER SURVEY

It is often hard to trace where an idea originally came from, and who thought of it first. With hindsight perhaps we are prone to impose later experiences on original explanations. Certainly the idea of a further user survey had been around for a while before we decided to repeat the exercise. It is likely to have come out of a renewed sense of concern on the part of some of us about whether the methods we were using were helping us to relate more adequately to our users. There was also enough energy and interest in the team to undertake the task of a further survey. In 1988, two years after the first survey had been completed, we decided we wanted to repeat the process and ask a further sample of users some of the same questions that had been used two years earlier, as well as introducing some new questions which were important to us. Would we receive the same answers as before? Had our practice changed sufficiently to be reflected in the answers that users gave? Why had we not thought of asking users about how they had felt about going to the referrer in the first place? Would they have preferred to self-refer, and why did they not do so, as many other users had done?

If we look at Figure 2 we can see how original issues in our own minds had gone through a long process of leading to some change in practice. We could now see the idea of carrying out another study as an opportunity for completing the circle.

In 1988 Paula Ford, a social work student, undertook a placement at the Chippenham Child and Family Guidance Centre. She was willing to help us undertake a further study and it seemed like a good opportunity to obtain some more views from users about the service. There were some snags though. Time was more limited and we had no research supervision, but we were keen to keep the spirit of research alive.

We decided to use the original interview schedule, but to leave out those questions which seemed to have been of little interest to the original respondents. We also had two new questions to add – one about feelings about approaching the referrer, and the other about whether users would have preferred to self-refer. If we look at the research–practice cycle again we can see how the circle was now becoming complete. Our practice was encouraging us to re-examine users' opinions, both to see how far a new set of respondents would raise similar or different concerns about therapy, and also to see how they would respond to new questions.

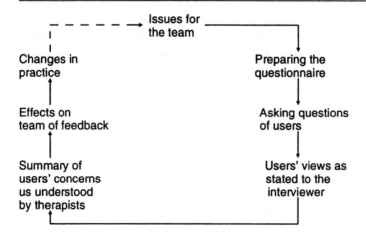

Figure 2 The research–practice cycle after the first user survey

THE SECOND SURVEY

In all, 19 parents were interviewed in their homes: 14 mothers, 3 fathers and 1 couple. We will start by looking at the two new questions together since they are closely linked.

Q.1 How did you feel when you first spoke to [the referrer] about the problem?

4 users said they had felt comfortable.
13 users said they had felt uncomfortable.

Q.2 Would you have found it easier or more difficult to have contacted the Centre directly?

11 users said it would have been easier.
3 users said it would have been more difficult.
3 users said they were unsure.

Most of the respondents had found it difficult going to see the referrer. Of the 19 respondents, 17 had been referred to the service by another professional – 14 of them from primary agency staff like health visitors, general medical practitioners or teachers. Users' familiarity with such agencies, however, did not appear to have diminished their sense of discomfort at having to seek help. The most commonly expressed emotions were those of embarrassment, inadequacy as parents, and fear of inquisitiveness on the part of professionals. Mrs Field had been to her GP, but had not felt he had been sympathetic:

I felt silly. The GP didn't take us very seriously, but we felt desperate. He suggested we might try you.

Not surprisingly, Mrs Field said that she would have felt more in control if she had referred herself. She could have asked questions about the service, but, like most of our respondents, she had not known of the existence of the service.

Mrs Parsons had also felt uncomfortable about asking for help when she saw her health visitor, even though she had been listened to sympathetically:

I felt very emotional . . . nervous and embarrassed, I suppose, to have to tell someone outside the family.

Mrs Parsons would have liked to have contacted the Centre directly, in common with many other users, had she known about it, but she worried about possibly having to complete a referral form because she had difficulty in reading and writing.

Mrs Stanton was also embarrassed, but was glad to have someone to get in touch with the Centre on her behalf:

It would have been difficult. The health visitor explained to the clinic about my problem before I went and this helped me. I'd have found it very hard to explain it all there the first time.

Mrs Owers had been referred by a social worker, but had not been keen on the idea at all:

I didn't want to talk to anyone about it. I felt they were nosy . . . would ask too many questions.

In fact, several users made the point that making a self-referral would have been easier because it might have avoided their feeling pried upon and also have helped them stay in control. For others, however, it seemed equally difficult, whichever way they sought help. The sense of failure was still there – as with Mr Simpson, for instance:

I felt grossly inadequate . . . like I had done something wrong. I would have done anything to try and resolve the problem.

Q.6 In what ways were you expecting to be helped?

7 users expected to be given practical advice.
6 users were unsure about what to expect.
5 users expected to talk and to be listened to.
2 users expected the child to be talked to by the therapist.

These results roughly confirm the findings from the first survey. Because respondents often give brief answers to direct questions, especially at the beginning of an interview with a stranger, it is important not to treat these answers as definitive. Answers to other questions suggested that some of those who had wanted advice had also expected to be listened to, and those who wanted to talk also expected advice. Take Mrs Pitt, for instance, who answered:

To tell them all about it. For them to give me a solution. To get it confirmed by experts that what I was doing was OK.

There are at least three different messages expressed here. In fact, after one session Mrs Pitt felt that it had been helpful to talk and to have her parenting style affirmed. There also seemed to be a number of messages within Mrs Baker's reply:

... someone to talk to. A stranger's view of the problem would be clearer.

In having a number of interlocking expectations, rather than just one, some respondents did seem to regard therapy as an interactional process, and one involving some flexibility on their part about what might be the central issue at any one time. Although a small group, they had all felt happy about the help they had received, and I wonder whether that flexibility may have helped them (and the therapist) to get the most out of therapy.

Q.4 Before you went for your first visit, can you remember what your feelings were about going?

6 users felt generally optimistic about going.
9 users felt generally uncomfortable about going.
4 users had very mixed feelings.

Again, this pattern of responses is similar to what we found in the first survey, but this summary masks the sheer diversity of worries which users had when they first came to see the therapist.

8 users were afraid of being blamed.
7 users were anxious about not knowing what to expect.
6 users felt that they were failing as parents.
5 users were afraid that their children would be taken away.
3 users were unsure about whether they wanted outside help at all.
3 users were concerned about having their private world pried into.

As we can see, some respondents expressed a number of different concerns, and we can imagine how some users who are referred may never even attend the first session because their anxieties are greater than their wish for help. Mrs Barlow expressed some of this diversity of feelings:

... nervous, unsure of being helped, but hopeful. I didn't know what to expect.

Mr Barlow was also concerned:

... apprehensive about family details and background being brought out. It felt like a last resort. We didn't know where else we could go for help.

Q.9 Can you say what was most helpful about going to the Centre?

Q.10 Can you say what was least helpful about going to the Centre?

10 users had found it helpful talking and being listened to.

6 users had found their parenting approach affirmed or had been helped in working more closely together as parents.

3 users thought that they now saw the problem differently.

3 users had been helped by being told that they were not to blame.

3 users had found therapy intrusive.

3 users had missed not being given advice.

Interestingly none of those who had felt they had been helped used the term 'advice', but some, like Mrs Walters, seemed to see advice-giving in a very general way:

They made you see how to do it. Picked what you said and made suggestions out of it. Then it all seemed so simple . . . why hadn't we seen it for ourselves?

The lack of advice-giving troubled Mrs James:

Although I talked alone with the therapist no one listened to what I was saying. They seemed to be saying 'there, there, never mind', but they didn't suggest any practical solution.

The mismatch between user expectation and therapy had left Mrs James unhappy. Mrs Field felt that this mismatch had changed somewhat in the light of later experience:

She pushed things to a head. It seemed to make things worse, but afterwards things got better, so that may have been helpful in the end.

Intensification (e.g. pushing users to face issues they normally avoid) is one technique in structural family therapy and some users obviously find it difficult. Mrs Owers did not see the value of similar structural techniques, in this case enactment:

. . . having to practise [in the session] telling my daughter not to do something. It felt like on my driving test . . . I knew how to do it, but it was unnatural to do it there, like that . . . I felt awkward and embarrassed.

Mrs Owers was a single parent who had recently moved to the area, was socially rather isolated, and admitted that she was not one to tell the therapist if she was not happy about the therapy. Perhaps the therapist was being rather ambitious in using enactment in the first session, but it is worth noting that in other respects Mrs Owers had felt well cared for and positive, both about the process and the outcome of therapy.

Q.18 At the time did it seem helpful or unhelpful to use the video?

The video had been used with 8 out of 19 families.

1 user had found it helpful.
3 users had found it unhelpful.
4 users had mixed feelings.

We can already see how much less the video was now being used than at the time of the first survey, but some people were uncomfortable, like Mrs Charles:

We couldn't relax. It was like being in the cop shop.

Mrs Latham said:

. . . unhelpful. . . . We were very wary of what we said or did.

These two respondents had very little else in common, and neither was amongst those who had found it most difficult to come to the Centre. One thing both had mentioned, though, was that they felt very uncomfortable about the therapist delving into their family history. They might have experienced the video as a part of such a process.

Those who had expressed mixed emotions were people who had initially been uncomfortable but had soon forgotten about the video. The one person who had been enthusiatic was Mrs Taplow, who had seen an excerpt from an earlier session:

. . . very helpful to look back and see how I'd been with the kids and how they'd reacted to me. To be able to discuss this at the next session . . . I couldn't believe it was me sometimes.

Q.24 At the time did it seem helpful or unhelpful to use the one-way screen?

The one-way screen had been used with seven families.

3 users thought it had been helpful, but only to the therapist.
1 user was uncertain about its usefulness.
3 users thought it had been unhelpful.

Since the earlier survey the use of the one-way screen had been reduced. Some users who initially had mixed feelings had come to feel more comfortable after a period of discomfort. Even so, Mrs Williams had disliked the screen:

. . . unhelpful. I felt I had to be on my best behaviour at first. Not saying what I really meant . . . it made me feel strange, difficult to say what I felt at first. After a few times I got used to it.

Discomfort can mean different things to different people and does not automatically mean that a particular approach should be abandoned. Mrs Carter was very concerned that she might be blamed as a parent, and saw the usefulness of the screen in terms of the children:

[I felt] under the spotlight. At first it was very embarrassing, but then we got used to it and didn't notice it too much after a time . . . it was helpful when the children were there.

Q.28 Did you feel that the person you talked to at the Centre understood how you felt about the problem?

12 users thought that the therapist had understood.
7 users thought that the therapist had not understood.

Some of the users felt that the therapist had understood how they had felt by showing some degree of self-disclosure. Mrs Carter said:

Yes, she'd obviously been through things with her own kids.

Mrs Latham, however, had not found the therapist's statements about himself helpful:

Yes, he knew what we were going through. He had kids of his own. They had problems, but he said they'd nipped that in the bud, sorted them out early on. It was all right for them to talk.

Mrs Viner's view was more complex:

She [the therapist] didn't show she understood. But she must have, I suppose. It's her job. They're probably trained not to show their emotions . . . it's run of the mill to them, isn't it? They must see hundreds.

Mrs Williams expressed her views about therapist understanding more succinctly:

Yes, they shouldn't be doing the job if they didn't.

FURTHER IMPRESSIONS

A survey such as this one inevitably throws up a large variety of issues, but it is hard to draw general conclusions which fit all or even most users. There are, however, two issues which stand out for me partly because they were brought up so frequently and in different contexts and partly because they are issues which commonly arise in the family therapy literature. One has to do with the control of therapy and the problem of child abuse, and the other with the balance between advice-giving and helping users arrive at their own conclusions.

Who's in charge?

We have already seen how many people feel powerless when they approach a professional and ask for help with personal problems. Fortunately many of them are able to move towards a more powerful position in time. But even people like Mrs Stanton, who had felt greatly helped, had been through a variety of feelings about therapy:

It was like a magic cure to me. Tough at times, but now I understand – they helped me . . . she [therapist] was different. Young and no kids. At first I did wonder. My parents said, 'How can they know anything if they don't have kids?' But I knew they were trained, seen hundreds of kids . . . [although] I was too scared to say too much at first in case they took the kids.

Mrs Stanton's final remark brings to light a menacing side of the therapeutic relationship. This study gave us an incidental but important insight into the profound worries which many users had about therapist power. These worries extended well beyond the general idea of expert authority. User after user told us of how they had worried that their children might be taken away. Both Mr and Mrs Barlow said that they had felt inadequate before they came, but desperate enough not to give up. What was more striking was Mrs Barlow's comment:

Might we be putting the family at risk? Might they see us as bad parents and take the children away?

Mrs Carter referred to the media as she expressed herself in almost the same words as Mrs Barlow:

They might say we were bad parents, might even take the children away.

Unfortunately parents do not usually articulate such fears directly to their therapist, particularly during initial sessions.

If we are not aware of the depth or the extent of such worries, we probably depend on a combination of good sense and good fortune to help make for a good therapeutic alliance. This may have been the case with the Carters. The one-way screen had been used and they had felt put under the spotlight, but 'we met the person behind the screen – that was nice – we knew who it was then'. They had been surprised that the therapist had wanted to see the whole family, but had found her different from what they had expected:

She was not abrupt like the doctors. She was helpful and had obviously been through things with her own kids.

We can almost feel the balance of meanings being experienced by this family as they opted in favour of staying with the therapy. Personal aspects of the therapist, like friendliness and the use of self-disclosure, seemed to have made an important difference to some of those who had worried about losing their children. Mrs Owers had found the therapist friendly, but had had profound worries before going to the Centre:

. . . they'd check the kids for bruises etc., looking to see if I ill-treated them.

Mrs Martin had particular reason to fear losing her children:

Our first child ended up in care. We were afraid this could happen again.

In the circumstances it is not surprising that they were also worried about the use of the video. They had not been convinced that no one else would see it, and they even thought that their social worker was behind the one-way screen, although it was not being used. The only thing that finally convinced them of confidentiality was when the court report was shared with them:

He [the therapist] worked with us, not against us.

Although one respondent had contacted the Centre directly for help after seeing a TV programme which gave a positive view of therapy, we gained a clear impression that many people had been worried by the portrayal of child care services in the media. The Cleveland Inquiry had taken place a short time before this study, and had acquired huge media publicity. This inquiry had followed a brief period during which a large number of children in Cleveland had been removed from their parents following paediatric examinations which had suggested that the children had been sexually abused. This had been a very different inquiry from the many earlier public inquiries into the deaths of children through physical abuse. As Esther Saraga (1993) points out:

Whereas Maria [Colwell]'s death was seen as a 'failure' of the social and welfare services, in the Cleveland case medical and social work professionals were accused of 'gross over-reaction'.

We have no doubt that the public, including our users, are influenced by media portrayals of child care services (and often of therapy, by implication), and I can give a small example of this. The week following the screening of the family therapy interview in the soap opera *EastEnders* (referred to at the beginning of Chapter 2) I had first interviews with three families. When they saw the one-way screen, members of two of the families referred to the *EastEnders* episode, and we used discussions of that experience as a basis for discussing how and what we were going to do together might be similar or different. With the third family I raised the subject of *EastEnders* (assuming by now that everyone watched it), but they had not even heard of it!

Listening or advising?

In this study, as in the earlier one, we found that the two main expectations of therapy were to be listened to and to receive direct advice. Users tended to say that they had wanted one or the other, and often judged their experiences of therapy by how far their expectations had been met. Mrs Taplow had wanted to talk about the problem, but had also wanted practical advice. She felt that she had received such advice, and had thought that both the video and the one-way screen had been useful because they had helped the therapist give the best advice available. The problem did not get better in itself, but:

> It helped me not to react as I had been. I understood what was going on. When things were difficult I thought about what they had told me.

Mrs Taplow had been particularly impressed by a follow-up visit from the therapist at home:

> I thought I'd just be another file thrown in the corner, but that showed they really cared.

Mrs Viner, on the other hand, was extremely critical of the service, apparently because of the lack of advice:

> Nothing [was helpful]. There was no suggested course of action, no practical advice, nothing constructive. They just wanted to talk . . . they could just as well have pumped us full of sodium pentathol and got on with it basically . . . they didn't tell me anything I could *do*. They weren't supportive . . . just asking questions.

Mrs Viner was a person who claimed to be outspoken. She had had no problems about asking her GP for help. She had wanted something done about her problem, and knew that she was not to blame. She accepted both the video and the one-way screen without any worries but she had found the whole experience clinical and useless.

Both Mrs Taplow and Mrs Viner had wanted practical advice rather than simply to be listened to. Or perhaps the only way they felt they could be adequately listened to was if they had first received what they saw as practical help. I suspect that there are quite a few users who are unable, or unwilling, to engage in a deeper interchange of experiences until they can first see some demonstrable progress, perhaps as a sign of therapist competence and caring.

Mrs Queen was one of the people who had come hoping to be listened to as well as to understand. Unfortunately the therapist had focused in the first session very clearly on her children's behaviour and the 'attempted solutions' adopted by the family. In doing this she had come across as critical; which, as we know, is a poor foundation for positive change:

> I was very disappointed. I felt I was being criticized in everything I'd tried . . . it made me feel inadequate, and I got so tense the words came out back to front. She said I should have tried longer or 'that was not a good thing to do' or 'you shouldn't have done that'. When I came again she told me to bring my husband, not the kids. How could I manage that – leaving the kids – my husband taking time off work?

Mrs Parsons, as we have heard, found it difficult to seek help outside the family. She said that she had worried about how to tell her story:

> It eased me really. It helped me . . . myself. When I went at first I was depressed, drinking, and couldn't cope with the children. Talking with a

stranger, who really listened, I could let it all out. It was a relief . . . helped me cope with the kids. They saw the kids on their own and that helped too.

The research questions themselves may have encouraged respondents to express their expectations in clear-cut ways. In fact, if we look at the details of the responses it appears that users were hoping for a combination of various types of help at different times. To judge by the overall responses, the thoughtfulness of the therapist and the flexibility of the users provided a good enough fit more often than not. It may have been impossible to have helped some of the users, but some might have been helped better if the therapy could have been more openly custom-built, with therapist and users constantly monitoring how their expectations and experiences of each other matched or failed to match.

FURTHER CHANGES TO PRACTICE

We had made a number of changes to our practice as a result of our first survey, but it was becoming disappointingly clear how difficult it is to be consistent in sustaining such changes. Some respondents had still not been adequately prepared for therapy. For example, at least one family had not been introduced to the team behind the screen and another had felt pushed into accepting the use of the video. There was, therefore, scope for further scrutinizing the changes in our practice. In addition, other important issues to do with the use of team and video which had already been apparent in the first survey were becoming clearer and would need to be taken more seriously. The first was the use of the telephone between the observation and interview rooms. Many users had found that the calls had interrupted their train of thought and did not provide them with many useful ideas. We therefore started using the telephone more sparingly, and when we did, it was less to give directives to the therapist than to share some thoughts or perceptions. The conversations on the telephone tended to become fewer but longer, and would not necessarily involve the therapist in repeating questions verbatim to the family.

These changes were prompted not so much by theoretical developments but by listening to user feedback. Almost imperceptibly the feedback began to alter the nature of the relationship between team, therapist and family. Elsewhere other family therapists were also making changes to their practice but these parallel changes seemed to have been developed because of changes in theory. Tom Andersen (1987) and his colleagues, and subsequently others, had for some time been developing a theoretical framework resulting in the use of reflecting teams. This might involve asking the family whether they would like to listen to the observing team talking amongst themselves. Following this, the family would be asked whether they would in turn like to comment on this conversation. In terms of open communication, such a practice clearly has a user-friendly aspect, but I am not aware that specific research, monitoring users' experiences, has played any part in the development of reflecting teams.

On the basis of our research we would argue that some families would find the reflecting team method uncomfortable, so the blanket introduction of such a method is clearly not user-friendly. Too often therapists are fascinated by innovations in family therapy theory and practice – but they forget that it is *users* who really have to cope with such innovations.

We ourselves were not using reflecting teams nor Cecchin's (1987) ideas of curiosity at the time. Our thinking was much less sophisticated, but it had the advantage of being grounded by our surveys of users' experiences and this gave us some confidence in our changing practice.

Another change which we adopted was in the use of video. We were already using the video less than before, but, as we have already seen, many of our respondents were worried both about surveillance and about the risk of losing their children. Some of us began to think about the question of 'ownership' of therapy – a fashionable word used widely in social work at the time. If we were to take the user's voice more seriously we would have to consider who 'owned' not only the therapy, but also the technology which was supposed to be helping the therapy.

There seemed to be a simple logic that if the video was such a useful tool to the therapist, and if families were not simply 'resistant systems' that needed to be outwitted for their own good, then there might be direct benefit for some users in observing video recordings from their own earlier sessions. My own increasing use of video feedback, and that of my team colleague Sally Noble, came directly out of the concerns of users in this study, and has at times provided a solid platform for discussions with users about important matters like therapist–user relationships, gender issues in therapy, and comparing the present with the past. Again, the theoretical foundation was basic, although the practice of Alger and Hogan (1971), established many years earlier, did act as an inspiration.

So far in this chapter we have seen how two user surveys influenced the practice of family therapy in the Western Wiltshire Child and Family Guidance Service. They demonstrate how salient research questions can be asked in order to allow the therapist's behaviour to change. There has, of course, been a major development in second-order thinking about the importance of therapist change (particularly well articulated by Goolishian and Anderson, 1992), but what we hope to have shown is how asking users about their experience of therapy can provide a firm grounding for changing therapeutic practice. We would hope that the changes that we have made have been prompted by our desire to see therapy as an encounter between people – albeit labelled 'users' and 'therapists'. Through our eyes, too many of the developments of family therapy seem to take place because therapists are fascinated by theory. Concentration on theory can lead them to forget that users' experiences are of paramount importance. Theoretically derived innovations in family therapy are obviously important but it is equally important not to create family therapy equivalents of the mad surgeon syndrome, i.e. the operation was a technical triumph but the patient died. A family therapy equivalent would be (albeit in milder form): the reflecting team did a magnificent job but the family was so overwhelmed by their sophistication that they did not return.

A good example of such a failure to custom-build can be found in my work with a family, where the mother had really only come to check whether her son's behaviour was 'normal'. Keen to try using a reflecting team approach, I introduced a team of three people to the family near the end of the first session. I never saw the family again!

THE THIRD SURVEY

Questions breed answers that breed further questions

In therapy it is quite common that users give answers to questions which have not been asked and do not answer the questions which have been asked. I used to think that either people did not understand my questions or were deliberately 'detouring' by avoiding giving answers. I am now more inclined to think that people sometimes give answers to questions they are interested in or preoccupied with, but which have not yet been asked. Anderson and Goolishian (1988) have written extensively about the 'not yet asked question' within their second-order framework, and some of the questions we asked seemed consistently to bring forth heartfelt answers, whereas others did not. Also, because our respondents were interviewed face to face they would often add asides – answers or comments which suggested to us certain new questions. Similarly the researcher might at times depart from the interview schedule and follow a line of thought which emerged from the discussion.

During the two years following the second survey, some of these new ideas and questions were doubtless lying fallow and I eventually became aware that one question we had not systematically asked was about the experience of coming to therapy *as a family*. A second question which occurred to us had to do with endings. We had occasionally received unsolicited comments about the ending of therapy from users in the two surveys, but I was aware of how much attention family therapy literature had given to issues of convening and engagement – as had our surveys – and how little to termination. For our own part, we had asked whether people would return for further sessions in the future if they needed to, but not specifically about the experience of ending therapy.

Anderson and Goolishian's (1988) claim that therapy is complete once the problem-determined system dissolves overlooks the psychological implications of the dissolution. The people involved in these systems, of course, do not dissolve. They say goodbye, good riddance, or drop out, and are likely to retain many unspoken or spoken thoughts about how their therapy has come to an end. It was thoughts like this that prompted us to undertake a further study, retaining much of the existing questionnaire but adding important new questions. The arrival in 1990 of Mark Weekes as a social work student on placement in Trowbridge provided the opportunity to undertake the study, since Mark was very willing to contribute to the project. In all he interviewed adults in 21 households: 17 women and 6 men (details of the questionnaire he used are to be found in Appendix 1).

Once again we cannot possibly repeat all the results from the questionnaire, so we have selected a number of key questions that produced results which contributed most to changing our practice.

Q.6 In what way were you expecting that you might be helped?

12 users came expecting advice.
7 users were expecting to find someone they could talk to.
2 users were unsure about what they were expecting.

These brief summaries conceal a variety of actual phrases used. Some talked of wanting advice, and others used words like 'ideas' and 'suggestions', although some wanted no less than a cure. Those who wanted to talk used words like 'understanding', 'throwing light on the problem' and 'getting an outsider's view'. In fact, the idea of the outsider was important to many people, expressed forcibly by Mrs Abbott:

> ... talking and knowing you weren't burdening a friend, although I did see her as a friend. I couldn't unload on a friend.

Q.4 Before you went for your first visit, can you remember mainly what your feelings were about going?

15 users felt apprehension or anxiety.
4 users felt relief.
2 users felt a mixture of feelings.

On the basis of replies to the second survey we had discovered that a number of users had felt worried about their children being taken away from them. The third survey produced direct evidence for similar worries. For example, we received a specific reply about this worry from Mrs Keating:

> I felt anxious because of the Cleveland case. I felt they may have the right to take children away. I told Clare [her therapist] who put us at ease.

Mrs Illingworth did not mention Cleveland specifically but she had been worried:

> I didn't go to the first appointment, because I was afraid my child would be put into care.

Q.13 Can you say what was most helpful about going to the Centre?

15 users had found it helpful to be able to talk about the problem.
3 users found the direct advice helpful.
3 users said there was nothing they could remember being helpful.

As we might expect, although respondents might answer a question simply and unambiguously, answers to other questions suggested that their experiences were often quite complex. Mrs Faraday emphasized the usefulness of advice:

It was helpful having an outsider look at the family as often the family is too entangled to see objectively. An outsider is able to give practical advice on issues we had missed.

And yet Mrs Faraday was not beyond wanting acceptance from the therapist. She had felt very uneasy about coming the first time, and had felt relaxed by being put at ease.

Q.14 Can you say what was least helpful about going to the Centre?

5 users found the service generally unhelpful.
5 users said that nothing was unhelpful at all.
3 users had found it unhelpful not knowing in which direction the therapy was going.
6 users found it unhelpful having appointments during office hours or had difficulties with transport. (Volunteer drivers were in fact used extensively by the Centre, but their availability may not always have been well enough publicized.)

The most critical comment came from Mr and Mrs Gray:

They treated us like imbeciles. The phone kept going throughout the session and we felt we were being watched. The questions were inept, no advice was given, and all the ideas were expected to come from the family.

We will see in a moment how the one-way screen had particularly annoyed and upset this couple.

Q.28 At the time did it seem helpful or unhelpful to use the one-way screen?

The screen had been used with 14 out of the 21 families. (Such a high proportion was not typical at that time.)

9 users had found the screen helpful.
4 users had found the screen unhelpful.
1 user was undecided.

Mrs Abbott had thought it was a good idea, with one reservation:

They could pool the advice and help calm things down if we became too heated. . . . I didn't bother, though I felt like sometimes talking to the person behind the screen.

As we have seen, Mr and Mrs Gray had major concerns about the screen:

We felt uncomfortable, and didn't feel we were offered any choice. I don't think it achieved anything, I felt I was sitting in a cage, and it made me feel self-conscious. Why couldn't they sit in the room?

They had been introduced to team members but were critical of the fact that they had not been invited to shake hands with them.

Q.22 At the time did it seem helpful or unhelpful to use the video?

The video had been used with 7 out of the 21 families.

   4 users had felt it was helpful.
   3 users had felt indifferent.

Significantly none of the respondents reported that the video was unhelpful. Although the sample involved is very small these results do suggest that a shift in our practice had occurred. A number of users commented how the video had made them feel uncomfortable at first, but it seems that at least with this group of users our way of introducing it may have been careful enough to help them make sense of the video, and this in turn may have helped them accept the video as useful. Even Mrs Keating, who had at first worried about the video, said:

It is used to assess you, though some people would worry it could be used against you. . . . I felt self-conscious about being watched, and awkward about my reactions being observed . . . it was helpful . . . I didn't bother about it after the first few sessions. I still feel it is helpful.

This is no small shift for a person who had come worrying about her children being taken away.

Q.32 Did you feel that the person you talked to understood how you felt about the problem?

   20 users said yes.
   1 user said no.

Of the users who had felt understood, Mrs Richards was the only one to add a qualification:

I had a good inkling, though no one can entirely be in someone's head.

This was a person who had felt afraid and isolated at first and had found the one-way screen unhelpful. What provided an important balance for her was the fact that she felt that the therapist had been very friendly, had not pushed her views, and above all had listened.

Looking back on the common questions in these three surveys we have to be cautious about drawing any sweeping conclusions, but it does appear that, despite initial worries about being blamed or losing their children, users were coming to see the use of the one-way screen and the video as making some sense, even if it was not going to be of immediate use to themselves. Both the video and the one-way screen were being used more sparingly and judiciously by the therapists, and there was a greater sense of both being negotiated in a more egalitarian way than in the past.

We will now move on to two new sets of questions which had struck us as particularly important. The first set related to being interviewed as a family.

Q.8 Were all the family seen together at the Centre?

Q.9a Were you expecting to be seen together or not?

Q.9b What did it feel like being seen together as a family?

Q.9c Did being seen together affect how you saw the problem?

In all the cases users had been seen as a family, although frequently with modifications. With four families, non-referred siblings had not been seen, and in one instance the father had not come. In over half the cases there had been other interview combinations, with the child being seen individually, and the parents on their own.

12 users said that they had expected to be seen together.
15 users said that they felt it was positive being seen together.
5 users said that they had not liked being seen together.
1 user was uncertain.

Some, like Mrs Sackville, had felt awkward at first about being interviewed with her family, but the benefits had become clearer:

Yes, it helped me see my daughter more as an individual.

Mrs Upworth said:

It made everyone realize what the problem was, and put it in perspective.

Mr and Mrs Faraday seemed to be saying something similar:

It was all right – it was better once the children understood what was happening.

Did being seen as a family affect how they saw the problem?

No, as we knew what the problem was, though it allowed different aspects to be worked on.

Mr and Mrs Gray, however, had some reservations:

It was just an open discussion . . . but it did hinder my daughter.

Some said they appreciated the fact that they had been seen in different combinations. Mr and Mrs Abbott had met the therapist on their own, but their daughter had also come for some sessions.

It made her aware of the effect [of the problem] on the family.

Mr and Mrs Jones, who were foster carers and had children of their own, had attended under pressure from their social worker. They did not themselves feel that there had been a problem, and were relieved at having met the therapist on their own first before a family session. They had found it helpful that the therapist had accepted their view that they did not have a family problem and had found it particularly helpful that he had said this in a letter to both their social worker and themselves afterwards. Although adamant that they did not have a 'problem', they said that they periodically reviewed their family life at home in the light of their experience at the Centre, which they had found interesting.

Q.34 How many times did you come to the Centre?

Q.35 Did that seem enough or not enough appointments?

Q.36 What do you feel about the way in which your contact with the Centre ended?

The number of sessions varied between 1 and 20, the mean for the sample being 6.5, and the mean for the whole year 5.5. All except two respondents had felt that they had received enough sessions. All those who had attended for one or only a few sessions felt that this had been enough, either because the problem had improved rapidly or because they had come to realize that they were not going to receive the kind of help they needed. What seemed more important than the actual number of sessions was the way that therapy had ended. Mrs Abbott, who had attended with her family for 20 sessions, had at times felt exhausted, but was keen to have the door left open after the last session:

It hasn't fully ended because we can contact them again if it's ever needed.

Mrs Abbott had experienced counselling before and had fitted into the family therapy way of working with ease. Mrs Partridge had also felt positive about therapy, but was keen to finish after six sessions, possibly worrying that she might become dependent on the Centre:

We were relieved for a while after it was over . . . to see how we'd get along without talking to someone.

Although the problem had improved, she had wanted to keep in touch:

I've felt like ringing up since to say how things have gone along.

Nearly all the respondents said that they knew that they could choose to return in the future if they needed to, and most said they would if further problems occurred. This included some who had said that the problem had not improved, or where any improvement had been short-lived.

In fact, we were quite surprised by how philosophical some users had been about the lack of improvement. The majority would recommend the service to someone else – and a number had already done so. Some said that the fact that their problem had not improved did not mean that therapy might not work for someone else.

Two people had clearly felt quite bad about what they saw as a premature ending suggested by the therapist, and one mother who only came for one session felt guilty that she had not accepted the therapist's suggestion of further sessions, even though the problem had greatly improved.

What was striking about nearly all of the rest of the respondents was that they felt that the ending had been left open, and that they could take the initiative to resume therapy again in the future, if they needed to. Mrs Richards said:

> [the ending] was all right. We could go back. It ended on a good note and it was left in our hands.

As a mother, Mrs Richards had originally felt herself to blame for the problem and had felt very isolated. In fact she did re-refer herself and her family shortly after terminating the first time.

SUMMARY

The three studies discussed (in the preceding chapter and this chapter) have demonstrated some changes in therapeutic practice. These changes were influenced mainly by the comments of a number of users about their experience of therapy. We have seen that users make many demands on their therapists to be sensitive, flexible and versatile. We have also seen an amazing tolerance, generosity and flexibility on the part of many users, and this has given us the confidence to make a number of changes within our work, but also to continue with our existing practice where this seems, after due consideration, to be well grounded.

It is difficult for us to estimate how you as a reader have responded to our discussion of these surveys. You may wonder why we have focused so little on outcome, dwelling almost entirely on the 'softer' and less easily quantifiable experiences of therapy. In fact we did ask users about whether 'the problem' had improved or not, and the results are shown in Table 2.

The seemingly 'hard' figures in Table 2 require further explanation. Many respondents gave complicated answers to the question about changes in the problem that brought them to therapy. For example, some users said that some problems had improved whilst others had stayed the same, that the problems had at first improved and later deteriorated (and vice versa). Others replied that, despite no substantial behavioural change, there had been an important improvement in their understanding of the problem.

Table 2 Users' views on the outcome of therapy

	Problem improved	Problem stayed the same	Problem deteriorated	No problem acknowledged
1st study (N = 22)	12	9	0	1
2nd study (N = 19)	13	5	1	0
3rd study (N = 21)	12	7	1	1

We do not want to criticize the idea of outcome studies (and we ourselves had, after all, never intended to undertake one), but we would make the crucial point that successful experiences of being in therapy may be as important to many users as any measure of behavioural outcome. We appreciate that this point may be an anathema to many readers but we do not subscribe to the idea that therapy is necessarily about cure. As Donald Schön (1991) has pointed out in his important book *The Reflective Practitioner*, the idea of cure is predicated on the idea that discrete, easily solvable problems exist. Many of the situations that users (and ourselves for that matter) face are not problems. They are, to use Schön's term, 'messes', which are not readily 'solved' by 'interventions'. For many users the essence of successful therapy is to gain new insights which enable them to live with their predicament. Sometimes changes (including changes to do with family and individual life cycles) do occur but some users are prepared to continue stoically to live in situations which other people would find intolerable. A GP-like model of therapy is perhaps most helpful to users like this. They welcome the idea of long-term, but very intermittent, support from their therapist, who only becomes engaged when certain crisis situations occur.

As far as the evidence for changes in our practice is concerned, you may feel that the evidence is rather slim, but, in our defence, we would say that it was the concerted effort to keep monitoring users' experiences that prompted a shift. The ultimate test of our user-friendliness must be, once the dust has settled and the research reports have been filed away, how far we have internalized a much more reflexive approach (based on consideration of users' experience of family therapy) which combines the most positive aspects of research and practice.

Our final chapter explores, in some detail, how my own practice has changed. The survey results influenced many of the changes but theoretical developments within family therapy also played their part. When the original study was designed by Carolyn White, she undertook a preliminary literature search which was valuable in designing many of the questions, but with hindsight we should have kept updating ourselves as the subsequent surveys were undertaken. The literature we have been able to collate is like a jigsaw with a substantial number of pieces missing. We hope our own study has filled in a few pieces, but it is itself unusual in that it does have an action–research component which is noticeably missing from most other studies, as we shall see in our next two chapters.

Chapter 8

Reviewing consumer studies of therapy
Social work and marriage guidance research

Andy Treacher

INTRODUCTION

In this chapter, we will review studies that have examined many aspects of therapy which, although not strictly relevant to family therapy as such, have made crucial contributions to developing ideas about user-friendliness. It seems to us that the social work tradition has contributed significantly to the development of user-friendly ideas but we will also review studies of marital therapy undertaken in marriage guidance settings. Such studies have also made a similarly important contribution because of the client-centred emphasis of the approach. As a footnote, it is also worth pointing out that client-centred models of family therapy do exist (see, for example Nathaniel Raskin and Ferdinand van der Veen's (1970) discussion of their Rogerian-inspired approach), but these models seem to have been marginalized by the expert models which became fashionable in the 1970s. Fortunately, Eddy Street has been commissioned to write a book which will help to re-establish this important tradition which has a great deal to contribute to user-friendliness (Street, 1994).

SOCIAL WORK STUDIES

Carolyn White's unpublished study (White, 1988) had originally attempted to summarize the field but it was clear from her review that users' experiences of being in family therapy had received very little specific research attention. Consumer surveys of experiences of social work were noticeably more numerous, and had perhaps been prompted by the work of Alice Overton, who had commented:

> There is no question about the value to us of client observations of social work methods . . . our clients can tell us more about how they are influenced or pushed away. They can suggest more effective stimuli for change. They can – if we develop better methods of asking!
>
> (Overton, 1960; cited by White, 1988)

One major study to take Overton's plea seriously was the much cited study by John Mayer and Noel Timms called *The Client Speaks: Working Class*

Impressions of Casework (1970). Significantly the first chapter of the book, entitled 'The neglected client', includes a survey of casework research which revealed that (1) clients were rarely asked to appraise the effectiveness of the services received, (2) if services were evaluated then it was professional judgements that were used as the basis for evaluation and (3) the very few studies that utilized both client-based and professional-based evaluations revealed wide discrepancies between the two evaluations. Similar conclusions could also have been applied to the psychotherapy literature of the time, because users' experiences were equally ignored. Mayer and Timms's own study was concerned with exploring users' experiences of help offered by a British charity, the Family Welfare Association. Their findings, which have been confirmed by many later studies, draw attention to the possible clashes of perspective particularly between users who were seeking practical help and social workers who were wanting to offer counselling.

Three years later, Noel Timms (1973) edited another important book that eloquently reported users' experiences of 'social help for children'. The book contains brief reports of parents' experiences of adopting children, children's experiences of being in either a child psychiatric unit, a children's home or a foster home, and a single woman's experience of offering foster care. These accounts are invaluable because they act as an antidote to more traditional forms of research which give professional accounts of different forms of care. Unfortunately, we have only been able to find one user account of family therapy (Strømnes, 1991), which we will review in the next chapter. Family therapists have obviously not encouraged their ex-users to publish accounts and yet such accounts are crucial to the development of user-friendly approaches.

Ian Shaw (1976; 1984) has provided useful general summaries of consumer evaluations of personal social services, but it is Diana Merrington and John Corden's more specific summary of users' experiences (1981) that we find most useful. They make a number of basic points about social work studies which we will now summarize:

1 Users have little knowledge of, and are uncertain about, what to expect and what kind of help they will receive when they approach an agency.
2 Users mostly anticipate the help they will receive as being practical and concrete – either material help or definite advice delivered in an authoritarian way.
3 Once contact has been made with an agency the value of having a sympathetic ear (a friend to show concern or a chance to ventilate) was valued by consumers even when the material aid or direct intervention (that they had initially expected) had not been received.
4 Users place great importance on the personal qualities of their workers, so their willingness to please, to be cheerful, to be empathic and to be friendly rather than formal or professional are universally reported as positive.

These findings will be largely confirmed by the specific studies that we will now review. Because of our own survey concerned with a child guidance setting, we will review two British studies of child guidance settings which provide some interesting further clues about users' expectations. Neither of the studies specifically studies family therapy in detail but they do provide an insight into how parents experience coming to a clinic. We will then summarize the important work of Maluccio before reviewing studies of marital counselling.

Burck (1978)

Charlotte Burck studied 10 families who attended a child guidance clinic. Seven of the families interviewed did not have any realistic idea of what the clinic did. Parents on the whole expected their role at the clinic to be a non-existent or a passive one (e.g. receiving information or being asked questions) but clinic staff expected parents to be much more actively involved. Five of the families came to the clinic with very specific expectations but none of these was met. Burck demonstrates that there was a noticeable degree of mismatch between clinic staff and users concerning the helpfulness of the clinic. Termination was equally complex with staff and users once again often disagreeing about the reasons for termination and who had initiated it.

Burck's overall conclusion stressed that it was important for clinics to develop new methods for preparing clients for therapy and alternative methods of treatment for users who did not fit the clinic's usual approach. However, the study was not an action-orientated one and it is not clear whether the clinic responded to her feedback.

Lishman (1978)

Interestingly, another social worker, Joyce Lishman, also published a follow-up study in 1978. The method she adopted in order to undertake the study was as follows. She examined her already completed files belonging to 12 families whom she subsequently interviewed. She analysed her file information under three headings: (1) Intake: problem at referral, social work assessment, goals set. (2) Process: length and kind of contact, treatment process. (3) Outcome: symptom removal, child's general functioning, parental functioning, estimation of whether parents were satisfied or dissatisfied. Lishman then tape-recorded interviews at home with the parents of the families she worked with, asking them questions relevant to the three areas outlined from her files.

On comparing the two sets of data, Lishman records a mismatch between herself and her users:

There is no evidence from the files about my perception of clients' feelings at this stage. My impression is that I under-estimated the confusion, guilt and anxiety, and that because seeing clients is for me an everyday occurrence, I become blunted to the uniqueness of it for them. Most clients . . . although uncertain about what referral meant were open to the possibility of help i.e. with a potential for satisfaction. By the end clients had strong feelings of dissatisfaction and satisfaction. Can one identify within the contact what 'set' these feelings?

(Lishman, 1978, p. 304)

Lishman is able to make some important suggestions about how the therapeutic work unfolded either satisfactorily or unsatisfactorily. For example, four sets of parents shared her assumption that they should be actively involved in helping their child. But three either did not expect to be involved or they thought the focus was too much concerned with them and too little with their child. Contract-making also emerged as being crucial. Lishman believed that she had made clear assessments and set shared goals in eight cases, remaining unclear about the other four, but her users mostly disagreed. . . .

She also adds some very intriguing thoughts about links between contract-making and satisfaction and dissatisfaction:

[E]xpectations about parental involvement linked strongly with subsequent satisfaction. Three of the four dissatisfied families did not want or expect any focus on them, but on their child, whereas the four sets of parents who expected to be seen were all satisfied.

Secondly, the same three dissatisfied families also felt that my assessment, where clear, was wrong. Their perception of my assessment was that they were being blamed or criticized . . . satisfied clients at this stage merely felt confused. . . .

From the files it is clear that, with these dissatisfied families, my goals focused on problems and confrontation e.g. 'facing a family with impact of father's illness'. Valuing and supporting strengths are not mentioned as goals. *In contrast for each of the six satisfied families one of my explicit goals is valuing and support.*

(Lishman, 1978. Emphasis added by SR and AT)

Lishman next examines the helping process itself. Five out of six satisfied families experienced positive support, and four positive insight. But four out of six dissatisfied families felt that they had gained no support or insight. Lishman felt herself that she behaved more or less similarly to all users, 'with slightly more support and less insight to the dissatisfied clients'. However, dissatisfied clients perceived Lishman as being totally unhelpful in any area.

Lishman's summary of the significance of her results is intriguing and explains why she chose to entitle her paper 'A clash in perspective'. She felt that her work was successful when her users and herself shared a common framework. She viewed her dissatisfied users as more vulnerable and suspicious but admits that her behaviour 'was equally, if not more important' in determining the outcome. Despite this interesting statement, there still remains an unanswered question: Why, if dissatisfied users were more vulnerable, did she respond with confrontation rather than attempting to be more supportive?

Interestingly, Lishman does not explore the possible counter-transference issues involved. Instead, she outlines a five-point plan for improving her practice which involves: (1) increasing her personal awareness of (a) the overwhelming impact on clients of referral and initial contact and (b) the initial openness and potential for being helped that users bring to their first contact; (2) spelling out more clearly at the beginning how the clinic works; (3) creating a more shared approach to goal setting; (4) reviewing goals and achievements periodically; (5) giving more feedback about her own perceptions of what is happening and avoiding a blank screen approach which invites workers to give no information about their thoughts, feelings and ways of working.

We have explored Lishman's work in depth because we believe her approach provides a potential model for busy practitioners. Clearly, her work goes much deeper than Burck's type of study. A case-by-case approach which attempts to match users' and therapists' perceptions is clearly very valuable and can perhaps influence clinicians more than survey studies which do not tend to link therapists and users directly.

Maluccio (1979)

Tony Maluccio's *Learning from Clients – Interpersonal Helping as Viewed by Clients and Social Workers* (1979) is an important book which went rapidly out of print and, despite its significance, was not reprinted. The study focused on exploring user and worker views regarding three phases of therapy: getting engaged, staying engaged and becoming disengaged. Data was generated by in-depth, semi-structured, face-to-face interviews with a small, randomly selected sample of users and their social workers. The latter worked for a Catholic voluntary organization; most clients interviewed were white middle-class women seeking help with personal or relationship problems.

Getting engaged

Users' memories of their own feelings and reactions to their initial session were vivid. Their workers, on the other hand, tended to focus on their observations of the client's problems and their efforts to engage each user in a treatment relationship. Or, as Maluccio himself says, 'There was the suggestion that, for the workers, the content of the interaction in the initial session was more significant, more lasting in their memory, than the process. For the clients, the reverse was true.' He pays close attention to the factors within the user's network of relationship which prompt referral to the agency, but his summary of the significance of the initial session is most relevant to our discussion in this chapter:

> In the initial session, a great deal of client–worker activity is directed toward a decision as to whether or not they should *get engaged*. This decision is influenced by their success in coping with various tasks that seem to be critical

in the beginning phase: (1) opening up the prospective client's life space; (2) assessing need and appropriateness of service; (3) establishing an emotional connection; (4) mobilizing the prospective client's motivation; and (5) reaching a beginning working agreement.

Each of these tasks involves complementary functions and responsibilities for both parties. For example, 'opening up life space' is dependent on the client's willingness to share of himself or herself, as well as the worker's readiness to provide encouragement and support. In most cases in the study sample, client and worker were able to resolve these tasks satisfactorily, and therefore went on with subsequent contacts. In some cases, the prospective client agreed to go on even though the tasks had not been adequately resolved. In these instances, the person's distress or pressure from external sources continued to be sufficiently strong as to force him or her to go on despite dissatisfaction with the worker and/or the initial encounter.

(Maluccio, 1979)

The middle phase: staying engaged

This phase involved the problem focus of the sessions being expanded – users seemed able to share more of themselves as their relationship with their worker developed. There was also a high degree of congruence between both sides in terms of problem definition. However, while both sides agreed that talking was the main problem-solving activity utilized, main clients (except college-educated ones) doubted its value in solving their problems. Listening was also construed in the same way – it was valuable but how did it help solve the problem? All users (irrespective of class background) expected their worker to have a more active role in the helping process (through expressing opinions, giving advice and offering suggestions), so all were frustrated to a greater or lesser degree.

Despite this clash in perspective, most users stayed in therapy and reported that they got help and were satisfied with the service. A minority clearly proceeded in order to save face but in the majority of cases other factors helped both sides to overcome disparities in their perceptions and expectations, or, as Maluccio says:

The key variables were the client–worker relationships, the interactional environment and the contracting process. The latter was especially prominent. Although workers and clients reported that they were not consciously or systematically involved in contract negotiation and renegotiation, their recollections suggested that much of their activity and energy went into this area. They were often involved in efforts to define their tasks and roles, to deal with their divergent expectations, and to explain or clarify their ideas in such areas as problem definition, desired goals, and treatment methods.

In about two-thirds of the cases, there was evidence of ongoing negotiation and re-negotiation between clients and workers that served to facilitate their interaction. In the remaining one-third, incongruent perceptions or expectations and other issues around contracting also emerged over and over. However, they were not handled adequately. Instead, in these cases there were indications of inability or reluctance on the part of client and/or worker to share their questions or differences openly with each other, resulting in considerable mutual frustration. As differences between clients and workers were not reconciled and there was insufficient complementarity between them, in the majority of these cases the clients eventually withdrew.

Two typical patterns emerged in these unsuccessful client–worker transactions. In one, the client and worker were aware of their differences in respect to choice of target problems or treatment objectives, but did not explicitly discuss them. In the other, they discussed their different views, but did not openly confront the issue of whether they should continue or not. They simply went on for a while with their contracts, despite their obvious dissatisfaction.

(Maluccio, 1979)

The ending: becoming disengaged

Users could be classified as falling into two groups: the 'planned termination' group and the 'unplanned'. The former were middle-class users, generally satisfied with the worker and the service, while the latter were working class and had either been pressurized to go to the service or became dissatisfied with the worker and the service. In most cases of planned termination, the user and worker concurred, were actively involved in discussing their ending and made plans to do so gradually. Not unexpectedly, unplanned terminations were more problematic, as Maluccio himself summarizes:

In cases in which termination was unplanned – that is in which the client withdrew – clients ended either because they felt that they had gotten what they were looking for or because they were dissatisfied with the service. Often, there was evidence of lack of openness between client and worker and lack of clarity or agreement in respect to their roles, goals, and expectations. These were cases in which problems in client–worker interaction were evident as early as the initial session. In contrast to those in the planned termination group, clients and workers in these cases had a vague sense of what would be happening in treatment, were unable to establish an emotional connection between them, did not actively engage in contract negotiation, and ended the first session with marked vagueness and uncertainty about future plans. Thus, there were various predictors or 'early warning signals' that should have alerted the worker to the need to clarify the focus of the service and/or confront the client's ambivalence.

(Maluccio, 1979)

Interestingly, Maluccio's research also revealed a striking difference in the emotional aspects of termination:

The termination phase provoked multiple and intense reactions in workers as well as clients. Most clients, especially those who ended by plan, expressed their feelings openly and directly about termination, bringing out such themes as dependence on the worker, investment in the relationship, ambivalence about ending, and loss of support. Workers, on the other hand, described extensively their *clients'* feelings, but were hesitant to bring out their *own* reactions to termination. Their feelings emerged indirectly, however, through frequent references to their disappointment in not having helped the client further, dissatisfaction with the degree of change that had taken place in the client's situation, concern over the client's continuing problems, or doubts about his or her capacity to deal with future life crises. These responses occurred even in cases in which client and worker agreed that mutually formulated goals had been achieved, and that the client was ready to terminate.

(Maluccio, 1979)

Needless to say, user and worker evaluations of outcome could also differ significantly. There was an overall agreement between users and workers that two-thirds of users had benefited from the service and one-third not. The main areas of improvement concerned change in either 'self or other individual family member' or 'in family relationships'. However, workers were much more pessimistic than clients in assessing the significance of the users' problems and weaknesses than the users themselves. Satisfaction assessment also differed, with users being satisfied with having obtained help in relation to specific 'problems of living' while workers were concerned (from their psychoanalytic viewpoint) with overall 'care' or broad changes in a user's situation or personality structure.

Maluccio's summary of the factors influencing outcome is so important that, once again, we will quote him directly:

The client–worker relationship was generally evaluated positively by both parties. Client–worker interaction was influenced by a number of qualities that clients and workers perceived in each other. Workers described two-thirds of the clients as having positive qualities and one-third as having negative qualities. The preferred client was someone who was open, responsive, and capable of emotional insight, while the least-liked client was presented as rigid, resistive, and nonverbal. The preferred client seemed to evoke a sense of competence and fulfilment in the worker, while the non-preferred client provoked feelings of self-doubt, inadequacy, and frustration.

Initially, clients talked in generic terms about the workers describing them as kind, friendly, likeable, warm, caring, and so on. As I probed further, however, they were able to spell out their views in more discriminating terms. Various worker qualities, such as empathy and genuineness, were especially important in influencing the client's views as well as the change process. However, there was no simple or linear correlation between worker qualities and outcome of the service.

From the clients' perspective, some qualities were more important at some points of the helping process than others. A number of clients suggested that the worker's age or empathy made a positive impression on them initially, sufficiently so that they became engaged with the worker and were optimistic about the contact. As the encounter progressed, however, the same clients would not continue to be satisfied unless the worker displayed other qualities, such as competence.

In addition, the same quality was evaluated differently by different clients. Thus, some clients considered a worker's 'low-key' approach as positive, while others viewed it as negative. Some clients reacted negatively to a worker's 'formal' or 'professional' bearing, while others reacted to it positively. It may be that a changing cluster of worker qualities influences the client's attitudes toward – and satisfaction with – the worker at different points in their engagement, depending on the client's changing life space and consequently changing needs and perceptions.

There was also some indication that the factor of social distance between client and worker was correlated with client satisfaction with the service; in general, clients felt more positively and were more satisfied with the service and its outcome the closer they were to their workers in respect to characteristics such as age, family status, and sex.

Clients and practitioners agreed on certain features of their interaction that influenced its outcome, specifically, *client qualities, worker qualities* and *client and/or worker activities*. They disagreed, however, on the relative importance of these features, with clients tending to emphasize *qualities of the worker* and workers stressing, first, *activities* and, second, *client qualities*.

(Maluccio, 1979)

Interestingly, Maluccio specifically discusses why workers did not seek to transfer users to other workers when it was clear that the therapeutic relationship had broken down. He felt that it was the worker's fear of failure that prevented a transfer from taking place.

Finally, Maluccio also makes some intriguing comments about the role of 'external' influences in determining outcome and satisfaction. Under this rubric he includes the user's social networks, the user's life events and experiences, and the agency environment:

Clients, more than workers, pointed to the positive influence of friends, relatives, and informal helping agents in the community. Clients tended to view positively their relationship with members of their kinship system, whereas social workers tended to define the same relationships as problems and obstacles in the client's functioning.

Although the majority of these clients had initially sought help from the agency because of dissatisfaction with people or resources in their environment, after having been involved in treatment they reported more positive feelings toward significant members of their networks. The suggestion was that, at least partly as a result of the service, they were better able to identify and/or use available supports and resources.

Both clients and workers mentioned natural life experiences and events (such as a job change) as factors influencing the outcome of their engagement; however, clients mentioned more of these factors in *positive* terms, whereas workers mentioned more of them in *negative* terms.

Clients and workers also referred to the positive influence of the agency's social environment (especially the role of the receptionist) and the negative influence of its physical environment (particularly its location). But workers did not assign as much importance to the environment as the clients did; they suggested, instead, that the client's personal relationship with the worker was more meaningful than the affiliation with the agency as an institution. Unlike workers, many clients also commented about the agency's 'operational environment,' that is, its policies, regulations, and procedures. In general, clients recommended greater flexibility in relation to such aspects as timing and location of interviews and use of diverse treatment modalities.

(Maluccio, 1979)

We have reviewed Maluccio's work at some length because it is one of the most coherent and thoughtful accounts of users' experiences of therapy that we have discovered. Many family therapists, particularly those who incline to working strate- gically, will no doubt seek to dismiss the significance of his work, arguing that it is of little relevance to family therapy work because the model of therapy adopted was psychoanalytic. However, we take an alternative view. We believe that working with users requires a 'both/and' approach not an 'either/or' approach. That is to say, in order to develop therapies that are experienced as both satisfying and effective by users, it is necessary to pay attention to both the relationship and instrumental facets of therapy. Therapists need to concentrate on relationship-building skills but they must also be aware that they require to contribute skills that actually facilitate change in areas that are valued by users themselves.

Maluccio's study is rather difficult to categorize from our point of view. It is not strictly a study of marital therapy since so much of the work undertaken involved individual therapy but nevertheless marital issues were tackled. Some- what arbitrarily we have chosen to place Maluccio's study at a transitional point in our review.

MARITAL STUDIES

Since our main interest in this book is users' experiences of family therapy we will not attempt to review comprehensively studies exploring users' experiences of marital therapy. However, we will briefly summarize three British studies that have produced interesting results which we would not want to ignore in attempt- ing to develop a more user-friendly approach to family therapy.

Brannen and Collard (1982)

Julia Brannen and Jean Collard's book *Marriages in Trouble: The Process of Seeking Help* is a mine of interesting information concerning couples' ways of seeking help when their marriages are at the point of breakdown. The authors (both sociologists) are very aware of the complex routes that users take in their attempts to find help for their marriages.

> Some of the characteristic stages which emerged in our data were: the perception of something being wrong; the interpreting and labelling of a problem as of a particular kind; disclosing or turning to a significant other over the problem; the decision to seek help from a particular agency; and finally the approach to the agency itself. At any stage in the process an individual could change his or her view of the situation and short-circuit the process. At the first stage it was characteristically wives who first appear to have felt that there was something wrong in their marriages, and characteristically husbands who denied or chose to ignore their wives' complaints, sometimes by diverting attention on to individual health problems which were located in their wives. Thus, the help-seeking careers of husbands and wives appear from their very beginnings to have diverged.
>
> (Brannen and Collard, 1982, pp. 232–233)

Movement on to the next stages in the career of being a help-seeker involved interpreting the problem. Sometimes a critical event clearly prompted this but in other cases the causation was less clear. However, once a problem was interpreted more clearly, the person involved selected a particular agency which was thought to be the most appropriate to consult. Typically, it was women not men who were more likely to consult and even when men did approach an agency it was at the prompting of their wives.

Brannen and Collard attempt to understand the movement of individuals through their help-seeking 'careers' by researching how their respondents describe their own actions, but as structuralists they are prepared to provide additional explanations that do not coincide with their respondents' accounts. We are partly sympathetic to their approach but since our emphasis in this chapter is on listening to users' accounts we will focus our attention on those aspects of Brannen and Collard's work that emanate clearly from a user perspective. For example, the issue of disclosure of personal issues was clearly very important, and once again, divided women from men:

> Women respondents were more disposed towards disclosure than men although they stressed the risks and consequent needs for safeguards. . . . Men seemed to fear losing their self-esteem most of all whilst women were more afraid that their disclosures might adversely affect others and their relationships with them; characteristically, wives more than husbands were concerned about being disloyal to their spouses if they disclosed what they regarded as discrediting information about their marriages.
>
> (Brannen and Collard, 1982, p. 235)

The significance of social networks in providing different forms of support when a marriage is in trouble is stressed by Brannen and Collard but they once again emphasize the gender differences that permeate such support-giving:

> The fact that wives tended to utilize their social networks as sources of help and support to a greater extent than their husbands testifies to their need for support. In other kinds of unequal relationships, the observation can be made that it is always subordinates and not superordinates who tend to complain first and most of all. Thus if it is accepted that men's and women's experiences are distinctively different in our society and that this is underpinned by an unequal distribution of power, both in marriage and in other key areas of human activity, it is not unreasonable to hypothesize that their careers as clients will also be different. In our study, gender did indeed emerge as a key factor in the understanding of respondents' action and interaction.
>
> (Brannen and Collard, 1982, pp. 235–236)

Brannen and Collard's important stress on the significance of gender factors in determining help-seeking behaviour is mirrored by their stress on their role in determining what we might call 'help-offering behaviour'. As part of their analysis, the authors examined how users' help-seeking behaviour was influenced by the structure of the agency that offered help. In particular, there seemed to be an important dichotomy between medical and non-medical agencies:

> Overall, doctors were seen by clients as offering highly specialist knowledge and competence, which clients perceived as largely unintelligible and inaccessible to themselves and as being generally inappropriate to the understanding of problems in personal relationships. Nonetheless, respondents as patients appear to have behaved towards their doctors with deference: they seem rarely to have questioned their pronouncements or even to have criticized the absence of information given to them. Women patients especially seemed to fear a dismissive reaction from doctors (of being thought silly).
>
> By contrast, clients of Marriage Guidance, and women clients in particular, were more likely to expect counsellors to perform a generalist role, expectations which we would argue are fostered within their social networks and are reinforced by their experience of counsellors as unpaid female volunteers. Women clients described counsellors as unbiased friends and even as allies and, if the counsellors did not act thus the desire was expressed that they should do so. There was a tendency amongst men clients to expect and to desire a directive approach from marriage counsellors, an expectation and wish broadly similar to the perception of the doctor who tells his patients 'what's wrong' and 'what they should do'. Allied to this was men's disappointment with, and their denigration of, the Marriage Guidance counsellor–client relationship as another example of 'women talking'.
>
> (Brannen and Collard, 1982, p. 240)

Brannen and Collard stress that users' perceptions of, and prescriptions for, user–practitioner relationships are related to models of power which are derived from both public and private domains, but another part of the equation also has to be considered. Agencies also shape the behaviour of their users. For example, they argue that the 'house style' of marriage guidance counsellors places emphasis on users talking and seeking to work co-operatively. Medical practitioners are concerned with priorities such as diagnosis and identifying appropriate treatments, and the user is regarded as the *object* of the practitioner's work. The question of the status of therapists also arises at this point. Brannen and Collard argue that high status *curative work* ('on or to people') is dominated by professional élite groups which are predominantly male. *Care work* ('with or for people'), on the other hand, is always considered low status and therefore is left to be performed by women. Marriage guidance work neatly conforms to this division of labour because it was performed (at the time of the study) predominantly by unpaid middle-class women.

Brannen and Collard conclude (amongst other things) that a series of crucial research questions need to be posed in order to explore these important issues further. These questions include: (1) How far do particular kinds of practitioner make their *knowledge accessible to lay persons and clients?* (2) To what extent is the model of help which is offered congruent with a traditional model of help in the domestic area. (3) How far is the practice of practitioners focused on working with or on clients? (4) In what ways are the goals of practice defined and by whom?

These are essentially user-friendly questions that help define the nature of any therapy that is being practised. Clearly such questions must be asked when evaluating the degree of user-friendliness of any therapy.

Timms and Blampied (1985)

This small-scale retrospective study investigated the experience of groups of users who attended two Catholic and one non-sectarian marriage guidance councils. In summarizing the results of the study we will once again concentrate on the findings concerning users' experiences while neglecting to pay attention to the counsellors' views, which are also richly summarized by Timms and Blampied. In their chapter on client expectations, the authors group their findings under a number of useful headings which can be used to summarize their findings.

Client expectations

While no single generalization covered all the responses, Timms and Blampied are able to offer the following summary:

> Some clients fear that as a result of making contact with the agency they, individually, will be blamed or reprimanded in some way by the counsellors or by their partners. Some hope for a safe place in which they can meet a

referee or neutral person, though they are anxious about talking or afraid that the counsellor will be 'too sugary' or 'feel too sorry' for them. Some come prepared to do anything that will save their marriage. Most come because they want to see or understand what has gone wrong.

(Timms and Blampied, 1985, p. 47)

Interestingly, Timms and Blampied comment that the user's desire to see why things had gone wrong was often very strong and yet counsellors did not often recognize this expectation. Factors that helped keep users in counselling included a sense that counsellors could be impartial and neutral unlike relatives and friends. Expertise was also attributed to counsellors (more so by men than women) and there was an appreciation that it would take time for issues to be resolved.

Termination was also studied by Timms and Blampied. Users expressed confusion about how and why termination occurred but that may have reflected the style of counselling. Their difficulties concerning termination are seen by Timms and Blampied to reflect the complex nature of counselling which contains an in-built difficulty – that counsellor and user struggle to be working on the same agenda at the same time (and to be aware of the fact).

Users' experience

Turning to the crucial question – what do clients experience as beneficial, Timms and Blampied report that there are three major elements that account for the positive judgements that clients report.

1 Gaining the counsellor's regard

This is such an important and complex finding that we will quote the authors specifically:

Counsellors talk easily of the counselling relationship but nothing resembling what counsellors might call a therapeutic relationship emerges from clients' descriptions of counselling. This is not to say that personal factors do not figure in these descriptions nor that certain relationship factors are not mentioned. These are seen, however, more in terms of regard than of a means of gaining understanding.

The word most commonly used is 'friendship' though the limitations and indeed the complexities of this term are also recognised. It is clear from the interviews that strong mutual attraction does develop between them and at least some clients. Counsellors do not describe this in terms of friendship. For clients, it seems the best single term but they also recognise that it fails to cover certain essential aspects: one described it as 'formal friendship' while another saw the development of friendship as a sign that counselling should come to an end, 'counselling is not meant to be enjoyed'.

(Timms and Blampied, 1985, p. 53)

2 Obtaining a version

Users wanted to obtain a version (or story) of what had happened to them. They either expected that they would be offered a version or that their version would be confirmed ('getting a picture' was another term offered by a user). When a new version was desired, then counsellors were seen as contributing expertise in two ways – they could either pursue a particular view of the user's own history and its active influence on the present or encourage a process of deeper consideration of the present situation by questioning or by becoming a kind of model for the user.

3 Counselling as official conversation

Under this heading are discussed all those features of counselling which provided users with a safe, official but confidential setting in which issues (normally avoided and not adequately discussed) could be discussed. Clearly, users valued this aspect of the counselling process but the issue of whether counsellors should offer authoritative advice was also an issue for some users.

Timms and Blampied's work is very detailed and is therefore difficult to summarize adequately but we feel we have dealt with their major conclusions as far as their data concerning users is concerned. However, there is one remaining aspect of their work that provides food for thought for anybody developing user-friendly services. This issue concerns the notion of agency function:

> One of the main conclusions to be drawn from our research . . . [is that] . . . discussions of marriage counselling . . . until now lacked an essential ingredient. They have not entertained any notion of agency function. . . . As we have seen counsellors go to some pains to distinguish their activity from that of social workers, and some are sceptical of adherence to any theoretical school. . . . However . . . the idea . . . [of agency function] . . . does encapsulate many of the themes discussed in this monograph. Agencies are public forms of service interested to realise certain broad purposes, such as the maintenance of satisfying marriages. . . . The achievement of such purpose is made possible through the provision of a preserved and authorized 'space' which is safe and unconnected with a client's social network. It is also achieved through authorized personnel, knowledgeable about marriage and able to help in the realization of a version of the problem, legitimized through causal or moral attribution. Above all, agency function can be appreciated by both counsellors and clients as they realize central elements of sociability and of solidarity. Ambiguities in the talk of counsellors and of their clients may be interpreted less as matters of faith or of psychological ambivalence, and more as difficulties in the full appreciation of function.
>
> (Timms and Blampied, 1985, p. 63)

As we will see in Chapter 11, such a statement does cause difficulties for family therapists who have adopted epistemological stances that have abandoned notions of objectivity. Personally we would support Timms and Blampied's notion of safety being a crucial dimension of users' expectations. If we ourselves were distressed, then we would want to work with a counsellor who had the ability to offer a sense of containment and strength which would enable us to feel able to work on the issues that were confronting us. The nature of the agency employing the counsellor would clearly enter into our estimation of whether that sense of containment could be established.

Hunt (1985)

Patricia Hunt's study of the work of marriage counselling contributes further findings which are very much in step with the previous two studies reviewed by us. Her sample was made up of 17 men and 34 women from 42 marriages. In-depth interviews were undertaken, with most respondents being interviewed individually. Again, we cannot do justice to the overall complexity of the findings, but we will summarize the main points concerning the users' experiences of counselling.

In fact, Hunt's results were very clear-cut. Users who said that they had got on well with their counsellor felt that they had been helped and were satisfied with the service provided. Dissatisfied users all reported that they had got along badly with their counsellors. Crucial to the success of counselling was the establishing of an understanding which involved the counselling being empathic. But this was a more active process than many counsellors appreciated because, as Hunt argues, it involved both a careful checking of the nature of the problem and the making of an explicit agreement about the aim of counselling. Many counsellors neglected actively to explore these two dimensions of counselling, so, as Hunt argues:

> As I transcribed the tapes I noted the degree to which the counsellor and the client 'connected'. Sometimes it seemed as if they were on two parallel tracks throughout counselling, although with the best intentions, just missing each other and in their understanding of each other and in their perceptions of what they were working on. It is difficult to give specific examples of how clients and counsellors misunderstood each other because the misunderstanding and the misconception seemed to run through the whole of the research interview.
> (Hunt, 1985, p. 49)

Hunt stresses that it is the active quality of the therapeutic alliance that is crucial to successful therapy. A therapist who cannot successfully negotiate clear work-able goals with her users is doomed to failure. This point is well illustrated by Hunt in discussing the experience of dissatisfied clients:

> [M]any of the dissatisfied clients experienced misunderstandings both over the goals of counselling and the means of achieving these goals. Most often the client wanted advice but the counsellor was aiming to promote insight. The

client wanted some concrete action and suggestions but the counselling method was to stay with exploring the problem areas. However, both satisfied and dissatisfied clients as well as some counsellors found it hard to be specific about the kinds of goals or aims that had been agreed in counselling and no client actually remembered the counsellor explaining their method of working either in the initial interview or once counselling was underway. Where counselling was successful it seems that the aims of both the counsellor and the client coincided in some way and the tacit method of achieving those aims was acceptable to the client. Some of these misunderstandings about the nature of counselling could have been minimized if some kind of properly negotiated contract had been made in the initial interview. None of the research clients remember a specific agreement or contract being made in that initial interview, although occasionally later in the counselling, an agreement was made more specific, usually concerning the aim of the work and the number of sessions.

(Hunt, 1985, p. 52)

Interestingly, Hunt is crucially aware of how quickly both transference and negative counter-transference issues can intervene to disrupt the therapeutic alliance. For instance, she was aware, in undertaking one of her research interviews, how her first question, 'How did you come to know about Marriage Guidance', evoked an explosive response from a husband being interviewed. He clearly thought the question was belittling and this seemed to reflect a process going on in his marriage.

Hunt's discussion of her respondents' overall experiences of therapy are very detailed, but we will pick out the principal points grouped under three main headings.

Point of entry

Users experienced having to wait for therapy as a disaster – a finding that confirmed the research of Orlinsky and Howard (1978).

First interview

Given the tension that built up because of having to wait and because of the users experiencing unresolved difficulties, first interviews were often disappointing and traumatic. However, overall, the response to the first interview was very complex as the following points indicate: (a) the act of ventilating, confessing, 'getting it off the chest' and expressing feelings of distress was the main memory of the first interview, but not all users reported it as useful; (b) counsellors were seen as being attentive listeners and while some users found this useful and supportive, others felt that the counsellors should have taken more control and offered more (for them the session was an anti-climax); (c) several users would have liked more information about what to expect; (d) users who were hoping for specific advice or a solution felt particularly disappointed, questioning the value of 'just talking'; (e) some users, puzzled by not receiving advice, felt that this was deliberate policy and that subsequent sessions would offer advice because they assumed that there was a body of knowledge that could be used to give them guidelines on what to do (interestingly, Hunt reports no class difference on this dimension); (f) although only approximately 35 per cent of the clients felt relieved or happier or just different after the interview, 80 per cent elected to continue counselling.

Counselling skills and management

Under this heading Hunt summarizes several diverse but important aspects of therapy.

Setting   Users had very complex responses to the physical nature of the setting. Some disliked the allegedly relaxed atmosphere with comfy chairs; they would have preferred upright chairs and a table, reflecting the fact that they had come for advice. Inadequate soundproofing also put some users off.

The duration of the interview   Many clients felt that the first interview length (50–55 minutes) was too short to allow them to have adequate time to deal with everything they wanted to. They felt attended to but hurried because the counsellor controlled the time.

Not knowing anything about the process of counselling   This (once again) emerged as a crucial factor as reported by users. Lack of a guiding map about what counselling could offer was a drawback that caused dissatisfaction and confusion.

Counselling skills   Users were mostly very perceptive in detecting the skills they were offered but often reported that 'just talking' or 'just listening' were not sufficient to the task of helping. Giving active feedback was valued but some users also wanted to be controlled and not allowed to chatter. The idea that counsellors should 'push' for change was also accepted.

The timing of interventions   Timing was also commented on by users. Some felt that they had been pressed to make decisions too early.

Counsellor empathy   Users also stressed empathy as being important, but the more active stage of setting goals and supporting the user to achieve goals was similarly emphasized by users who experienced it.

This last finding is of crucial interest, since, as Hunt points out, marriage guidance counsellors are not usually trained to utilize such skills because the accepted model is a non-directive one. (In family therapy it used to be accepted that such skills were necessary for successful outcome: cf. the key paper by Alan Gurman and David Kniskern (1978), which is cited by Hunt.)

The final sections of Hunt's chapter on users' experiences of the counselling process deal, amongst other things, with endings, agreements and contract-making, and the need for advice. Her findings are very similar to those reported by Maluccio and Timms and Blampied, so we will not summarize them here. However, her section on the different responses of men and women to counselling does require comment, since she specifically compares and contrasts her results to those of Brannen and Collard:

> Brannen and Collard also found that men were more critical and less committed to MG counselling than female clients. However, I did not find such a marked difference. Proportionately the responses of the sexes were quite similar. The 17 men interviewed were indeed more critical of the counselling they received initially and found it more difficult to accept the value of 'just talking'. However, half of them persisted and eventually found that counselling helped them. Of these 17 men, six were satisfied with counselling, three were predominantly satisfied but wished it had been more directive, and eight were dissatisfied and definitely felt that more direction or action was needed and were disappointed with what they felt to be the reflective, more passive approach. However, several of those who were satisfied acknowledged that they had had to learn to use and appreciate the reflective approaches to their problems. Several mentioned that they had not felt satisfied in the first interview, but had obviously struggled through their initial doubts and part of the counselling process for them had been learning the value of talking about their feelings.
>
> (Hunt, 1985, p. 63)

Interestingly, Hunt points out that the discrepancy between her findings and those of Brannen and Collard could be explained in terms of the point at which users were interviewed. (Brannen and Collard interviewed their users at a much earlier stage in counselling.) She also stresses that many women also found the lack of advice a problem. Two-thirds of the men hoped for more direction, advice or action but so did 50 per cent of the women. Although more of these women were converted to the value of exploring their problems and discovering their own solutions, many remained equally as disappointed as the men.

Hunt's overall conclusion summarizing these findings is very clarifying so we quote it in full:

> Perhaps this research suggests that there may be a case for using a different kind of intervention or approach with some clients, both men and women, who find the client-centred approach difficult to accept, even when it includes a

more active component. For people who see the value in 'just talking', a task-centred (behavioural) approach may be more appropriate from the outset. This would at least involve making a contract with the client on some kind of plan or action involving task-setting and reporting back, which is the approach used in marital and sexual therapy. Discussion in counselling sessions would centre more on what happened and how it happened – the more concrete aspects of behaviour in addition to how the clients felt. The immediacy of this kind of approach often seems more relevant to some clients, and, of course, usually provides exactly the same kind of material to work with in counselling that 'just talking' provides. The skill, of course, would be in deciding which clients required which approach and implicit in this suggestion is that counsellors should feel relatively skilful and comfortable with a number of counselling approaches or interventions, which is not the case at the moment. Certainly this research indicates that the client-centred approach cannot be universally applicable to all MG clients.

(Hunt, 1985, p. 79)

We have quoted Hunt's interesting comments at length because, as we will see later in this review, a family therapy researcher, Ian Bennun (1989), dealing with a similar issue of gender difference in relation to the outcome of family therapy, arrives at a rather different conclusion about the significance of the gender difference he discovers.

SUMMARY

The studies that we have reviewed so far are all important to us because they make important contributions to clarifying our notions of user-friendliness. Clearly there is a common thread running through all the studies – the importance of the therapeutic alliance between user and therapist is documented in similar terms, but each study also contributes other important pieces of the jigsaw. Many family therapists, and particularly those trained to dismiss the idea that there are crucial continuities between different forms of therapy, will find these studies uninteresting because they are not centrally concerned with family therapy and involve models which mostly avoid therapeutic intervention in the technical sense of the word. However, we take a different stance. Therapists, from their professional viewpoint, may think that therapy is a technical interventionist endeavour but clearly users are not so convinced. Gender differences are important, with men tending to want therapy to be more instrumental and advice-giving, but we found Brannen and Collard's discussion illuminating because it stressed a crucial point – that initial attitudes of a user are not necessarily fixed and immutable. Therapy is an interactional process during which mutual learning ideally needs to take place.

Family therapy has until recently been dominated by men (as theorists and trainers), who have tended to value instrumentality to the detriment of other dimensions of therapy. Marriage guidance counselling (a much less well established profession of mainly women) has taken a very different path, at least in this country. Client-centred or psychoanalytic ideas stressing the importance of the therapeutic relationship have taken centre stage. Ideas about advice-giving or creating 'interventions' are criticized within this tradition because they challenge the reflective nature of the approach. These two approaches are very different from each other, and in this country there has been remarkably little contact between family therapy and marriage guidance counselling. Historically, this has been very damaging but we believe that both traditions have a lot to learn from each other. In particular we believe that family therapists need to be more aware that the significance of the therapeutic alliance (stressed by the marriage counselling approach) is almost universal and permeates most forms of therapy, as our review of family therapy studies in our next chapter will help to confirm.

Chapter 9

Reviewing consumer studies of therapy

Family therapy research

Andy Treacher

INTRODUCTION

In order to qualify for inclusion in this chapter, the focus of the study needed to be on users' experience of therapy, rather than on demonstrating the efficacy of a particular family therapy model. The literature concerned with users' experiences of therapy is quite difficult to organize coherently. However, we have chosen to divide the studies into five groups: large-scale studies, small-scale studies, individual case studies, studies aimed at unravelling specific features of therapy, and studies utilizing second-order methodologies. The last group utilizes ethnographic interviewing techniques which purport to be free of the positivist frameworks that permeate more traditional research.

LARGE-SCALE STUDIES

Woodward *et al.* (1978)

This project by Cristel Woodward and her colleagues was part of a comprehensive McMaster Family Therapy Outcome Study. The number of families who answered their family therapy satisfaction questionnaire (279) was impressive, but as in many large-scale studies, the results were rather global and difficult to relate to practice. Overall, 64 per cent of all family members were satisfied or very satisfied with the total services received. However, only 56 per cent felt that the services were comprehensive and adequate. Satisfied families were also likely to have been noted by observers as having changed during the course of therapy, as having a good prognosis, as feeling better with regard to the presenting (child-focused) problems and as having attained or exceeded their goals. They also tended to have sought additional help less than dissatisfied families during a six-week follow-up. Dissatisfied families could not be summarized so easily. For example, some families undoubtedly did change positively but that did not overcome their feelings of being dissatisfied. Overall the prime source of dissatisfaction for all families concerned was the focus of treatment (i.e. the family) and patient–staff interactions.

Frude and Dowling (1980)

Neil Frude and Emilia Dowling also used a postal questionnaire design in their study of 102 respondents (from 42 families) who had attended the Family Institute in Cardiff. Their basic findings were as follows:

Experiences of treatment sessions

Fifty-one per cent of users found sessions uncomfortable at least sometimes; 47 per cent reported feelings of embarrassment; 31 per cent felt anger towards the therapist; 90 per cent felt affection towards the therapist; 95 per cent felt that the therapist was caring; 76 per cent felt at least somewhat close to the therapist.

Therapeutic effectiveness – the original problem since therapy

Fifty per cent found family therapy 'extremely useful', 39 per cent 'somewhat useful', and 11 per cent found it 'not at all helpful'. Seventy per cent said the original problem was 'better', 23 per cent 'the same' and 7 per cent 'worse'. Fifty-two per cent reported no problem substitution, but 14 per cent said there had definitely been substitution, and 29 per cent thought that perhaps there had been.

Therapeutic effectiveness in family life since therapy

Sixty-nine per cent said life had 'improved', 25 per cent that it was 'unchanged' and 6 per cent that it was 'worse'. Fifty-four per cent said family talk had 'somewhat improved' and 21 per cent that it was 'much improved'. Thirty-two per cent reported that they understood themselves 'much better', 54 per cent 'somewhat better' and 15 per cent 'not at all'; 31 per cent reported understanding others 'much better', 51 per cent 'somewhat better' and 18 per cent 'not at all'.

Users' attitudes to the Institute

Fifty-seven per cent would 'definitely' return with another problem, 30 per cent 'perhaps' and 13 per cent 'would not'; 73 per cent of users would 'definitely' advise a friend to contact the Institute with a problem. Interestingly, the study also contains data about the efficacy of family therapy in terms of the model practised: 39 out of 65 users who received structural family therapy found it 'extremely' helpful, whereas only 3 out of 19 who received strategic family therapy found it helpful. Another interesting finding (emerging from the more complex statistical analysis undertaken) was concerned with a general factor that Frude and Dowling call a 'favourable impression of family therapy'. The following responses contributed to this factor: (a) finding family therapy helpful, (b) original problem now better, (c) family talk improved, (d) feeling affection towards the therapist, (e) understanding other family members better, and (f) would return with another problem.

Examining the reported feelings of the users during therapy, there was no evidence that feelings of anger or embarrassment were a useful part of the therapeutic process. However, some users who did report frequent feelings of anger or embarrassment also claimed that the treatment had been highly effective. Significantly, those who felt anger towards the therapist seldom felt affection towards the therapist. Affection towards the therapist was even more strongly related to feelings that the therapist was caring. Judgements concerning the therapist being caring were also related to a low rate of reported anger feelings; clients who felt close to their therapist rarely felt sessions to be uncomfortable.

Frude and Dowling also examine several user-friendly questions – for example, did family members (men vs women vs children) experience family therapy differently? In fact, they found few differences, but interestingly while only 20 per cent of parents felt they understood themselves better as a result of therapy, the comparable figure for children was 50 per cent. Generally the degree of consensus about therapy between husbands and wives was high, except in two areas: 'understanding themselves or others better' and 'relationships outside the family had improved since therapy'.

Overall, we find Frude and Dowling's results very intriguing. The very marked difference in user satisfaction according to whether they received structural or strategic family therapy is very striking, and it is worth noting how Frude and Dowling interpret these results:

> About half of the clients claimed that family therapy had been extremely helpful but an even greater number reported that the original problem had improved and this discrepancy is interesting. It could be taken to suggest that clients sometimes attributed changes to factors other than therapy or were claiming the 'spontaneous remission' of a problem, but also raises the intriguing possibility that there is a positive reluctance among some clients to attribute improvement to therapy. This is supported by further analysis showing that the tendency to report symptom improvement while maintaining that family therapy was of little benefit was considerably greater (just short of statistical significance) in those treated 'strategically' than in those treated 'structurally'. In many of the strategic cases paradoxical injunction was used and in such cases we might expect symptomatic change to occur and to be recognised by the client but *not* to be recognised as an effect of the specific treatment. Thus the evidence obtained is in line with the theoretical prediction and underlines the special problems associated with the status of clients' reports as evidence where paradoxical methods have been employed.
>
> (Frude and Dowling, 1980, pp. 160–161)

No doubt Frude and Dowling's methodological point is valid but what about the ethical and professional issues raised by the discrepancy they observe? If users are helped by covert or paradoxical methods, but cannot themselves identify that they have been helped by them, what are the long-term results? Do they recommend other potential users to attend the Institute? Do they criticize the Institute so that its reputation is sullied? And what if they run into a similar problem – do they feel empowered to return for help? Strategic therapists must surely be embarrassed by these questions because they expose the fallacies of an expert model which cannot empower users by the genuine sharing of skills and knowledge. Strategic therapy may well be effective but such results are clearly opportunist and are just as potentially disempowering as, for example, the use of psychotropic drugs in psychiatric treatments (as previously pointed out by Andy in Treacher, 1998a).

Bjørgo and Due-Tønnessen (1992)

Målfrid Bjørgo and Bernt Due-Tønnessen's study explored users' experiences of attending a family counselling service in Norway. A clear majority of users were satisfied with the service, particularly if they had individual therapy. Those who came as couples were the least satisfied overall, reflecting the fact that it was usually one partner who was seeking help and the other more grudgingly agreeing to attend. The majority of users felt accepted, listened to, and offered new perspectives but there were significant differences concerning advice-seeking. If users attended for couple therapy, then 61 per cent of them wanted direct advice. If they attended as individuals, then the comparable figure was 49 per cent. If as family members, then the figure was 27 per cent. Curiously, the authors take a remarkably non-user-friendly approach to this issue of advice-giving. They argue that since advice-giving clearly does not fit the ideology and thinking of therapy, 'a challenge for the future will be to communicate some of this thinking more clearly in our meetings with clients'.

Of greater interest to us is the fact that they monitored gender difference as recorded by the 163 women and 134 men in their sample. They report little difference in satisfaction scores and little difference in terms of help-seeking behaviour in the future, or as they themselves comment, 'The somewhat hesitant or sceptical attitude of men to therapy (which is different from outright un-willingness) does not mean that they are less satisfied with the service since they have started' (a finding that confirms a point made by Hunt (1985) in her paper). This rather complacent comment leads them to conclude that their service did not need to be more 'man-friendly'. Instead they suggest that they needed to concentrate on communicating the fact that they had a good service to offer.

Another difference reported by the authors does require further comment. Women tend to describe the presenting problem as having lasted a long time (54 per cent) and being very difficult (67 per cent). The comparable figures for men were both 42 per cent. It seems that women find family situations more difficult as they feel both dominated and treated unequally in comparison to men. They also seek greater intimacy.

SMALL-SCALE STUDIES

Merrington and Corden (1981)

Diana Merrington and John Corden (1981) studied eight families referred to a child guidance clinic. Families mostly felt uncertain about what to expect and were surprised that their worker proposed to meet them as a family for several sessions. The idea of meeting for one family session was not unexpected but parents expected sessions to be held with their child and with themselves but separately. This type of clash of perspective was also demonstrated by other findings. For example, four families did not change their view of the presenting problem despite receiving a family therapy input that challenged that view. Interestingly, most families felt that their perception of their problem had been accurately recorded by their worker but very few could be sure how the workers had seen the problems themselves. Six families recalled that their worker had been explicit about the proposed length and duration of contact and none had any difficulty with the language used by their worker. Four families had either not understood or had disagreed with some aspects of the treatment but more recalled that they had asked for clarification.

Overall, all the families found their workers friendly, warm, approachable and genuinely concerned. All expected advice to be given but four felt that more advice could and should have been given. Families' views about outcome were equally positive – one family considered their problem completely resolved while six felt that treatment had been quite helpful. One felt it had been unsuccessful though not a waste of time.

Interestingly, and very much in line with our own results, families had views about the use of additional individual sessions. Most felt they would have been useful because they would have enabled both children and parents to speak more freely about difficult issues. Many parents still felt, at the end of therapy, unsure about whether their children should have been involved so much in therapy. Six families felt that the referred child had found the sessions an ordeal. And some parents wondered if younger children could not have been more actively involved since the discussion probably went over their heads.

Merrington and Corden summarize their own thoughts about engaging families as follows:

> In suggesting family therapy as the treatment of choice . . . the worker is asking the family to take a substantial risk, and make a conceptual leap of some magnitude. . . . In this study, the families seem to have been positively influenced by the warmth and genuine concern communicated by the workers. Families were also impressed by the workers' rapid grasp of how different family members experienced the problem. On the other hand, some families would have liked clearer information about how the workers themselves viewed the problem. It is likely that the workers deliberately refrained from assuming an 'expert' role, to ensure that the family continued to wrestle with

their problem and possible solutions, and did not abdicate their responsibility
to the workers. Could clearer feedback be given without undermining the
family's responsibilities? After the family therapy had been terminated, half
of the families agreed that it was not the workers' role to give advice, whereas
they had all originally expected the worker to provide directive advice. This
may be seen as a recognition by some families that their problems could not
be resolved without the involvement and commitment of family members.
They began to understand that solutions could not be imposed from outside the
family.

(Merrington and Corden, 1981, pp. 258–259)

Russell and Leyland (1986)

Jacqui Russell and Maureen Leyland's study of 18 families attending a child
guidance clinic covers very similar ground to the previous study but evidence of
gender differences in expectations are also documented in the study. Having
reported the classical finding that mothers initiated contact in the majority of
cases, the study shows that it was mothers who had the most complex feelings
about coming to the clinic. Asked to rate themselves on eight dimensions, the
number of mothers responding compared to fathers was as follows: anxious (3:1),
relieved (2:0), desperate (2:0), hopeful (6:1), curious (1:1), reluctant (0:2),
sceptical (3:1), frightened/defensive (1:1).

Some of the nitty-gritty of therapy was also monitored by asking families
about the advantages and disadvantages of team participation and using video. In
both cases families' responses were complex and ambivalent. Significantly, users
also expressed difficulties with attending daytime sessions and suggested that
evening sessions needed to be organized. Some specific comments were also
made about features of the family therapy on offer. One or two families thought
the team were 'blank and dead pan in appearance' or unemotional. Split messages
from the team caused two families some consternation but a third had found the
technique very useful in prompting discussion at home. Phone calls by observers
tended to confuse family members who had often thought that something they
had said had prompted the call.

SINGLE CASE STUDIES

Jackson (1986)

Sue Jackson invited a family to return to her clinic for a follow-up interview one
year after they had completed therapy. The early stages of the interview were
relatively unstructured so that the family could retain the initiative in identifying
key aspects of the therapeutic process. Unfortunately Jackson's attempt to match
the family members' views of what was significant in therapy with her own is not

particularly successful, largely, we think, because she is too anxious to theorize about what happened. A less complicated method of presenting the paper would have involved presenting the family members' accounts in greater detail. Her own account could then be compared with these accounts. However, despite this criticism, the paper is both interesting and significant.

Jackson clearly shows that the initial process of engagement was crucial. The father of the family was initially very hostile to her because he was convinced that the presenting problem (his daughter's anorexia) was medically caused. Crucial to the engagement was a process whereby the parents could admit that 'we are not that perfect after all'. Jackson also stresses that her strategic/systemic style of questioning seemed to be useful in helping the family to reflect about what was happening. The mother of the family particularly recalled the value of the questions at the follow-up interview.

Jackson also attempts to tease out three other dimensions in the therapeutic process which she felt were significant in producing change. Two of these dimensions, validating the daughter's uniqueness and triggering a determination to change in the daughter, were quite specific, but the third dimension, changing the family's belief system, was very general. Jackson's documentation of the significance of these dimensions is rather uneven and she often cites examples of the family's responses from the therapy sessions rather than the follow-up interview which we think creates methodological problems. However, we are persuaded that a major shift did occur in relation to what theorists like Rudi Dallos (1991) and Harry Procter (1984) would call a core construct. From the recording of the interview, Jackson is able to demonstrate how the father changed his attitude to being perfect. Commenting on the fact that he and his wife had believed that they were perfect and did not fight, he adds: 'until you [the therapist] eventually destroyed the myth and had us being perfectly normal and fighting just like everyone else. . . . I remember we started off as God's family put on earth . . . all pure, all loving . . . I think that's the way we tried to portray ourselves . . . but we ended up being perfectly normal.'

Jackson's work is very stimulating and she herself suggests that follow-up interviews of the type she organised could feasibly be incorporated into routine practice. Therapists could benefit from this approach, but Jackson also suggests that it gives families a chance to give something back to their therapist – hence redressing the power imbalance which always seems to place the family in debt to the therapist.

Strømnes (1991)

Helen Strømnes's study is the only one we have discovered that deals with the user's perspective as recorded by the user herself. The author was the recipient (with her now divorced husband) of family therapy. Strømnes debates many issues in her paper – including the fact that family therapy (whether it likes it or not) can often either increase or create guilt among family members. She also debates the issue of personal responsibility and the role of personal factors in contributing to problems. She asks whether all problems do have to be construed as joint problems – can there not be individual factors? Strømnes's point is very challenging to conventional family therapy ideas and the force of her argument is clearly illustrated in the following quotation:

> We are constantly not only *tempted* to misidentify problems but also *encouraged* to do so. The implied cause and effect of family problems so often becomes a self-fulfilling prophecy of the problem family. Family therapy has a lot to offer, but the timing must be right; if not, the timing may itself suggest that the family is at fault. The 'experts' need to know roughly what type of therapy is right at what time. We patients have begun to talk, not just *during*, but also *about* therapy. We are bringing up independent thoughts which do not need interpreting by therapists.
>
> (Strømnes, 1991)

Strømnes's account is both powerful and unique but it is a real reflection on family therapists that we have singularly failed in encouraging our ex-users to record and publish their own accounts of what it is like to be in therapy.

STUDIES THAT EXAMINE SPECIFIC FEATURES OF THERAPY FROM A USER'S POINT OF VIEW

Piercy, Sprenkle and Constantine (1986)

This study by Fred Piercy, Douglas Sprenkle and John Constantine is the only major study we have discovered which focuses specifically on families' experiences of video and team supervision. Piercy and his colleagues studied 75 family members drawn from 32 families attending sessions at a university marriage and family therapy clinic which had a structural–strategic orientation. Respondents filled out the Purdue Live Observation Satisfaction Scale, which has a series of questions which are rated on a scale using five categories – strongly agree, moderately agree, neither agree nor disagree, moderately disagree, strongly disagree. By comparing the combined first and second and the combined fourth and fifth categories it is possible to get a global sense of the rates of satisfaction and dissatisfaction derived from the 10 questions which are relevant to our discussion in this chapter.

Inspection of these scores reveals the overall satisfaction level to be favourable but it is worth commenting on the percentage of users who were *not* satisfied with the package offered: 21.4 per cent of users felt the therapist was too often interrupted by the observers (the remaining 78.6 per cent were either neutral or were positive about interruptions); 13.3 per cent felt uncomfortable that the therapist left the room to talk with the observers; but while only 5.3 per cent felt that the observers' ideas were unhelpful, 32 per cent would have liked to talk with the therapist without being observed; 23.8 per cent were actually bothered by people observing and 17.3 per cent felt that observers made therapy less effective, although only 5.4 per cent felt that the therapist paid too much attention to the observers; 8.7 per cent felt that they could not be themselves while being observed but only 5.3 per cent felt the therapist spent too much time outside the room talking to the observers; finally, 17.3 per cent felt they had less confidence in their therapist because he or she could talk with the observers.

Clearly, despite quite sizeable overall satisfaction rates, there was a minority of users who did not like central aspects of therapy. Unfortunately, despite the methodological sophistication of the study (with great care being taken to establish the reliability of the questionnaire), the authors made no attempt to use correlational or linkage analysis techniques. These could hopefully have yielded a profile of users who tended to be satisfied and those who tended to be dissatisfied.

Interestingly, Piercy *et al.* also provide data relevant to the use of phone-ins as supervision: 93 per cent of users were either positive or neutral about phone-ins; 87 per cent about the therapist leaving the room to take supervision; and 84 per cent about phone-ins resulting in observer conferences. Users' response to videotaping was very positive with only 5 out of 37 reporting any negative reactions.

Confirming at least partially the results of Frude and Dowling reported earlier, Piercy *et al.* found no differences in satisfaction scores between male and female users or between children and adults. However, therapist gender did prove to be highly significant. Irrespective of whether users were male or female, they reported higher satisfaction with the live observation/supervision process if their therapist was a woman rather than a man. A number of explanations for this phenomenon are offered by the authors. They suggest that women may (because they tend to be socialized to be more nurturing and accommodating than men) generate more family trust and hence more satisfaction with a team approach to supervision. Alternatively they suggest that since women have generally been forced to hold less authoritative, lower status positions they may, as therapists, feel more comfortable with being supervised and therefore be better able to develop team relationships among themselves, their observers and the user families.

Finally, viewing the situation from a user's point of view, it may be that families may have seen it as more natural for a woman to receive supervision than a man, so that they may have felt that a supervised man was incompetent. On the other hand, user families may have felt pleased that their woman therapists had back-up in the form of a team, given that women are (in terms of the results of lay surveys) seen as less authoritative, knowledgeable, competent and independent than men.

Piercy and his colleagues (all men) obviously come close to sexism in offering these explanations, and we are left wondering whether there were other explanations. For example, in order to achieve the same status as men (given the sexist biases against them), women have often to be more competent than their male colleagues. Perhaps this was true of Piercy's sample, although no results are presented that can confirm or disconfirm this point.

Surprisingly, Piercy and his colleagues make no observations about the implications of their study for family therapy practice. They seem lulled into complacency because the majority of users were either positive about the 'technology' of family therapy or were neutral about it. In fact, as we have demonstrated, there was usually a significant minority of users who did have objections to aspects of therapy. Clearly, their figure of 32 per cent who disliked having observers cannot be shrugged off by anybody who adopts a user-friendly approach.

Mashal, Feldman and Sigal (1989)

Meeda Mashal, Ronald Feldman and John Sigal designed an ambitious study to unravel a treatment paradigm – specifically the Milan approach (MFT) to family therapy. Fourteen families and five couples who had received MFT were interviewed by telephone a minimum of a year after the completion of therapy. The outcome measures for the study were intriguing, with a marked discrepancy between parents and identified child users. The former reported a 56 per cent improvement in family functioning; the latter 89 per cent. Better self-functioning figures also showed differences, with 56 per cent of fathers reporting improvements, 67 per cent of mothers and 78 per cent of identified child users. However, these positive results have to be set against other figures recording that a high percentage of families reported that at least one family member sought further therapy after completing MFT (68 per cent of fathers reported this, 59 per cent of mothers and 58 per cent of identified child patients).

The study also explored the user-friendliness of the approach. Strikingly not a single respondent replied with indifference when directly questioned. Fifty-six per cent of mothers disliked it, compared with 47 per cent of fathers and 44 per cent of identified child patients. Curiously, spontaneous comments about therapy, which were also scored, revealed a slightly different pattern. Fathers were strongest in the condemnation of treatment, 37 per cent voicing strong condemnation (11 per cent making positive comments). The comparable figures for mothers were 25 per cent and 6 per cent, and for identified child users 40 per cent and 10 per cent.

Fortunately the study provides correlational data about like/dislike of therapy and specific aspects of treatment. For the identified child users, no significant relationships were found but, for parents, the results were often significant. Dislike of the group behind the mirror correlated with dislike of therapy in general for both mothers and fathers. For fathers, dislike of therapy correlated with a dislike of the time interval between sessions. The mothers' response was similar but results did not reach significance. Scores relating to videotaping also yielded insignificant results. Length of treatment satisfaction scores directly related to fathers' enjoyment of treatment, i.e. treatment experienced as too long was associated with disliking therapy. The results for mothers were not significant.

Mothers who enjoyed the therapy experience tended to report family improvement and self improvement more strongly than fathers, although in neither case did the results reach significance. Seeking further treatment correlated with disliking therapy for mothers but not for fathers or for identified patient children.

Scoring spontaneous comments provided additional support for the idea that dislike of MFT correlated with seeking further treatment. The more negative the mothers' and fathers' spontaneous comments, the more likely it is that at least one family member would seek further treatment. However, it was also demonstrated that families with the most severe difficulties (as rated by the researchers) did tend to seek further treatment.

In commenting on the significance of their results, Mashal *et al.* stress the value of their documentation particularly of families' responses to the group behind the mirror. While many positive responses were forthcoming – in terms of the group's value in helping users 'to take stock of themselves' and to be heard, and to give feedback to the therapist – there were also a number of sharp criticisms, reflected in the following comments:

I would have liked to know the purpose of the group. The whole thing was couched in such secrecy. When I asked for information about the objectives of the group my questions were answered with other questions. . . . I never felt so used and guinea-pigged in my whole life!

They were a bunch of kids! Students who know nothing . . . given to extremes. They were ridiculous. We ignored it. My wife and I were exasperated.

The group was not for our benefit, [the] group was only there to learn [about therapy].

I didn't like it all. I like to see the people and their reactions. It was very impersonal.

(Mashal *et al.*, 1989, pp. 466–467)

Families were equally strong in voicing their views about their therapists:

It was incredible. [Dr. X.] seemed to have nothing to do with it. He seemed like a puppet. It was very disconcerting when [Dr. X.] was called out in the middle of [an] emotional sequence and then comes back and repeats mechanically what [the] group says.

(In contrast to previous therapies) [Dr Y.] said very little. No one-to-one feeling . . . at arm's length . . . very impersonal.

I didn't like [the] attitude and way [Dr. Z.] operated. She turned me off. She wouldn't answer questions.

I was very impressed by how well it was done . . . very professional, but it was very cold.

((Mashal *et al.*, 1989, pp. 467–468)

Mashal *et al.*'s paper is significant because it is the first paper that we have discovered that clearly records problems that users are likely to have with an approach that relies heavily on circular questioning. Mashal *et al.*'s own discussion of this crucial issue is very much in tune with our own thinking, as the following important quotation reveals:

> [C]oldness and lack of empathy are the opposite of the ingredients shown to be effective in the treatment of individuals (Frank, 1971; Garfield, 1973; Strupp, 1973; Truax and Mitchell, 1971) and in the prevention of family therapy drop outs (Gurman and Kniskern, 1978). . . . Our finding that superior outcome was reported by parents who had a more positive feeling about the treatment, though it does not establish a causal link, is consistent with this hypothesis. Contrary to the suggestion by the [original] Milan group that creating disequilibrium in the family, even to the point of anguish, may be needed to produce change (Palazzoli *et al.*, 1978) negative responses seem to inhibit therapeutic change.
>
> Results from a recent examination of research on the effectiveness of paradoxical interventions suggest a further amendment to one's view of what produces change in families. On the basis of a (statistical) meta-analysis of 12 studies . . . Shoham-Salomon and Rosenthal (1987) found that paradoxical interventions were indeed therapeutically successful . . . but the effect was exclusively due to prescriptions based upon *positive* connotations; they found that prescriptions with neutral or negative connotations were ineffective. . . . It appears that the affective context within which the disequilibrium is created is relevant, as is the families' perception of the affective tone of at least some of the disequilibrium creating interventions. What remains unknown is the mechanism by which the family's affective responses bring about change in this model of family therapy. It appears that, even with the Milan approach to treatment, the therapist must make some attempt to join the family system (Minuchin and Fishman, 1981) . . . in order . . . to foster a positive attitude toward the treatment team and the treatment procedures for the most favourable results.
>
> (Mashal *et al.*, 1989, pp. 467–468)

Mashal *et al.*'s comments are salutary but, and in fairness to MFT, it is important to stress that many of the innovations made by Boscolo and Cecchin have addressed the issue of coldness and distance as we shall explore in Chapter 11. Karl Tomm's work on interactive interviewing (Tomm, 1987a, 1987b) is particularly crucial in this respect as Mashal *et al.* point out. Tomm's work demonstrates how the use of elegant, thought-prompting questions can be productive in helping users to re-think their attitudes both generally and specifically.

Reichelt (1990)

Sissel Reichelt's Norwegian study explores the issue that effective therapy can only occur if therapists adopt a custom-building approach. Reichelt, impressed by the findings of Stanton and Todd's (1979) study of structural-strategic work with drug misusers, decided to explore users' experiences of receiving similar treatment. She concludes that a structural-strategic approach did not suit all the families who experienced it. The approach fell short particularly where families had come across experts in the past and felt hopeless and guilty. Reichelt arrives at the basically user-friendly conclusion that the true task of the therapist is to find the right model for the right client at the right time.

Crane, Griffin and Hill (1986)

Russell Crane, William Griffin and Robert Hill (1986) were interested in exploring what characteristic skills make therapy effective from a user's point of view. Crane et al.'s careful reviews of individual psychotherapy literature prompted them to select five dimensions of therapist activity which were central to their study: (1) therapist level of experience; (2) therapists' 'knows how to deal with user problems; (3) level of concern of the therapist; (4) therapist confidence level; (5) therapists' ability to 'fit' the treatment approach to the user's perception of his or her own specific needs. Using step-wise multiple regression analysis of variance procedures, they were able to discover which of these factors were most indicative of successful outcome for a group of 102 users attending marital and family therapy clinics.

The results of the study (a postal questionnaire) were very clear-cut. Only one variable, 'fit of treatment', was found to predict users' ratings of treatment outcome. A second analysis of the relationship between perceived therapist competence (i.e. being well trained or not) and other therapist variables revealed that competence was judged predominantly in terms of the therapist's exhibiting concern.

Commenting on their results, Crane et al. stress that it is the therapist's ability to present therapy as consistent and congruent with user expectations that is important to the client, at least as reported retrospectively in this follow-up study. They suggest, therefore, that the engagement work of the therapist must focus on the therapist selecting a treatment approach that matches those expectations:

> Attention must therefore be paid to each user's unique view of the family. The therapist also needs to use 'the language and symbols of the family, constructing a common therapy agenda or pacing therapy at a rate so as to be understood by clients. . . . In terms of perceived therapist competence, the most important therapist skill was that of appearing concerned. The influence of this variable is suggestive of the importance of establishing a positive therapeutic relationship. To help acquire this skill, beginning therapists might best be coached in such skills as establishing a 'collaborative set' (Jacobson and Margolin, 1979), 'joining' (Minuchin, 1974) and 'relationship skills' (Alexander and Parsons, 1982).
>
> (Crane et al., 1986, p. 95)

Zimmerman-Tansella and Colorio (1986)

Some of the points that Crane *et al.* make about fit of treatment are echoed by the Italian study of Christa Zimmerman-Tansella and Constanza Colorio (1986). The study explored results from 17 families, who were interviewed after they had dropped out of MFT treatment provided by a state-run clinic, after just one session. When asked the straightforward question, 'Why did you not return?' 23 per cent answered evasively; 19 per cent could not remember why; 30 per cent reported that they thought treatment had been concluded after one session; 21 per cent dropped out because the situation had improved; but only 9 per cent reported that they had found the single session no use at all. However, 38 per cent of users reported that they looked for professional help elsewhere after the family session.

Users' attitudes to the sessions and to their therapists were complex: 69 per cent found the sessions embarrassing but only 17 per cent felt angry with the therapists. Fifty-nine per cent felt they received affection from the therapist; 79 per cent remembered the therapists as impartial, 88 per cent as interested and 90 per cent as active. Seventy-four per cent reported that treatment had been helpful, 78 per cent that their problem had been understood correctly, and 79 per cent reported satisfaction with the family approach. Seventy-one per cent said that they would advise a friend to seek help using the family approach.

Zimmerman-Tansella and Colorio were clearly puzzled by their results. The actual drop-out rate from therapy – 37 families out of 109 (i.e. 34 per cent) – apparently does not cause them great concern, as they state that several other researchers have reported similar levels (Shapiro and Budman, 1973; Sigal *et al.*, 1976; Slipp and Cressel, 1978). However, the fact that nearly a third of users had considered the treatment to be concluded after just one session is difficult to explain. There are some clues in their data, however, as they themselves report. Interestingly, 85 per cent of the users ascribed the problem which brought them to therapy as belonging to the identified patient. However, a clear majority of family members judged the family session as least useful for the identified patient and more useful either for themselves or other family members. This mismatch could explain why drop-out occurred.

Bennun (1989)

Ian Bennun's interest, like our own, is in how users' perceptions of their therapists may influence therapeutic outcome. He studied 35 families presenting with a variety of problems ranging from alcoholism to childhood disorders. A 'perception of therapist 'questionnaire measuring three factors – positive regard/ interest, competence/experience and activity/direct guidance – was answered by the respondents. Results from this scale were correlated with satisfaction with outcome measures. The orientation of the therapists was either MFT or problem-solving.

Considering the ratings collected from fathers – two factors (competence and direct guidance) correlated significantly (at the 0.01 level) with positive outcome whether or not the father was the IP (index patient). For IPs, ratings of positive regard and direct guidance correlated with outcome. However, none of the factors rated by non-IP mothers showed correlations (significant at the 0.01 level) with outcome. For IP mothers, activity/direct guidance emerged as an apparently significant factor. On the basis of these findings, Bennun concludes that, 'when mothers' ratings are taken as a whole their perception of the therapist has little bearing on outcome unless she is an IP whereas perceptions held by fathers, whether IP or not, interact with outcome' (Bennun, 1989, p. 247).

There are several comments that need to be made about this conclusion. Firstly, since the data is correlational and derived from a relatively small sample, it is extremely dubious to make a causal inference. Secondly, it seems to us that Bennun overstates his case – the correlation coefficients relevant to mothers' ratings on two variables (positive regard/interest and activity/direct guidance) were demonstrably significant at the 0.05 level, so a less partisan reading of the results would draw attention to the fact that the results were more complex than Bennun allows.

Admittedly, Bennun is on firmer ground when he utilizes an alternative form of analysis. He divided his sample into two groups – one reflecting the best 10 outcomes and the other the 10 worst outcomes. These two groups were then compared on the original three factors. Statistical analysis revealed that there were highly significant differences between the two groups on three therapist factors (competence, activity/direct guidance and positive regard), as rated by fathers; mothers' ratings did not produce significant results but IP ratings did, though only in relation to the positive regard factor.

Bennun undertook one further analysis which also requires comment. He was able to demonstrate that there was an interesting difference between parents who reported a positive clinical outcome and those who did not. Unsurprisingly, the greater the discrepancy between the parents' ratings, the worse the outcome.

To us, Bennun's interpretation of the gender differences he discovered is similar to a football commentator insisting that a given team's victory is due to the skills of the forward line. The forwards may indeed have scored the goals and 'won' the match but such an analysis can easily overlook the fact that the defence may have contributed to victory equally, by stopping the opposing team from scoring goals. We would argue that a genuinely user-friendly approach to therapy prompts therapists to be aware that they must find ways of working with both constituencies. As Bennun argues, fathers, when they do attend, tend to remain disengaged, show higher drop-out rates, are less willing to self-disclose and are less likely to be active in the treatment process. They also have a much higher threshold vis-à-vis problem identification before attendance for therapy begins.

Clearly therapists faced by the difficulties are forced to concentrate a lot of attention and skill on engaging them. Bennun cities research reviewed by Heubeck et al. (1986) indicating that men prefer active, structured therapists who offer advice and goal-setting. They tend to stay in therapy if the therapist also offers a positive prognosis and demonstrates a liking for the family. Research by Kerr and McKee (1981), cited by Bennun, reports that mothers were more reliable informants about family matters but were less powerful in determining the outcome of any therapeutic encounter involving the family although they initiated help-seeking more often than fathers. These facts are a sad reflection of sexism in a society dominated by men, but unfortunately therapists have to learn to work with such imbalances.

STUDIES UTILIZING CONSTRUCTIVE METHODOLOGIES

Finally, and before attempting to summarize the findings of this chapter, it is necessary to review briefly two studies that utilized ethnographic interviewing in order to establish users' experiences of attending family therapy where the presenting problem is adolescent drug abuse.

Kuehl, Newfield and Joanning (1990) and Newfield, Kuehl, Joanning and Quinn (1990)

These two papers essentially cover the same ground and report findings from more or less the same sample, so we will review them together. Neil Newfield, Bruce Kuehl, Harvey Joanning and William Quinn argue in their paper that ethnographic interviewing is an important methodological innovation which can challenge therapists' tendencies to view therapy as a therapist-dominated process.

Ethnography is a branch of anthropology that is concerned with describing individual cultures or aspects of cultures in ways that avoid using interpretations based upon the investigator's frame of reference. The ethnographer adopts the position of a learner who needs teaching or informing about the subject matter that is being explored. Interviews are conducted on an open-ended basis, with the informants being prompted to lead the researcher into an understanding of how they perceive the situation. At first only very general questions are asked but then further questions are prompted by the answers elicited by the first questions, so ideas used by the respondent are incorporated in new questions. In this particular study a number of domains or areas of discourse were elicited in the course of the interview. These included: (1) expectations of 'counselling'; (2) types of 'psychos' and 'shrinks'; (3) the setting; (4) individual versus family therapy; (5) ways to make therapy work; (6) the behaviour of the counsellor; (7) kinds of weak spots or family problems; and (8) 'ways of being picked on in meetings'.

It is, in fact, extremely difficult to summarize the two papers, because it is precisely the detailed reponses of the informants that are the substance of the approach, but it is noticeable that the responses elicited are very similar to those in the more traditional studies that we have already reviewed. For example, looking at the domain 'expectations of therapy' and listening in to what parents have to say about advice-giving, it seems that they were often confused by their structural-strategic therapists' tactics. For example, Newfield *et al.* comment:

> [Parents often] . . . approached the family therapists in the same manner they would approach a physician for treatment. However, what the informants experienced was that when they asked a question about how to solve the problem the therapist in many instances turned the question around by manoeuvres such as asking the client what she/he thought the answer should be. Such manoeuvres sometimes seemed like ludicrous game playing to desperate parents seeking answers from an 'expert' who has years of education and experience dealing with these problems and who often had a group of 'experts' with which to consult behind the mirror.
>
> (Newfield *et al.*, 1990, p. 65)

Such findings clearly match the findings of more traditional studies that we have reviewed earlier but the strength of the work of the group relates specifically to the methodology adopted by them. Their much more user-centred approach means that the voice of the user is heard in a more convincing way. From these accounts the reader becomes far more aware of the complexities of therapy seen through users' eyes. Lishman's 'clash of perspective' therefore becomes enriched by the idea that users and professionals clash in many subtle and complex ways which traditional, research-driven interviewing methods often conceal.

Summary

The studies we have reviewed in this chapter lack coherence when compared with the studies reviewed in the last chapter, and it is more difficult to arrive at an overall conclusion. However, we believe that the importance of the therapeutic alliance does once again emerge as crucial. Therapists who neglect the relationship aspects of therapy in their pursuit of interventions that induce change run the risk of creating considerable dissatisfaction as far as their users are concerned. Users, on balance, seem to need and seek a varied and multifaceted relationship with their therapists. Active elements of therapy (e.g. advice-giving, intensity of interventions) need to be combined with reflective and supportive elements. It is also clear that therapists need to understand that therapy (which to them is an everyday, relatively matter-of-fact way of earning a living) is a unique, challenging, often threatening experience to their users. In many ways it is David Howe's (1989) study (which we reviewed in Chapter 2) which summarizes these aspects of therapy best, but it is important to stress that when therapy goes well (and the therapeutic alliance is truly built), then both user and therapist can unite to face issues that can be deeply challenging or disturbing.

Chapter 10

Social policy, the family and family therapy

Is there a meeting point?

Sigurd Reimers

In describing our own studies and examining those of other authors, we have so far talked about family therapy as if it treated the miseries of families as exclusively matters of private concern. It is easy to adopt a simple logic that if there are relationship problems within families, then it is within families that solutions are to be found. However, this position overlooks the fact that there is a long line of authors, both within and outside family therapy (see Hoffman and Long (1969), Jordan (1981) and Kingston (1979), amongst others), who have reminded us of the importance of highlighting the *public* aspect of relationship problems.

Many of these public aspects are ambiguous or easily overlooked by therapists, and in this chapter I want to examine how social policy issues in particular can affect users' experience of family life, and indirectly their experience of family therapy. It seems to me to be particularly urgent that therapists maintain such an awareness at a time when users of therapeutic services are increasing in numbers and to an increasing extent becoming disadvantaged by the effects of government policies.

I will start by looking at how the apparently private and everyday concerns of family members are affected by public issues like poverty, housing, education and health, and put these within the context of recent social policy changes. I will then move on to examine how the structure of the family itself has been changing during the last two decades, and how social policy has related to many of these changes – often in ways that have made a large number of people, including many users, increasingly vulnerable.

But first let us be clear about why it might be helpful for a user-friendly therapist to address the effects of social policy. Firstly, users can feel more valued and better understood. Secondly, essential information about help provided by other services can be passed on. Thirdly, the therapeutic service offered to users can be more custom-built, more respectful of their needs, and less driven by the often narrower conceptions of therapists about what is the purpose of therapy and what is not. Phil Kingston's explanation that a discussion of the provision of material resources can be a useful part of therapy (Kingston, 1979), is a valuable reminder that professional views about what constitutes therapy rarely address the fact that many families are in need of material, as well as psychological, help.

Perhaps we could develop a link between people's experience of the loss of material resources and their experience of lack of stability in family life if we extend Kenneth Gergen's concept of 'the saturated family':

> The ordinary, daily confluence of multiple lives within one household makes for a sense of fragmentation, as if the members of the family were being scattered to the centrifugal force of postmodern life.
>
> (Gergen, 1991, p. 29)

Gergen was talking about the enormous number of external impulses which confront individuals these days, and the confusing effects these impulses have on one's sense of identity as a member of a family. He was not particularly referring to disadvantaged families, but perhaps we could also include within the idea of 'saturation' a form of family life which, more and more, is having to shoulder the conflicting responsibilities for dependent members – whether they be older adolescents or elderly or disabled relatives on low incomes – and for longer periods of time because of progressive reductions in public services. Many of these responsibilities are now undertaken without the formal and informal networks that used to exist in the past.

SOCIAL AND FAMILY POLICY IN BRITAIN UNDER THATCHERISM

We need to remember that in the United Kingdom we cannot properly talk of *family* policy because there is no tradition in this country of policy-making around the family, and there are very few public institutions that are specifically concerned with families. Some countries have comprehensive family policies, including ombudsmen and ombudswomen, ministries for families and children, and other specifically focused institutions. In Britain we have at most *social* policies, each usually based on a single issue, like income maintenance, law and order, or education. These policies may be carried out by a variety of agencies or departments in a more or less co-ordinated way. However, although the 'family' component may be hidden or only implicit, the policies are no less powerful in their influence on family life. This has certainly been true for families in Britain since 1979, when there was a profound movement away from all forms of state provision. Margaret Thatcher, the incoming prime minister, made an early promise of 'less government, not more government'. This proved to be true as far as providing public resources was concerned, but ironically the state has at times had to *increase* its activities in order to make sure that its privatizing policies are strictly adhered to. The policy of so-called 'less government' has, for example, involved central government in keeping a close check on local authorities, by imposing penalties such as rate- or charge-capping, to make sure that they keep within nationally dictated budgetary limits. This policy has led to substantial cuts in local welfare and related services, on which many, if not most, people have come to depend. The declared purpose of such central government restrictions is partly economic – to limit public expenditure and reduce the risk of inflation. However, behind this economic policy also lies a set of strong beliefs which directly relate to the family. These can be expressed as follows:

1 Consumer choice can best be promoted, and wastefulness avoided, through competition, even within the field of health and welfare provisions.
2 The 'family' is the cornerstone of society. Social problems can to a large extent both be explained in terms of failures within the family, and should be solved within the family.
3 People should be encouraged to be self-reliant. A 'dependency culture', encouraged by the state, undermines families and individuals in their willingness and ability to care for themselves and their relatives.
4 Family life should as far as possible be a private activity – protected from public 'interference'.
5 Within the family it is the role mainly of women to care for children and other dependants, and the role of men to be the main breadwinner. It is the duty of parents to provide a responsible model for, and to take responsibility for, the behaviour of their children.

Such beliefs will not always be found explicitly stated in social policy pronouncements, but they nevertheless permeate the hundreds of fragments of legislation or – more likely these days – statutory regulations that combine to form the patchwork of 'family policy'. The effects of these beliefs are twofold, first on how social policy is directed at family life, and second on the way people think about their families.

EFFECTS OF SOCIAL POLICY ON FAMILY LIFE

The overall trend in social policy is away from state-run facilities and resources. This move is commonly referred to as privatization – mistakenly, we believe, because in this process resources are frequently removed rather than transferred. Even when the private or voluntary sector does take over responsibility from the state it, too, may have to give up – as numerous charities have discovered – because of withdrawal of grants and lack of other forms of support. This will in turn lead to greater pressures on many families. Where the state does continue making provisions, it is likely to narrow its ambit, as a few examples may illustrate:

Income maintenance

Maintaining an adequate income has become a greater struggle for some of the most vulnerable people in our society. Between 1979 and 1991 the standard of living of the wealthiest 10 per cent of households rose by 62 per cent in real terms, whilst that of the poorest 10 per cent (involving 3 million children and 2.7 million adults) went down by 14 per cent.

In 1993 Wages Councils were abolished. These had fixed the minimum wages of 2.6 million of the lowest-paid workers in the country, 80 per cent of whom were women. This policy of abolition was in clear breach of the European Community Social Chapter, but the United Kingdom was the only country not to sign the Chapter, because of its government's beliefs in free market forces.

The National Child Development Study, in one of the world's largest longitudinal studies, found that a large underclass of women is emerging, trapped in a downward income spiral. Typically these women are bringing up young children on their own, and are either working at low hourly rates, or are not able to go out to work in the first place because of the lack of affordable child care facilities. The United Kingdom is at the bottom end of the league table when it comes to public child care facilities for children under three (2 per cent compared with Denmark's 48 per cent). At the time of writing, Prime Minister John Major has just made a speech in favour of state funding for nursery schools – 'when we can afford it'. Margaret Thatcher made a similar commitment when she was Education Minister in 1972.

The failure of many fathers to pay maintenance following divorce has been held up by the government as a major cause of family poverty. As a result, the Child Support Agency was set up in 1992 to recoup unpaid maintenance, partly to ensure regular payments to the mothers, and partly to reduce the burden on the state of Income Support to the mothers. Mothers are now obliged to disclose the name of the father to the Child Support Agency – or risk losing benefit. New problems are now developing as most divorced men go on to make new family commitments, and one of the effects of the policy of the Child Support Agency is to shift the financial burden from first to second families.

Housing

The move to make Britain a 'property-owning democracy' may have opened new opportunities for some families, but it has also taken its toll. Council house rents rose by 119 per cent between 1979 and 1983 (compared with a general Retail Price Index increase of 55 per cent during the same period). This may have prompted a number of people to buy their own council homes. In the process many over-committed themselves, as the rise in interest rates and redundancies led to their falling behind with their mortgage repayments. Between 1981 and 1990 the number of repossessions doubled to 75,000 homes, and numerous families became homeless. Homelessness was further exacerbated by the removal in 1986 of the rights of 16- and 17-year-olds to claim Income Support in their own right. Strictly speaking, parents are responsible for this age group (and the Government is currently considering raising this age to 21). Unfortunately, many homeless young people come from homes where they have been abused or badly rejected, and therefore cannot depend on the goodwill of their parents.

Health

The National Health Service has proved a much more difficult system for policy makers to change – not least because of its broad popular support amongst voters. Nevertheless the service which the government said was 'safe in our hands' has for long been suffering from a crisis of funding. The amount of money spent on the NHS did not actually change very much in monetary terms during the period 1975–1988, which means that it declined in real terms, when inflation is taken into account. The crisis, however, has also been about rising expectations of, and demands on, the NHS, partly in line with advances in medical technology. The impact of an ageing population is also having an effect, as per capita expenditure on the 65–74 year age group is approximately twice as high, and on the 75+ age group is about four times as high, as on the rest of the population. Bids for available funding are therefore having to compete against each other more than ever before.

The introduction of market forces into the NHS, with splitting between 'purchasers' and 'providers', is currently in its early days, but there are real fears that health care decisions about how to allocate funding will increasingly be made on the basis of cost rather than assessed need. As demand outstrips supply, desperate measures may be used. The Citizen's Charter for the NHS requires, amongst other things, a published maximum waiting time for operations. This may be a positive innovation, but some hospitals, strapped for cash, have decided to deal with an impossible situation by introducing delays at the diagnosis-making stage instead, thereby still remaining within the terms of the Citizen's Charter. Although most of the NHS services are still free at the point of delivery, charges have gradually been brought in. Charges for optician and dental services and for prescriptions have risen faster than the general rate of inflation, and there is every reason to suppose that other direct charges will be introduced into other parts of the NHS in due course.

Education

Since rate- or charge-capping was introduced during the 1980s as a way for central government to control the independence of local authorities, there has been little scope for these authorities to increase the amount that is spent on education – particularly since education already represents by far the largest part of local authority budgets. As local schools have increasingly become grant-maintained, they have come to depend on grants from central government and such other funds as they can raise themselves.

Following government directives to increase school accountability and to promote 'parental choice', each school is now required to publish a prospectus, and will soon have to publish truancy rates and tables of examination results. Openness and accountability must be welcomed, but because the market philosophy which is accompanying these positive features is not being counterbalanced by local strategic initiatives to take account of overall local community needs, we can only expect that the inequalities in educational provisions will continue to rise, yet again to the detriment of those people who are the least competitive and have the fewest resources in the first place. These people will include children with a variety of special needs and their families.

Balancing the equation

The past 15 years have clearly been hard for many of our users. There have, however, been some positive changes as well. More open accountability on the part of public services had long been needed, wastefulness in the delivery of these services did need addressing, and changes like the Citizen's Charters – for all their smoke-screen effects – can also be seen as an attempt to give individual citizens specific guidelines about their rights of redress against some of the restrictive practices in public services (interestingly, private services are exempted from most of these requirements).

Equally, some legislation has been progressive, like the Children Act 1989. The Act was greeted by many as the most important piece of child care legislation this century. It stresses the importance of ascertaining the wishes and feelings of any child that is subject to its provisions. It insists that professionals must work in partnership with parents, and that court orders should be avoided, except where absolutely necessary. Questions of race, religion, language and culture must be taken into account at all stages of any work undertaken. In many respects the Act is empowering and respects the views of very vulnerable people. Yet, in other respects, it makes it clear that the state, as a matter of principle, does not wish to intervene in family life. In practice this means that the family must find more of its own solutions. The backdrop to this, as to the 1992 NHS and Community Care Act, is the effect of limited budgets. The Act has therefore sometimes been referred to as 'the privatization of misery'.

Other progressive legislation, such as the Sex Discrimination Act (1975) and the Race Relations Act (1968) – important earlier milestones that could create a new context for effective political interventions against sexism and racism – is further limited by the fact that other policies undermine such possibilities. For example, because black people find it hard to enter the work force in the first place, the Race Relations Act could be seen as another piece of liberal law-making which obscures the savage oppression which black people experience. Similarly, at work women are supposed to be treated equally to men. One of the many problems in implementing such a policy is the fact that, as I pointed out earlier, the United Kingdom has refused to sign the Social Chapter of the EC (now the EU), which lays down specific rules about minimum pay, maximum working hours, and the employment rights of pregnant women.

Overall, we must conclude that despite some positive achievements in terms of legislative changes during the past 15 years, the verdict has to be that many of the users we meet are worse off in many ways than they used to be.

THE INFLUENCE OF DOMINANT BELIEFS ON HOW PEOPLE THINK ABOUT THEIR FAMILIES

Government ideologies about what constitutes family responsibilities do not only affect the practical delivery of services to families. They also become a common currency for general public debate. Michel Foucault's seminal term 'discourse' is used by him to refer to influential and widely held (although not necessarily universal) beliefs that permeate society. Dominant social discourses take their power from the fact that they set the agenda for what we think and how we think about social issues, even if they can never achieve a total monopoly. However, during the 1980s and early 1990s the dominant discourse of Thatcherism has not been effectively challenged by alternative discourses. We probably have to go back to the mid-1940s to find an era when a comparably strong discourse about social issues could be found. At that time the very legislation which is now being dismantled was being created. The 1944 Education Act, the 1946 National Health Service Act and the 1948 National Assistance Act effectively created the backbone of publicly owned social provisions. That 'welfare discourse' was a reformist social democratic one which held that state intervention was the only way to correct the deep crisis stemming from the Wall Street crash and the Second World War. We are now reaching a stage that is the dialectical opposite of that period, where cutbacks are not just made reluctantly: they are also believed by many to be right. In their eyes, private now becomes good, and state becomes bad. The 'badness' of the state is frequently backed up with references to the waste of public resources (through lack of competition), and the failure of institutional solutions, like children's homes, psychiatric hospitals and elderly persons' homes, where abuses may admittedly occur and where people are sometimes forgotten and neglected. The badness of the state also subtly becomes linked to how we think about those who are dependent on the state, like single parents and young offenders, and not least to how they think about themselves. In such a discourse 'care in the community', 'family values', 'parental choice' and similar slogans will seem, by comparison, to be relatively attractive – certainly to those who do not believe that they will need to use public services themselves.

Users of family therapy are not exempt from the practical or moral force of dominant discourses, any more than their therapists are. Whether or not we approve of these discourses, we are obliged to acknowledge their impact on both users and ourselves. We need to acknowledge that the role of being a therapist is becoming more complex as families are forced to carry more challenging burdens. Many family members feel increasingly uncertain about the future as unemployment remains high, job prospects are poor, and the safety net of the state becomes weaker. The income of a small part of the population may have risen under Thatcherism, but for one-third poverty is an everyday experience that is health-damaging and demoralizing. These developments may mean that therapy, in the traditional sense, can only be initiated after real attention has been paid to the welfare needs of users. Therapists may need to spend more time liaising with welfare agencies and ensuring that advocacy becomes a legitimate part of any therapeutic contract that is negotiated with users.

HOW DEFINITIONS OF 'THE FAMILY' ARE SHAPED BY SOCIAL POLICIES

We have seen how public policies affect physical realities (like how large a family's income is), as well as beliefs (like whether a family is 'deserving' or not). Let us now look at what definitions of 'the family' are created by social policies. As therapists, we are familiar with the idea that all human activities communicate some form of message. We would also suggest that it is impossible (intentionally or not) for social policy not to give some kind of message about family life. Exactly how each family member interprets such messages cannot be predicted, but it is quite clear to me that family forms which diverge from the nuclear family model are likely to have particular difficulties because the predominant message is so clearly that the nuclear family is the desired norm.

We will use some examples of recent legislation to illustrate how policy changes have had the effect of creating new definitions of family life, whilst at the same time reflecting Thatcherite ideas about the sanctity of individual responsibility:

Legislation	Messages about 'the family'
Children Act (1989)	'Parental responsibility' replaces parental rights. Parents cannot shed their responsibility for their children, even after the dissolution of the nuclear family or if the children are in care.
Child Support Act (1992)	Parents (fathers) have financial responsibility for their children whether they live with them or not. Separated mothers are obliged to disclose the name of the father to the Child Support Agency. The stereotype of the male bread-winner and female care-giver is strengthened.
Criminal Justice Act (1991)	Parents are responsible for their children's behaviour. In a court of law they can be bound over or required to pay their children's fines. The idea of poor parenting as the main cause of crime is reinforced.
Immigration Act (1988)	Immigrants sponsored by a relative already living in the United Kingdom cannot claim Social Security benefits and must be maintained by their sponsor. The message is one of being a 'guest' rather than a citizen.

Housing Act (1980)	Local authorities are no longer permitted to provide council housing at a loss, or by subsidy. Effective families are those who are part of the 'property-owning democracy'.
Social Security Act (1986)	16–17-year-olds cannot claim Income Support in their own right. Benefits to those under 25 are reduced relative to those over 25. Family dependency for this age group is confirmed as desirable.

Overall, families with two adults looking after their own children will be the ones who prosper most under the current dominant discourse, partly through being better off, and partly through the official state-sanctioned acknowledgement that they are a 'normal' family.

Nevertheless, as we will see from the next section, it has not been possible for social policy to halt the progressive decline of the nuclear family in the United Kingdom. So far it has only been possible for government policy to shame or to punish alternative types of families. Needless to say, these policies must be of grave concern to user-friendly therapists, who are daily confronted with families at the receiving end of such policies.

CHANGES IN FAMILY STRUCTURE

As family therapists, we often come across examples of what Coote *et al.* (1990) call 'the gap between what people think ought to happen in families and what is increasingly happening in real life'. Nevertheless, although many people feel their own family formation is not normal, there has been a clear and continuing trend away from the traditional nuclear family, and there is no evidence to suggest that this trend is likely to be reversed. The gap between social policy and the 'family values' ideal on the one hand and the reality of diverse forms of family composition on the other hand is currently increasing. This has to be taken into account by user-friendly therapists and trainers who often use methods and texts which assume that the nuclear family is still the standard format. We ourselves have had to revise our old assumptions about family hierarchy and boundaries, about life cycles and geneograms, and not least about who should be invited to 'family therapy' interviews. Let us look at a few statistics and examine in particular how these reflect some of the ways family life as it is actually lived compares with standard definitions of the nuclear family.

Marriage and divorce

In 1989 the United Kingdom had the highest marriage rate in the European Community, and yet was only exceeded by Denmark in its divorce rate. About 50 per cent of all divorces take place within nine years of marriage, long before most of any children involved reach adolescence.

A large proportion of people who divorce go on to remarry, and remarriages in 1989 formed 35 per cent of the total of all marriages. This is not a new phenomenon, and this figure had been stable for the previous 13 years. The Divorce Reform Act (1969) had made divorce easier to obtain (and it is worth noting that divorce proceedings are initiated by about three times as many women as men), and the Act may account for the large increase in divorces (and remarriages) in the early 1970s.

Although marriage is still popular, the proportion of women who cohabit with their future husband before marriage steadily increased from the early 1970s to about 50 per cent in the late 1980s.

Births outside marriage

Except during wartime, the proportion of children born outside marriage was very stable until the 1960s. But it was throughout the 1980s that this proportion really increased (from about 10 per cent in 1981 to 28 per cent in 1990). What is also interesting to note is that the percentage of joint registrations of such births has also increased (from 6.8 per cent of all children conceived in 1981 to 16 per cent in 1989), suggesting that many couples who are living together, but are not married, live in a 'stable' relationship.

Type of family

There are few reliable figures about the numbers of stepfamilies, but the increase in numbers of remarriages may indicate a substantial increase in the numbers of stepfamilies. We have clearer figures for single-parent households, which regularly cause concern for ideologies based on the importance of the nuclear family. As a proportion of all families with dependent children, single-parent households increased from 8 per cent in 1971 to 12 per cent in 1981 and 19 per cent in 1991. About 90 per cent of these households are headed by women, and 70 per cent depend on Income Support.

Elderly people

Whilst the number of people in the 65–79 year age group has remained fairly stable since 1981, and is not expected to change much for the next 12 years or so, the proportion of people aged 80 and over increased by about 30 per cent between 1981 and 1990, and looks set to increase by a further 25 per cent before the year 2006. In this context it is no surprise that the household group which is increasing the most rapidly is not single parents but the single-person household (6.3 per cent in 1971, 8 per cent in 1981 and 10.6 per cent in 1991). About 60 per cent of these single people are over pensionable age.

As we might expect during a period of 'privatization', the number of elderly people in local authority homes has decreased. Between 1981 and 1990 this proportion went down by 13 per cent, whereas in private homes it increased by more than 100 per cent during the same period. Under the NHS and Community Care Act (1992), there is now a clear policy to care for elderly people in their own homes where possible, and public funds for all forms of residential care have been cut back drastically since the Act was passed. Gallup polls have consistently shown that the majority of elderly people prefer to live in their own homes, but it is clear that without an adequate level of funding of public resources, including residential care where necessary, 'community care' will be an empty rhetoric and will leave many families overstretched.

Ethnic minorities

This chapter is being written at a time when right-wing politicians like Winston Churchill are once again attempting to raise public concern about the threat of ethnic minorities to the 'British way of life', partly because of their supposed numbers, and partly because ethnic minorities are apparently not integrating adequately. In fact, in 1987–1989 ethnic minority groups formed only 5 per cent of the population of the United Kingdom. Although the birth rate of ethnic minority groups, taken as a whole, may be higher than that of the white population, it declined by about 30 per cent between 1971 and 1990. In terms of the nuclear family ideology it is perhaps ironic that the percentage rate of births outside marriage is only about a third of that in white ethnic groups. These points are made in response to the supposed 'danger' of the British way of life disappearing. In reality, of course, there are considerable variations between and within all the various ethnic groups in Britain, including white groups.

SOCIAL POLICY, AGENCY FUNCTION AND FAMILY THERAPY

We have seen how social policies are dictated by certain ideologies or dominant discourses. Current policies, in turn, encourage a particular form of family life which is based on a clearly gendered division of labour, on differing assumptions about mothers and fathers, and on family responsibilities for dependent relatives which go well beyond divorce and coming of age, and also extending into old age. By contrast, we have seen how the way many people choose to conduct their family life increasingly conflicts with such an ideology, despite complex social, economic and practical consequences.

   It is an open question whether a user-friendly approach to family therapy can genuinely reflect the multiplicity of needs that are generated by the social and economic pressures that impinge on families. Psychotherapy is sometimes attacked as being a middle-class form of therapy which requires young, active, verbal and intelligent types of users in order to be successful. However, in Chapter 5 we briefly summarized the work of Lorion (1978), who has demonstrated that many forms of psychotherapy can be modified to be user-friendly and therefore appeal to users from a wide range of backgrounds. We also found in our own surveys that family therapy could be experienced as positive by users from differing backgrounds. However, we would never claim that family therapy, however user-friendly, can be a universal panacea.

In many ways it is a pity that the history of family therapy cannot be rewritten. Family therapy was developed initially mainly by psychiatrists working in clinical settings. It developed as a largely clinic-based form of therapy and therefore had a tendency to recapitulate the inverse care law later postulated by Julian Tudor-Hart (1971) (see Treacher (1986) for a further discussion of this issue). Notwithstanding the work of Minuchin and his colleagues with poor families in Philadelphia (Minuchin *et al.*, 1967), users from the most disadvantaged backgrounds were therefore likely to receive the least attention from family therapists. A genuinely user-friendly approach, which took the issues outlined in this chapter seriously, would attempt to find an organizational base which would better suit the needs of users. In Britain some family centres come close to achieving this goal since they are able to offer users a wide variety of services including advocacy, group work, support groups, individual counselling, and couples and family therapy (for some examples, see Koziarski *et al.* (1986) and Gill (1988)). Such centres are better equipped to provide a more comprehensive service to disadvantaged users than are, for example, child and family guidance centres staffed by professionals who have a narrower range of predominantly clinical skills.

Here our discussion moves beyond the individual practitioner and touches on the issue of agency function which we discussed in Chapter 8 when reviewing Timms and Blampied's (1985) study. It is clearly not possible for therapists to practise without reference to their employing agencies. Most agencies in this country which are concerned with families have been created directly by, or in response to, social policies, and do not themselves have a completely free hand when it comes to devising their own policies. This applies particularly to agencies which have statutory responsibilities.

Vernon Cronen and Barnett Pearce's (1985) model of multiple levels of context can be used as a way of illustrating how agencies form a link between social policy and therapeutic work with families. Cronen and Pearce claim that any one level of context will both offer meaning to and derive meaning from other levels of context. Figure 3 demonstrates one way in which the model could be applied to this link.

We would expect the strongest influence between the different levels to be 'downwards' (a contextual force in Cronen and Pearce's language), with agencies and practitioners frequently in a position to implement policies in ways which can respect their users and even give them hope.

Work with families can therefore never take place in isolation, because it is constantly influenced by meanings and beliefs at levels 'above' it. If there is any one message for user-friendly practice in this chapter it must surely be that we must take whatever opportunities we can to influence these 'higher' levels of context in the service of our users. Such an 'implicative force' is generally less

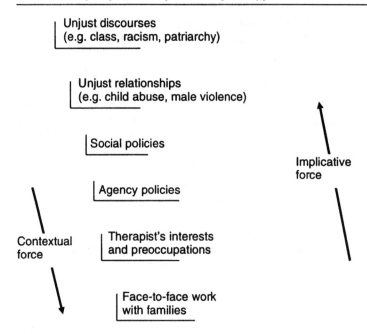

Figure 3 Multiple levels of context

powerful than a contextual force, but it can still be significant. For example, how willing are we as therapists to try and influence our managers and agency culture about issues which are clearly relevant to our users? These might include, at the very least, the provision of evening clinics, the availability of refreshments for families, refunding of fares, provision of transport and the geographical location of the service. It could also encompass user representation in agency policy-making, and the strengthening of links with other agencies which are more central in the provision of practical resources.

CONCLUSION

Much of our discussion in this chapter may still seem rather remote from the practice of everyday therapy. However, therapy is affected by seemingly remote policies in ways we gradually come to take for granted. Policies affect therapists as well as users. As resources decline, staffing levels may become more stretched, making therapeutic teamwork less common. Less time is available for multidisciplinary work. Time spent on therapy is more tightly audited. On the positive side, information about services is more readily available to the public, users have a right of access to their records, and it is easier for users to make complaints. These are the most obvious examples of the effects of changes in policy-making on day-to-day practice. At this point we must confess that we both work in settings which offer a relatively high level of autonomy, so there is genuine scope for innovation in our practice. However, we hope that the ideas we explore in this chapter do have relevance for workers in other agencies, but we acknowledge that a great deal of our thinking is of necessity influenced by the contexts within which we work.

Finally, an awareness of social policy issues and access to resources do not automatically create a good therapeutic alliance. There are also theoretical considerations, and these can come into conflict with our social awareness, as the following example demonstrates.

A short while ago I was working in a family therapy centre with Connie, who was a single mother living on Income Support with three children under the age of five. There had been domestic violence and possibly sexual abuse. Connie had sought help from the Centre because of extremely clinging and demanding behaviour on her daughter's part. It was known that the journey to the Centre was a long one, and involved a change of buses.

The possibility of offering help with transport was discussed by the team, but it was felt that this might give Connie the message that the therapist held a strong belief that she was in need of therapy and also that she was too dependent on welfare services to be capable of making her own independent arrangements. As we will see in the next chapter, some theories would support this as a perfectly valid concern. Some second-order models are concerned to avoid imposing ideas on already vulnerable users, whereas some feminist models would advocate a more robust approach to dealing with the practical disadvantages faced by users. Suffice it to say that in this case the user-friendly potential was lost because our dilemma was not discussed explicitly with Connie, and she was never involved in any decision-making about the issue.

As the reader, you may have your own thoughts about ways in which social issues relate to your agency, to your users, and not least to your own practice. We would encourage you to hold on to these thoughts as we move on to the next chapter, where we will look at the two theoretical models which, in our opinion, have been the most influential ones within family therapy practice during the past decade.

Chapter 11

User-friendliness and theories of family therapy
The contribution of second-order thinking and feminism

Sigurd Reimers and Andy Treacher

In the original plan of our book we set aside a chapter in order to review all the major models from a user-friendly point of view. However, this task has proved over-ambitious, so we have decided to limit ourselves to the two major influences within family therapy during the 1980s. As we have demonstrated in the opening chapters of our book, user-friendliness was primarily developed in order to address weaknesses in the way some of the original models of family therapy had been formulated. Family therapy has not remained static during the last 10 years, so it is necessary to ask the important question: have other models of family therapy evolved that can make a significant contribution to user-friendliness? Our preliminary answer to this question is that it is probably the 'second-order' models and models based on feminism that can contribute most to user-friendliness, but we also acknowledge that many other models (sadly unreviewed by us) are also capable of contributing important ideas.

SECOND-ORDER APPROACHES

From the standpoint of popularity (and extent of publication), it is second-order approaches that have taken pride of place within the family therapy movement. These models have been grouped together under headings such as 'second-order cybernetics', 'second-order thinking', 'post-Milan thinking' and 'the new epistemology'. These approaches, developed during the 1980s, challenged the older established models within family therapy and caused a great deal of controversy. They have been most clearly described by Lynn Hoffman (1985, 1990, 1991). Thinking about how the original first-order models had originally influenced her work she comments:

> From then on I only saw circles, timeless circles. They seemed to invade every sphere. Influenced by this metaphor, I subscribed to a theory of family therapy in which a symptom was described as part of a homeostatic cycle that stabilized the family. A therapist was a person who had the skills to disrupt that cycle and help the family get back to an even keel. . . . It has only been

gradually and with great difficulty that I have become aware of this lens and what some alternatives are.

(Hoffman, 1990, p. 2)

We will first summarize briefly some of the most important components of the second-order approach and then attempt to understand what might be the users' experience of such therapy. One of the key issues in second-order thinking is the questioning of the expert position commonly adopted by family therapists. 'First-order' family therapists traditionally tried to gain a 'meta-position' (*vis-à-vis* their users) by a variety of means, including not disclosing anything about themselves, using invisible teams and devising paradoxical interventions which allegedly could not be noticed by users. First-order therapists have also been accused of working to restructure families to fit therapists' norms, rather than accepting that there are innumerable ways in which families can function successfully. The idea of the expert position often carried with it the assumption that an outsider (or expert) can understand the reality of another person, and can instruct that person in how best to conduct her or his life.

Some of the major challenges to the first-order approach have come from outside family therapy. Best known perhaps is the Chilean biologist Humberto Maturana (Maturana and Varela, 1987), who claimed that 'instructive inter-action' is not possible. Biological systems, including human beings, are simply not designed to be able to influence each other in a direct way. Instead, systems are 'structurally determined' by their own make-up, and at most are able to 'perturb' each other, albeit in an unpredictable manner. The cybernetician Heinz von Foerster (1981) claims that human beings are not 'trivial machines'. Unlike pressing the button of a machine, one cannot tell another human being exactly what to do in a mechanistic fashion. Similarly Ernst von Glaserfeld (1984), who has a background in linguistics, argues that therapists and users can at best only hope to create a 'fit' (rather than an exact 'match'), that is, an understanding which is adequate for therapeutic purposes. These ideas are collectively referred to as a constructivist position. Although they have had a major influence on therapeutic approaches based on second-order thinking, they are clearly limited because they fail to acknowledge the fact that human beings are primarily *social* beings. We will return to this issue later in this chapter, when we attempt to evaluate the overall significance and validity of second-order ideas, but we now need to explore second-order developments which took place *within* the family therapy movement, particularly under the influence of social constructionism.

Beyond the expert role: developments within the family therapy movement

In order to trace the development of the influential 'non-expert' position within family therapy practice we will summarize the developments that took place in the Milan school, because it is this school that has been most closely connected with ideas stemming from second-order thinking.

Elsa Jones (1988) in a helpful and remarkably condensed paper argues that a key development in the Milan school was the split (*circa* 1980) between Luigi Boscolo and Gianfranco Cecchin on the one hand and Mara Selvini Palazzoli and Giuliana Prata on the other. (Prata later parted company with Palazzoli but this split was of lesser importance and will not be discussed by us.) Jones summarizes the reasons for the split as follows:

> It seems that the two groups separated as a result of profound differences in relation to concepts of neutrality, power and the therapist's membership of the system under observation, to the extent that Selvini Palazzoli can now be described as having made a 'creative U-turn' (di Nicola, 1984). Boscolo and Cecchin have continued to pursue the idea of a system's own capacity for self-regulation and the 'goals' of therapeutic neutrality, and 'curiosity' (Pirotta, 1984; Boscolo *et al.*, 1987; Cecchin, 1987). The effect of Humberto Maturana (Maturana and Varela, 1980; Maturana, 1983; Mendez *et al.*, 1986) on their work has moved them further in this direction so that their work has been influenced by the idea that any apparent 'reality' or description has been brought forth by the observer, that objectivity at best has an 'as-if' status ('objectivity in parentheses', Efran and Lukens, 1988) and that systems are primarily structure-determined and constantly evolving (Maturana and Varela, 1980; Maturana, 1983). A therapy session would therefore be best described as a conversation (Boscolo *et al.*, 1987; Tomm, 1988) in which the therapist hopes that the perturbation of his temporary membership of the family/therapist system, would create conditions in which the family may construct a new 'story' for themselves (Cecchin, 1987).
>
> (Jones, 1988, p. 327)

Jones is aware of how complex this passage is, so she immediately offers her reader an example to illustrate how the new method of working would feel if the reader were a consumer of it:

> I may talk to you and attempt in my talking to influence you and 'give' you certain 'pieces' of 'information'. What you make of what I say depends on you and your alertness or state of fatigue, interest in new or surprising or confirming aspects of my communication, attachment to your previously held views, and so on – and even more importantly, on your view of the relationship between us. Even if you believe what I say, it is unlikely that your version of what has passed will coincide with mine.
>
> In consequence the therapy sessions of Boscolo and Cecchin are characterized by more interest in the process of questioning within the session and less emphasis on an inevitable and powerful end of session intervention. There is more variability with regard to the session itself, length of intervals between sessions and the number of sessions. Their attention is directed particularly towards the therapist-family supra-system and in regard to families and

trainees, they are more concerned with stimulating a changed way of thinking and a co-creation of a new system than with working to a set method.

(Jones, 1988, p. 328)

The crucial difference between the two groups seems to hinge around the issue of neutrality which Palazzoli appears to have abandoned. In order to understand families with psychotic members she has developed the notion that such families are caught up in 'dirty' family games and therefore display 'subtle cunning, brazen lies, relentless revenge, treachery, manipulation, seductions', and so on (Selvini Palazzoli, 1986, p. 345; cited by Jones, 1988, p. 328).

It is also clear from Jones's account that the Palazzoli group does not share Boscolo and Cecchin's stance in relation to objectivity. Jones summarizes Palazzoli's position as follows:

> In her description of work with families and organizations other than families, she makes it clear that she is searching for truth, for classifiable patterns, and that she may regard this search as a struggle in which members of the system she is observing (with more claim to objectivity than Cecchin and Boscola would make) are doing their damnedest to baffle and outwit her: 'we will be forced to guess or infer the truth in the face of reticence, contradictions or even deception' (Selvini Palazzoli, 1984, p. 306).

(Jones, 1988, p. 329)

Palazzoli's new stance clearly has important implications for the therapist–user relationship as John Carpenter (1993) has pointed out. It may appear from our summary of Jones's work that the Palazzoli group have an aloof and de-humanizing approach to their users but the reverse may be true. Carpenter illustrates this possibility by drawing attention to the significance of a joint publication by Palazzoli and her son Matteo Selvini (Selvini and Selvini Palazzoli, 1991) which sheds a different light on this issue:

> Referring to the risks of dehumanizing the relationship between family and therapist, they warn against the artificial creation of distance and the strength of team spirit which treats the family as an 'adversary to be tamed'. The search for a detached 'meta-position' for the team they now consider to have been the result of a theoretical error, '. . . supporting the scientific illusion of having found the royal road to the study of the "objective reality" of the family'.
>
> Selvini and Selvini Palazzoli (1991) also consider the emotional detach-ment of the therapist to be a tactical error in that, in order to make a therapeutic impact, the therapist 'must be in strong emotional and cognitive contact with all members of the family'. This is in marked contrast to their earlier approach using the techniques of positive connotation, neutrality and paradoxical pre-scriptions which relied on emotional distance. They summarized their current position . . . [as follows] . . .

'We once tended to believe that emotional involvement with the family meant that we had fallen prey to the family game. But this is an arbitrary equation. The job of the team actually consists of allowing the therapist's maximum involvement whilst simultaneously guarding against the therapist supporting or even reinforcing a pathogenic family process. It is also absurd to consider the team as a whole as detached: teamwork needs to integrate two separate ways of maximum involvement, one for the direct therapist and another for the consultant (p. 43).'

Selvini and Selvini Palazzoli also discuss the subjectivity of the therapist, using the therapist's affective response on the importance of valuing the personal style of each of the team's members.

(Carpenter, 1993 p. 216)

We must admit that we are not entirely sure whether the new position is based on a respect for the individual differences between family members or whether it is merely a useful strategy for winning over the family to the therapist's point of view. Indeed, in contrasting Jones's and John Carpenter's accounts we are aware of the difficulties in summarizing the position of a school of thought which is evolving so rapidly.

It should also be stressed that there are some very real and practical difficulties that confront therapists who try to keep up with their unfolding work. Matteo Selvini (1991) has himself commented very frankly on these difficulties in a short paper replying to the research paper by Alan Carr (1991), which we cited in Chapter 2. In trying to articulate why his group has never undertaken a major research project, Selvini says the following:

In fact it is precisely the constant, rapid evolution in our way of working and doing therapy that is one of the main reasons which has discouraged us from carrying on at least one of the many quantitative follow-up projects we planned, and sometimes even started, in these last years: *our problematic pathology consists in a persistent and repetitive feeling that what we were doing a couple of years earlier was junk!*

(Selvini, 1991, p. 265. Emphasis added by SR and AT)

This admission may be both frank and honest, but it does put a question mark over the value of a team's work if they dismiss research so easily. There is also a worry from a user-friendly point of view. Is it the needs of users that are central to the innovations being made or is it the fascination for developing new theories and new methods that motivates the group? We also note that Palazzoli's main focus now seems to be in forming a therapeutic alliance with the parents of the adolescent who is presenting with psychotic behaviour. We would stress that the user-friendly implications of this are important because the views of the adolescents themselves may well be ignored in this process.

This criticism can also be made of the family management approach to schizophrenia advocated by Julian Leff *et al.* (1989), Ian Falloon *et al.* (1984),

Carole Anderson *et al.* (1980), and Ian Bennun (1993). These models have the advantage of being relatively well researched, although Lucy Johnstone (1992) has criticized the shaky theoretical underpinnings of the model. Their user-friendliness is explicit but one-sided – parents are offered specific help in dealing with the family member who is labelled as psychotic but the heavy labelling that this involves is worrying.

From a user-friendly point of view we are concerned that the therapeutic alliance between parents and therapist could easily end up as a therapeutic coalition against the family member who is labelled schizophrenic. We suspect that part of the popularity of such an approach will lie, not only in its 'effectiveness', but also in its attractiveness to Health Service managers eager to see concrete 'results' being achieved but by a service that does not challenge the medical model adopted by most psychiatrists.

The vexed question of neutrality

As we have already pointed out in Chapter 4, the term 'neutrality' was originally intended to encourage the therapist not to form an alliance with any one person within the family and not to show approval, disapproval or any form of moral judgement concerning family members (Palazzoli *et al.*, 1980). In order to help maintain neutrality, therapists were encouraged to adopt an interviewing style based upon the use of circular questioning. Circular questioning was later described by John Burnham as a means 'to gather information by asking questions in terms of differences and hence relationships. In addition to the usual direct questions, family members are asked, in turn, to comment on the thoughts, behaviour, and dyadic relationships of the other members of the family' (Burnham, 1986, p. 110). Vernon Cronen and Barnett Pearce claim that circular questioning has a number of other benefits: 'In a system troubled by too much clarity and rigor . . . it opens new ways of thinking. . . . In a system troubled by too much confusion . . . it provides a way of thinking which can replace unstructured "mush"' (Cronen and Pearce, 1985, p. 79).

Cronen and Pearce's view is subtly different from Burnham's, which seems to assume that the therapist should retain a role as a collector of information. As the therapist asks circular questions, the information is stored and utilized in devising interventions. Within Cronen and Pearce's framework, circular questioning is construed as interventive in its own right. The therapist is allegedly not a repository of privileged information. She can only ask questions and these will not have predictable outcomes. The process set in motion by circular questions is all-important since the answers to the therapist's questions form the basis for further questions. The term 'co-creation' is sometimes used (Harlene Anderson and Harold Goolishian, 1988) to describe this recursive process, but we would argue that this can be something of a misnomer if an approach dictates that it is only the therapist who is entitled to ask questions. The aim of circular questions is not to attempt to discover a user's point of view for its own sake but to enable users to co-operate with the therapist in exploring and creating new meanings and beliefs in relation to the problems they are describing. Although David Campbell, Ros Draper and Clare Huffington (1989) graphically demonstrate how beliefs and behaviour are interlinked, second-order thinking has encouraged a clear shift towards focusing on beliefs. Earlier schools of family therapy had tended to place greater emphasis on observable behaviour, and improvement was usually measured in terms of changes in behaviour.

Circular questioning, as originally devised, was often a powerful tool in the hands of the therapists, despite the adoption of a stance that attempted to play down the idea of power. Anyone who has seen video recordings of Gianfranco Cecchin's work in the early 1980s will have witnessed a skilled therapist firing off a battery of circular questions, sometimes at the rate of 11 questions per minute!

This form of questioning appeared to be both controlling, uninvolved and distant, but it must be added, in fairness, that there have been many modifications to the technique in the last 10 years. Thus, Benson *et al.* (1991) and Lee Combrinck-Graham (1991) talk of how circular questions can be used to good effect with children, who love the idea of creating new realities rather like stories.

Although most of the developments in circular questioning have concentrated on how to improve its effectiveness (see Peggy Penn (1982), Karl Tomm (1987a, b) and John Burnham (1986)), there has also been an increasing awareness of the reputation of the technique as rather cold and uninvolved.

Many therapists also came to regard neutrality as a form of non-involvement, or even lack of commitment, on the part of the therapist. In response to this Cecchin (1987) suggested that neutrality could encourage the therapist to develop a state of 'curiosity' about the family. Curiosity carries with it a greater sense of being interested in the user's views. The therapist adopting it as a stance would not become too attached to any one hypothesis or explanation of her own, but was able instead to engage in a conversation which would open up, rather than close down, new ways of perceiving difficult situations. Curiosity can become a stance not only for the therapist, but also for the family, and extends beyond what second-order thinkers would see as the limiting perspective of approaches based on behavioural change only, where the dangers of blame and counter-blame are never far away. Because the therapist is no longer seen as an expert on solutions to other people's problems, she can develop curiosity not only about issues within the family, but also about the limiting effects of her own attitudes and beliefs.

This last point brings us to a more sharply focused discussion of what role the therapist actually plays within second-order therapy. If the therapist is no longer an expert in a meta-position, but 'a participant manager of the therapeutic conversation' (Goolishian and Winderman, 1988), then she is no longer defined as becoming stuck in a 'pathological' family process, or sucked into an 'enmeshed' system. Anderson and Goolishian talk of therapy as a narrative, which is co-created by therapist and family, and which develops according to its own evolving 'rules' (Anderson and Goolishian, 1988; Goolishian and Anderson, 1992). The therapist is no longer on the outside. She can only be an insider.

SECOND-ORDER THINKING AND THE DEFINITION OF THE FAMILY

We have so far talked of the 'family' as if it were a clear and uncontroversial concept within second-order thinking. Carl Whitaker (1967) used to talk of the need for the therapist to win the 'battle for structure' by convening all 'family' members to the first session. Defining the family was not problematic and was considered to be the task of the therapist. Times have certainly changed – consider, for example, the alternative position of Jay Efran and Michael Lukens (1985), who insist that a therapist cannot speak to a family; he or she can only *think* about the concept 'family' while speaking to an individual or several individuals. In between these two positions – one based on certainty and the other on total relativism – a user-friendly therapist needs to arrive at an acceptable definition of how each family defines itself without imposing conventional ideas, based on notions of the 'household' or 'nuclear' family, on the users with whom she is working.

Second-order thinkers like Anderson and Goolishian (1988) have challenged the idea of any standard unit of treatment and have developed a different term, the 'problem-determined system'. They argue that particular problems create certain systems around them rather than that certain types of systems create particular problems.

They question the pre-determined idea of 'individual' or 'couple' or 'family' as a natural focus for therapy and prefer to work with whichever system can be defined to exist around a problem at any one time. The exact composition of this system may vary over time, but it needs to be established collaboratively, after due negotiation between users and therapist, rather than unilaterally by the therapist. It is important that the therapist adopts a 'not-knowing', rather than an expert, stance in relation to all outcomes. Indeed, once the problem is described as no longer existing, the system round the problem merely dissolves, according to Anderson and Goolishian.

On the basis of our rather condensed descriptions, second-order practice may seem rather un-engaging and mystifying and yet Lynn Hoffman (1991) claims that a second-order practice can be one that is less disrupting, less mechanistic and less pathologizing of the family than a first-order approach:

> As I began to search for a 'different voice', I became increasingly un-comfortable with this technocratic coldness. Actually I never entirely bought it. When unobserved, I would show a far more sympathetic side to clients than my training allowed. I would show my feelings, even weep. I called this practice 'corny therapy' and never told my supervisors about it. . . . I began to talk with other women and found that they too used to do secretly what I did and also had pet names for this practice.
>
> (Hoffman, 1991, p. 11)

Lynn Hoffman's comments are very intriguing because second-order thinking has enabled many therapists to recover methods of working with users that were outlawed because of the impact of first-order thinking. This is hardly new, though. The psychotherapy movement has for years been replete with user-friendly approaches (e.g. Kellyian and Rogerian psychotherapy) that have traditionally invited therapists to abandon the expert stance in favour of a much more down-to-earth, humanistic approach.

Having made her important point about 'corny therapy', Hoffman goes on to describe how her particular way of developing second-order practice was significant to her. It was most valuable because it encouraged her to make clients feel more comfortable, to share stories with them from her own life, to ask about expectations of therapy, and to invite questions from clients about her own work. She also found that the reflecting team (Andersen, 1987) made a major contribution to this way of working. She argues that, 'The professional was no longer a protected species, observing "pathological" families from behind a screen or talking about them in the privacy of the office.' With this came notions of collaboration and partnership, where the therapist, if not exactly neutral, would adopt a position of multi-partiality, or a willingness to sustain a variety of explanations at the same time.

There is, of course, always a risk that therapists become too attached to a few favourite theories and fail to appreciate the unique position of every user. Cecchin *et al.* (1993) make the point that systemic therapists risk becoming trapped by their models. They have therefore devised the term 'irreverence' to describe playful ways that therapists can utilize in occasionally breaking out of such a strait-jacket. Similarly, Brent Atkinson and Anthony Heath (1990) suggest that therapists may adopt 'wilful' behaviour like giving personal opinions to users, providing the aim is not to be normative, not to be too instrumental and not to become too attached to a particular outcome.

SUMMARY

Since our discussion of second-order approaches has been quite detailed, we will now briefly record two summaries of the approach before making some comments that assess the approach's contribution to user-friendliness. Anderson and Goolishian's (1988) summary is as follows:

1 The therapist keeps enquiry within the parameters of the problem as described by the clients.
2 The therapist entertains multiple and contradictory ideas simultaneously.
3 The therapist chooses co-operative rather than unco-operative language.
4 The therapist learns, understands and converses in the client's language.
5 The therapist is a respectful listener who does not understand too quickly (if ever).
6 The therapist asks questions, the answers to which require new questions.
7 The therapist takes the responsibility for the creation of a conversational context that allows for mutual collaboration in the problem-defining process.
8 The therapist maintains a dialogical conversation with himself or herself.

Hoffman summarizes the main points in a second-order therapy more briefly (Hoffman, 1985, p. 393):

1 An observing system stance and inclusion of the therapist's own context.
2 A collaborative, rather than a hierarchical, structure.
3 Goals that emphasize setting a context for change, not specifying a change.
4 Ways to guard against too much instrumentality.
5 A 'circular' assessment of the problem.
6 A non-pejorative, non-judgemental view.

Some limitations of second-order approaches

Elsa Jones in her review article (which we cited earlier in this chapter) has made some fundamental points about the weaknesses inherent in the radical constructivist version of post-Milan thinking:

> Cecchin and Boscolo have been criticised on the grounds that their approach is irresponsibly non-interventive, that their 'curiosity' resembles indifference and, instead of being value-free, has the effect of reinforcing the status quo (Colapinto, 1988). Golann (1988) refers to the risks of this approach as allowing 'therapists to float trial balloons and not take responsibility for them if it is expedient to not do so'. Concern has, in particular, been expressed with regard to the application of their ideas where abuses of power are enacted within families in physical violence, sexual abuse or the oppression of those, e.g. women and children, who have less access to power and rule making in our culture. . . .
>
> Taken to its logical end-point . . . [their] . . . approach would lead to quietism, the placid withdrawal of the Buddhist or the contemplative. If, as Maturana recommends, we give up our 'passion for change', if systems are constantly evolving and changing, anyway, if you can never step into the same river twice, if the joining of one system with another inevitably leads to (unpredictable) change, if families do what they do in response to perturbation and therapist contact, or the basis of their own structure-determined system and might as well change or not change in response to any other random event, the time may come for therapists to desist from taking money in return for setting themselves up as agents for change.
>
> (Jones, 1988, pp. 331–332)

Jones's comments are salutary but, from a user-friendly point of view, it is worth examining what the approach can offer if it is utilized in a modified form, as part of an approach rather than being central to it.

A second-order approach may help users feel that they are listened to by an attentive therapist who will not understand them too quickly, and jump to conclusions. What may also happen, in this painstaking process, is that the therapist may end up understanding too slowly. Chris Dare and Caroline Lindsey

(1979), writing about what were still called multi-problem families at the time, argued that there are families that require therapeutic work to be completed fairly quickly. The therapist has a brief period within which to establish her credibility, after which her welcome within the family will sharply diminish. A user-friendly therapist will recognize that, in some situations, families feel over-burdened, either directly by the problem behaviour referred, or as a result of their contact with other agencies with which they have, or have had, ambivalent and dependent relationships. Jo Douglas (1981), in applying behaviourist ideas to family therapy, also suggests that some form of behavioural success is essential for some families before they can enter a more detailed discussion about the meanings behind problems which may be maintaining them. There is also research evidence to back up this idea as we demonstrated in Chapters 8 and 9.

We would also argue that certain class and gender variables need to be considered. For example, Bennun's research (1989), as we noted in Chapter 9, documents a crucial finding that many men prefer to receive direct advice, something second-order therapists, in particular, try and avoid giving. Some cultures within British society stress the importance of authority, of experts, of leaders. However, therapists using second-order ideas, who are likely to come from social backgrounds which value words and ideas, may themselves find advice-giving crude, unsophisticated and ineffective. This is the type of clash of perspective that we commented on in Chapter 8. We would argue that therapists need to accept that a large proportion of users would not find a therapeutic style based exclusively on second-order thinking helpful, particularly on initial contact with an agency, when anxiety levels are very high and the desire to be contained and to be offered expertise is strong.

Laurie MacKinnon et al. (1984) have compared three major 'strategic' therapies (MRI Brief Therapy, Haley/Madanes Strategic Therapy, and Milan-systemic therapy), and have suggested that the original Milan model, with its emphasis on neutrality and non-directiveness, as well as long intervals between sessions, may not fit so well with what they call 'centrifugal' families, which are seeking authority and structure in therapy. In developing ideas of user-friendliness, we are cautious about typecasting families as centrifugal (or centripetal, or anything else), but MacKinnon et al.'s point still interests us. It could be argued that Cecchin et al.'s (1993) idea of irreverence might help a therapist adopt an uncharacteristically authoritative, structural and even expert stance, so long as she does not believe too strongly in it. But therein lies a snag. If a 'second-order' therapist spends half her time using such first-order methods, but without really believing in them, will this not create strains in the therapeutic relationship and confusion within the therapist herself?

We ourselves are comfortable with the idea that we can probably never completely act from a non-expert position, but we hope that we are not so tied by our theories that we could not openly share our concerns about therapy with the people we are working with. As Jay Efran and Leslie Clarfield (1992) suggest:

Therapists who have decided to adopt a neutral stance and to eliminate elements of hierarchy from their work have generally not consulted their clients about the matter. This creates an inconsistency between 'text' and 'subtext' akin to what happens when parents announce to their offspring that certain family issues will now be settled 'democratically'. This doesn't eliminate parental authority – it disguises it.

(Efran and Clarfield, 1992, pp. 206–207)

Second-order writers rightly emphasize that therapeutic questions can work in a liberating way. Statements can close down or limit thinking whereas questions can be facilitative. Nevertheless, we suspect that all forms of questioning, including circular questioning, may act in a mystifying way. As Ben Furman and Tapani Ahola (1988) point out, users must wonder what the purpose behind the questions might be and they can also feel placed at an arm's length from the therapist (as we established in Chapter 9). Karl Tomm (1988) acknowledges this point when he says, 'A therapist may, in effect, hide behind perpetual questions, and fail to enter the relationship as a real person.' He then goes on to suggest that a large number of questions, asked early on in therapy, can be experienced as distancing, non-empathic and even punitive. We would add that this possibility is always present, even later in therapy. Statements may indeed came across as equally judgemental, but it is naive for therapists to assume that questions cannot be construed as judgemental by users, who may be very sensitive to questions that probe areas of great hurt or embarrassment.

Clearly, persistent questioning, and (as we have seen in Chapter 9) the answering of *users*' questions with further questions, can create a poor therapeutic climate. The power of the therapist is, in fact, manifest in her ability to dominate the session through questioning. A genuinely egalitarian therapeutic alliance cannot be built solely on the basis of questioning. At times users want us to level with them, to offer thoughtful advice and express our own opinions, and we need to reflect their need for us to be genuine and honest with them.

We believe that there is an anachronism in the development of second-order thinking which needs to be addressed. We can readily support the criticism of the expert role and the idea of co-construction that the models support. But it is important to point out that the approach is not based on any concerted attempts to research what users actually want and need from therapy or how they experience therapy. In fact the literature search undertaken in order to write Chapter 9 yielded only one piece of research based on a second-order perspective. Bruce Kuehl and his colleagues (Kuehl, Newfield and Joanning, 1990; Newfield, Kuehl, Joanning and Quinn, 1990) have produced two interesting papers which utilized ethnographic interviewing techniques in order to explore how users experienced family therapy. Despite the methodological sophistication of these studies, we do not believe they have made a significantly different contribution to the literature. Perhaps future studies will make a more substantial contribution, but the dearth of studies is very striking, particularly as the approach stresses at a theoretical level that users' views are so important.

From our user-friendly standpoint there is much of value in second-order approaches but we worry about their idealist basis. They risk stressing the importance of changed ideas and concepts to the detriment of changed behaviour (or other aspects of physical reality) which can in turn change ideas. The model often comes across as dogmatic despite Cecchin's use of irreverence as a form of wild card which softens the monolithic nature of the approach.

We hope that a more elaborated model of therapy as a co-constructed project will eventually be developed by actually listening much more intently to users' experience of therapy. But such a development also needs to take account of sociologists, anthropologists, philosophers and researchers who themselves contribute understandings of the complexities of the therapeutic processes. Within family therapy it is feminist theorists who have perhaps contributed the most important antidote to the idealist position of second-order thinking.

The feminist contribution to family therapy

Feminism, by way of contrast with the restraint of second-order approaches, has brought a more direct, certain and down-to-earth challenge to family therapy. In particular it has challenged the failure to address seriously issues of power and inequality. As long ago as 1979, Phil Kingston pointed out that, within family therapy, there was a striking 'absence of a political perspective; or sometimes the presence of a desperate attempt to be apolitical.' Kingston used the term 'political' to mean any intervention aimed at changing or maintaining the balance or distribution of power.

During the 1980s a great deal was written about the particular problems of power experienced by women. It is striking that as recently as 1990 Jane Conn and Annie Turner were still able to say, 'Patriarchy, sexism, and oppression are terms which do not appear often in family-therapy literature, even in writing by women.' The crucial question for us, though, is the effectiveness of such a literature in altering the practice of family therapy. Power, after all, must be a central concern for anyone aiming to practise a user-friendly therapy.

In reviewing some of the feminist literature within the family therapy field, we will be looking at how this literature has contributed to the broadening and deepening of the theory of family therapy. Or, to quote the words of Deborah Luepnitz (1988): 'feminism need not be the *theme* of therapy; it must simply be its sensibility, its spoken or unspoken centre'.

Rachel Hare-Mustin (1978, 1986) is one of the pioneer writers from within family therapy who has most clearly articulated some of the basic differences between family therapy and other forms of therapy, such as psychoanalysis. In doing this she has made more visible the particular differences in power between men and women. She talks of psychoanalysis as suffering from 'alpha prejudice' in its tendency to make too sweeping and rigid a distinction between men and women. By contrast, she sees systems theories as being dominated by 'beta prejudice' because they overlook the differences between the sexes and treat all members of a system as similar. This blindness to gender differences means that the essential social differences between men and women (which tend to put women at a disadvantage in therapy) are overlooked. She also quotes a survey of family therapists which showed that the majority of them ranked creating independence and differentiation as the most important task of therapy. Caretaking was ranked as the least important. Needless to say, these preferences themselves demonstrate gender bias – it is the former characteristics that are associated with the male role, and the latter with the female role.

Jennie Williams and Gilli Watson have also criticized the way family therapy devalues women:

> Within family therapy there has been a systematic preoccupation with, and pathologizing of, women's power in families. Women have been consistently blamed for family dysfunction with reference to their over-centrality, over-intrusiveness, over-protectiveness, over-control and mind-reading.
>
> (Williams and Watson, 1988, p. 299)

They advocate a two-fold approach to correct the mistakes:

1 Taking 'power' into the room. This involves addressing power issues which are normally invisible and 'have no name'. For example, therapists may need to explore how basic decisions are made about which partner earns the money and which partner looks after the childen. They also need to explore another central question that is normally ignored in therapy – how far are domestic arrangements negotiated at all or are they regarded as natural or normal and therefore not in need of negotiation?
2 Taking therapy out of the room. This involves 'de-privatizing' the family (to use their term) by challenging oppressive ideologies within the family, and attempting to empower the family in its relationship with the outside world.

Unlike Williams and Watson, Jenny Pilalis and Joy Anderton (1986) refer to what they see as some of the limitations of using feminist therapy on its own. They suggest that it is possible to integrate feminist and systemic approaches, arguing that feminist family therapists should refuse the 'relative comfort of opting for one perspective or the other'. They urge family therapists to be clear and explicit about their own values, and to share and discuss these but without imposing them on the family. They also advocate the development within family therapy of skills in consciousness-raising, education, negotiation and advocacy.

Like Pilalis and Anderton, Marianne Walters et al. (1988) also feel that it is possible to cross-pollinate feminist and systems ideas. (Their own model is mostly a mixture of structural family therapy and feminism.) Like many other feminists, Walters et al. are concerned with explicitly addressing the inequalities manifested in family life and in treatment. They also seek to broaden the argument beyond the boundaries of the home, claiming that many of the problems and inequalities in the home reflect inequalities prevalent throughout society. Another important contribution made by them concerns the rethinking of several structural family therapy concepts which have been criticized as sexist. To illustrate their rethinking, we will briefly explore how the concepts of enmeshment and hierarchy are reconstructed by them.

Enmeshment

This aspect of relationships is usually viewed pejoratively by structural family therapists, who assume that a state of relative differentiation is more healthy. Walters *et al.* point out that the type of relationship that women seek (as opposed to men) may involve a greater degree of genuine intimacy, hence 'enmeshment' may actually be a valued experience of connectedness.

Hierarchy

Ideal family relationships are often portrayed by structural therapists in an authoritarian way as involving hierarchy, but Walters *et al.* argue that women utilize hierarchical relationships in a more consensual (although less obvious) way than men who exert power much more explicitly.

Another important contribution made by Walters *et al.* is a series of guidelines to help feminist family therapists keep track of the issues that need to be incorporated into therapy. This list is useful and we reproduce its headings below:

1   Identification of the gender message and social constructs that condition behaviour and sex roles.
2   Recognition of the real limitations of female access to social and economic resources.
3   An awareness of sexist thinking that constricts the options of women to direct their own lives.
4   Acknowledgement that women have been socialized to assume primary responsibility for family relationships.
5   Recognition of the dilemmas and conflicts of childbearing and child rearing in our society.
6   An awareness of patterns that split the women in families as they seek to acquire power through relationships with men.
7   Affirmation of values and behaviours characteristic of women, such as connectedness, nurturing, and emotionality.
8   Recognition and support for possibilities for women outside of marriage and the family.
9   Recognition of the basic principle that no intervention is gender free and that every intervention will have a different and special meaning for each sex.

(Walters *et al.*, 1988, pp. 26–29)

The crucial issue posed by this valuable list is: How is it possible to utilize these ideas in actual family therapy sessions? As Virginia Goldner (1991) herself has commented (in reviewing Rosine Perelberg and Ann Miller's (1990) book *Gender and Power in Families*), there is now a third wave of feminist books which have moved feminist thinking to a new stage. The 'first wave' of feminist commentary succeeded in creating a revised theory of families which, in turn, prompted a second wave of creativity, which produced a revised practice of family therapy. However, according to Goldner, there is a third wave or, as she says:

> 'Now as I read the rich and complex discussions that accompany the multitude of examples provided in this book, I see yet another phase of feminist project emerging: a revised *theory of therapy*. This is because in order to make room for gender in the consulting room the therapeutic conversation must expand to bring the larger world of macrosystems – material, social and cultural – into the intimate discourse of treatment.

> (Goldner, 1991, pp. 341–342)

Perelberg and Miller's book is particularly valuable because it contains many thoughtful examples of how gender issues can be used in therapy without users feeling at the butt end of issues which are crucial to their therapist but are marginal to them. Goldner's idea of expanding the therapeutic conversation is crucial to solving the difficulty. As we have seen from our review of research studies, there is often a clash of perspectives between users and therapists which can undermine the success of therapy. There may, however, also be a clash of perspectives between users themselves. As Charlotte Burck and Glynn Daniels have pointed out:

> Many women come into therapy with a wider brief . . . [than men] . . . often wanting (fundamental) changes in relationships in the family. Men, on the other hand, generally adopt the narrower view that there is simply a problem to be solved. . . . One can hypothesize (therefore) that women often come into therapy with a wish, however covert, for second-order change (wanting her partner to take more responsibility for child care) whereas the man may only see change in first-order terms, i.e. at the behavioural level (helping her out a bit more).

> (Goldner, 1991, p. 86)

It can be difficult enough for a family therapist to help the partners work towards a common agenda, if she is attempting to take seriously the diverse expectations of all family members. Still more problematic are situations involving couples where both believe that therapy should only be symptom-focused, but where there are also clear gender imbalances within the family. A feminist family therapist may wish to find a way of working on the initial concerns expressed by the couple, whilst looking at ways of expanding the therapeutic conversation to include wider gender issues. A user-friendly therapist, however, will have the added difficulty of considering how far she has the right to push her own views and interests onto users who have a much narrower agenda. There is no simple answer to such a dilemma, but in such situations it may be best for her to sharpen her awareness and share these dilemmas with the couple explicitly.

CONCLUSION

In this chapter we have looked at some of the main user-friendly aspects of second-order and feminist theories, since these theories have been, in our opinion, the most influential ones in family therapy during the past 10 years. Our own background has been in structural family therapy, and we still adhere to many of the fundamental tenets of that theory. However, we have also had to acknowledge some of its limitations, in particular its certainty, its expertness and its normative approach to what constitutes ideal family functioning.

Second-order thinking and feminism have influenced us in ways which have allowed us to develop an integrated practice, which hopefully avoids the woolliness of eclecticism. Feminism has helped us as male therapists to see more clearly the nature of male oppression and the structured abuse of power. We have been encouraged to work more closely and personally with users, particularly in examining gender and other power issues in therapy. We have also had to develop our own agendas (see Reimers and Dimmock, 1990) for looking at the issue of being men in therapy – whether as therapists or users – and we agree with Barry and Ed Mason that 'patriarchy damages men's quality of life as well as women's, that it constrains men rather than enabling them to develop' (Mason and Mason, 1990, p. 210).

By way of contrast, second-order thinking has influenced us in the direction of not taking any theories or beliefs for granted. This, in turn, has meant that we have been much more able to work alongside users, jointly drawing on a wider range of ideas and solutions in an effort to solve the problems that brought them to therapy. The different emphases of various theories like structural family therapy, second-order thinking and feminism inevitably involve some tensions. These tensions are potentially helpful and can prevent the monopoly of one line of thinking or action and can help us more sensitively to custom-build therapy with our users.

We will return to some of these issues in Chapter 13, since we will look at particular ways in which we have tried to develop a user-friendly approach with our users, using case examples to illustrate our points. However, in our next chapter we will attempt to draw the threads through our book and explore a series of guidelines which provide a framework for user-friendly therapists.

Chapter 12

Guidelines for user-friendly practice

Andy Treacher

INTRODUCTION

In this chapter we will explore eleven guidelines which we have developed in order to help us keep user-friendly concepts at the centre of our work. We have chosen to use the term 'working guidelines' to reflect the fact that we need to undertake a great deal of additional work in order to ensure that they actually perform their function. In the following sections of this chapter each guideline will be briefly stated before we attempt to summarize the experiences, research and theorizing that prompted its formulation.

1 User-friendly family therapy is based on the core assumption that therapists must accept that ethical issues are of primary, not secondary, importance in therapy. Therapy is recognized to be essentially a human encounter between participants who meet as human beings first, and therapist and users second, but the crucial power difference between therapist and user is recognized as a major source of difficulty and danger that must be successfully addressed. Failure to address this power differential opens the way to abusive practice.

Therapy is, unavoidably in our opinion, an encounter between human beings but it is an encounter in which the participants are unequal. The impact of systems theorizing in all its many hues has been so powerful in the family therapy movement that we still feel some sense of embarrassment in making a statement like this. The idea of co-constructing therapy apparently offers a different approach to these issues but we remain unconvinced because such theorizing, once again, leads therapists into thinking about therapy in a way which obscures the power differential between therapist and user.

To insist that ethics should be the cornerstone of therapy is still demonstrably a novel – even controversial – idea in family therapy. For example, if we once again examine the 'bible' of family therapy, Gurman and Kniskern's *Handbook of Family Therapy* (which plays a powerful role in defining the field), then we discover that Volume 1 (1981) contained no chapter on ethics and only one index reference to ethics. Volume 2 does contain an ethics chapter, by William Doherty and Pauline

Boss (1991), but this chapter is effectively little more than an addendum, tacked on to the end of the book. In fact, all the index references to ethics are to this chapter with the exception of one remaining reference, which is concerned (like the reference in Volume 1) with Boszormenyi-Nagy's contextual therapy.

Clearly ethical considerations are not at the forefront of the minds of most of the leading theoreticians within the field of family therapy. User-friendly family therapy, like contextual therapy, takes the exactly opposite view. Any theory of therapy that is based solely on allegedly value-free rational-scientific constructs is very vulnerable to criticism because such a theory is bound to hide behind a smoke-screen of scientific neutrality. In practice, all sorts of highly unethical, reactionary and chauvinistic frameworks are smuggled into therapy, as Deborah Luepnitz has clearly demonstrated in her book *The Family Interpreted* (1988). From a user-friendly standpoint, the crucial question to be answered is this: How can the observance of ethical codes become a cornerstone of the day-to-day work of practitioners? Doherty and Boss (1991) have very usefully summarized the main components of the code of ethics of the American Association for Marriage and Family Therapy but their discussion also includes an exploration of the somewhat different approach taken by the American Psychological Association. The AAMFT guidelines, which are regularly revised, cover five main areas: (1) responsibility to clients; (2) professional competence; (3) professional integrity; (4) professional development; (5) social and legal responsibilities. The Association for Family Therapy has also published a provisional set of ethical guidelines, which Sigurd helped to draft. Both sets of guidelines are invaluable in helping practitioners to map out how to practise ethically. However, as Andy has pointed out in a recent debate in the AFT magazine *Context*, professionals are notoriously weak at policing ethical codes (Treacher, 1993; see also Treacher, 1986, and Jennie Pilalis, 1984).

A user-friendly approach to this problem insists that an inspectorate needs to be set up in order to provide users with an independent body to which they can appeal if they feel they have cause for complaint. Treacher (1993) points out that teachers are regularly inspected in order to establish whether they are performing their role effectively (and ethically). A similar system could be devised in order to monitor psychotherapists. Government funding would be required in order to set up such an organization, but clearly such a body could be used both to monitor effective practice and to deal with complaints against practitioners.

Clearly such a system would also require a number of other innovations in practice. The first would be the publication of ethical codes which could be given to each user on first contacting a practitioner. The code would also need to contain a clear description of how a user can make a complaint. Ironically such a system could only work effectively if an independent ombudsman or ombudswoman were available to support the complainant in pursuing the complaint.

As a reader you may feel that our proposals are utopian but we firmly believe it is only the implementation of radical proposals like these which can create a safe context for undertaking therapy. If such a structure is not built then it is clear to us that Jeffrey Masson's criticisms of psychotherapy (reviewed in Chapter 3) will never be answered. We also believe that the issue of an ethically based practice can be tackled at a more personal level. For example, it is feasible to expect every therapist to translate their own values into an ethical code that they can then share with their users. Obviously the code would incorporate the main elements of the worker's professional code of ethics but such a code inevitably does not deal with all the issues that a more personal code could deal with. Writing one's own personal code would take time and effort but it would have the built-in advantage of being more personal and more meaningful to the practitioner – we suspect that the response from users would also be very worthwhile because all the research evidence we know indicates that users respond very favourably when therapists seek to clarify the basis on which they undertake their therapy.

As a footnote to our discussion we should add that we have found Mary Zygmond and Harriet Boorhem's (1989) exploration of ethical decision-making in family therapy very useful. They demonstrate how Kitchener's model of ethical justification can be used to clarify situations in which, for example, the AAMFT ethical code is difficult to utilize when making a specific decision about how to proceed in therapy. Clearly we badly need thoughtful articles like this which address the nitty-gritty of clinical decision-making from an ethical point of view.

2 A user-friendly approach to family therapy is based on the assumption that the building of a therapeutic alliance between users and therapist(s) is usually crucial both to the success of therapy and users' reported satisfaction with therapy.

In Chapter 8 we explored the valuable empirical work of Patricia Hunt (1985) but it is well worth returning again to her study because she usefully summarizes many basic points which we would wish to include in our discussion of the therapeutic alliance. In reviewing her results, she comments:

> It was the degree to which counsellors and clients could *collaborate* in working together which seemed to be the overall significant factor in whether counselling was successful or not. However warm the counsellor is or however motivated the client, the crucial factor is whether they connect and somehow agree together to work. The important factor then is whether the 'therapeutic alliance' is established or not. . . . Orlinsky and Howard's very thorough review of the research on all aspects of the processes of psycho-therapy . . . concludes that 'psychotherapy that is effective is distinguished most consistently by the positive quality of the bond that develops between the participants' (1978, p. 317). . . . Gurman and Kniskern's review of marital and family research comes up with similar conclusions, but they emphasize the therapist's responsibility for creating a good relationship. They also point to the fact that when deterioration occurs . . . 'it appears that the therapist variables, and the patient–therapist interaction, account for negative effects far more than patient factors alone' (1978, p. 884).
>
> (Hunt, 1985, p. 50)

Hunt also quotes the important work of the psychotherapy researcher, Hans Strupp, who sees creating a good therapeutic relationship as the challenge that every psychotherapist must meet:

> The professional therapist's stance of acceptance, respect, understanding, helpfulness and warmth, coupled with deliberate efforts not to criticise, pass judgement, or react emotionally to provocations, creates a framework and an atmosphere unmatched by any other human relationship. How to create a relationship and to turn it to maximal therapeutic advantage is the challenge facing the modern psychotherapist.
>
> (Strupp, 1978, p. 7)

Strupp's position is very close to ours but we dislike his use of the term turning the relationship 'to maximal therapeutic advantage'. It is better, in our opinion, to say 'to create a relationship which enables the user to feel empowered/safe/ supported so that she (or he) can then decide which issues can be explored'. Strupp's formulation is also, in our opinion, somewhat utopian. We would like to build into therapy the notion that a therapist cannot be all things to all people and that the most user-friendly approach available is to be empowered to take action which addresses the needs of users when therapy has got stuck. This means therapists need to be able to give themselves permission to fail. Not all therapist–user matches are workable. It is much better and much more respectful for both parties either to seek consultancy to unstick the relationship (see Carpenter and Treacher, 1989, especially Chapter 7) or, if this fails, to find a supportive way of transferring the users (if they so desire) to another therapist who is more sympathetic to them and therefore better able to work with them.

Hunt's own discussion of the therapeutic alliance is valuable because it explores the complexity of the relationship. Interestingly, she points out that Freud himself recognized that patient passivity was a pitfall – the patient needed to become an active partner who collaborates with the therapist. However, she does not cite Ferenczi's important work that addresses the issues more fundamentally through highlighting the dilemmas that a therapist faces (see Chapter 3 for an extended discussion of this point). We would argue that a family therapist who actively works at believing in the potential of her clients from a basically humanistic point of view can go a long way to overcoming the inevitable dislikes that she may have for certain users. At a practical level, the therapist needs to challenge herself with the question: What do I need to do in order to find ways of liking and respecting the users I am working with?

Sebastian Kraemer's discussion of the psychological impact of positive connotation on the therapist, which we explored in Chapter 5, is also worth remembering in this context. He points out that the discipline of actually formulating a positive comment that can be shared with a user begins to shift the relationship between the therapist and the user. Obviously support and supervision from colleagues can help but Ivan Inger (1993a, 1993b; Inger and Inger, 1992), who has paid very close attention to these problems, insists that it is essential to have conversations directly with users around these relationship issues. For instance, he suggests that apparently taboo questions need to be discussed directly in therapy. To ask clients directly about their sense of liking and trusting the therapist is one way that the therapeutic alliance itself can be placed at the centre of therapy. Asking such questions may seem to be extremely risky but if such questions are not asked (and answers mutually provided), then the therapy may fail anyway sooner or later. Bordin (1983) has summarized a number of studies of individual therapy that report that good therapeutic outcome was correlated with the ability of the therapist to pay attention to alliance-related problems and to intervene and repair effectively any damage to the relationship. Interestingly, passive registering of these difficulties by expressing interest or concern was not sufficient to prevent disruption in the alliance.

In a futher paper, with Windy Dryden, Patricia Hunt has provided a very useful analysis (based on Bordin's work) of the structural components of the therapeutic alliance:

> [T]he therapeutic alliance is made up of three major components . . . the *bonds* refer to the quality of the relationship between the participants, the *goals* are the ends of the therapeutic journey, while the *tasks* are the means for achieving these ends. Disruption to the therapeutic journey might occur because the 'travellers' (a) do not get on or have a relationship which is not conducive to the goals or task of therapy (weak or inappropriate bonding); (b) disagree on journey's end (non-agreement about goals); and/or (c) prefer different ways of reaching the therapeutic destination (non-agreement about tasks).
>
> (Dryden and Hunt, 1985, p. 123)

Elsewhere, Andy has argued (with John Carpenter) that family therapists need to learn the lesson of these general findings (Carpenter and Treacher, 1989). Some models (particularly Minuchin's structural approach, e.g. Minuchin and Fishman, 1981) have absorbed many ideas about the therapeutic alliance and have made significant original contributions to the literature. It is also important to update Hunt's argument by pointing out that Alan Gurman, David Kniskern and William Pinsof (1986), in a major review article, have once again stressed the importance of alliance-forming in all forms of therapy, including family therapy.

Under the general heading of the 'new process perspective' in family therapy, they stress that the significance of the psychotherapeutic alliance is a key development:

> The most exciting development in this realm has been that within the last decade [i.e. 1975–1985] . . . a number of psychotherapy groups in North America have developed a loosely listed network study of the alliance in individual therapy. . . . Currently there is tremendous excitement within the psychotherapy research community about the potential of the alliance as (1) a potent predictor of outcome and (2) an organizing and formal construct for subsequent process research. . . . Until very recently . . . [however] . . .

alliance theory and research have not emerged within family therapy theory and/or research.

(Gurman *et al.*, p. 600–601)

According to Gurman and his colleagues, it is primarily William Pinsof and his research group at the Family Institute of Chicago who have attempted to translate ideas about the therapeutic alliance into practical and serviceable measures which can be used to develop research and practice. Their research has spanned a number of research instruments, including the Integrative Psychotherapy Alliance Scales (IPAS: Pinsof and Catherall, 1984), which have been specifically developed in order to introduce alliance theory and research into the field of family therapy. IPAS itself consists of three self-report scales: one for individuals, one for couples and one for family members. These scales, which take approximately three to five minutes to complete, can be used at the end of each therapy session in order to monitor the development of the therapeutic alliance from the user's point of view.

The IPAS is based upon Bordin's multidimensional definition of the alliance which we have already explored. Pinsof and Catherall have introduced a number of other important dimensions. The Interpersonal System dimension monitors three aspects of the user–therapist relationship: (a) Self–Therapist (I and the therapist; (b) Other–Therapist (significant others and the therapist; (c) Group–Therapist (us and the therapist). Clearly these sub-dimensions provide crucial information about how the therapist is being viewed by users during the progress of therapy.

Gurman, Kniskern and Pinsof also review the important work of Gerald Patterson and his colleagues at the Oregon Research Institute. Patterson's group has developed a somewhat unfortunately named Client Resistance Code (CRC) which attempts to evaluate 'co-operative' and 'resistant' behaviours which either impede or facilitate therapy. A Therapist Behaviour Code (TBC) has also been developed in order to monitor therapists' verbal behaviour in sessions. Patterson and Forgatch (1985) were also able to demonstrate that certain therapist behaviours (e.g. 'Teach' and/or 'Confront') increased resistant behaviours (in a group of mothers) while 'Support' and 'Facilitate' therapist behaviours decreased resistance. They conclude that their research indicates that therapists need a wide range of skills to enable them to overcome the resistance elicited by their own teaching behaviour.

These findings will be of considerable interest to second-order therapists who may well feel that a more co-constructing approach might be preferable, but the research also draws attention to the contribution that users make to the therapeutic equation. Gurman, Kniskern and Pinsof report that the CRC is similar to the Supportive/Defensive Coding System of Alexander *et al.* (1976), which demonstrates that certain features of family functioning seem to determine whether a family can successfully engage in therapy. It is also important to add that the value of IPAS has been further explored by Pinsof himself (Pinsof and Catherall, 1986) and by other researchers, such as Laurie Heatherington and

Myrna Friedlander (1990), who report that its sub-scales seem to be valid and reliable and offer a real basis for meaningful research.

Gurman, Kniskern and Pinsof's review of research concerning the therapeutic alliance is significant to us because it has immediate implications for day-to-day therapy. Some of the measures being developed by researchers can clearly be incorporated into therapy in a user-friendly way, but such developments have a wider significance. The ability of researchers to translate the rather nebulous concept of the therapeutic alliance into tangible measures which are of significance to therapists and users is a considerable step forward and can be used to counter the research–practice gap that we have commented upon in previous chapters. (See also Schwartz and Breunlin, 1983.)

Finally it is important to add a corollary to the guidelines. We hope our view is firmly grounded but we need to acknowledge that there is a significant minority of users who would probably find our ideas about the significance of the bond between therapist and user bewildering, and user-unfriendly. Different folks want different strokes, and some folks seem to want virtually no strokes at all because they do not stop around long enough to engage in any relationship-building with their therapist. For example, parents dropping in to a drop-in service need a response from their therapist which matches their customerhood. They may be wanting quick advice or they may be wanting what we call an MOT – confirmation that what they are doing to cope with their child's difficulty makes sense to the professional too. On the other hand, they may be wanting to engage in therapy at a deeper level and have come to suss out whether the therapist or the service appeals to them or not.

What we are saying here amounts to a truism – the therapeutic alliance formed with different families needs to take many different forms, ranging from the minimal to the maximal. In a previous book with John Carpenter, Andy has attempted to explore this point in some depth (Carpenter and Treacher, 1989, pp. 60–98). In particular we drew attention to the important work of Weitzman (1985), who has summarized some important principles to guide therapists working with families whose commitment to therapy is difficult because of problems to do with their chaotic life style. Weitzman's thoughtful approach is a useful antidote to any grandiose thinking on the part of therapists who may well feel that engaging families is just dependent on the skills of the therapist. He argues in favour of a minimalist approach with some families – the therapist needs to set realistic goals and accept that working with all family members is usually impossible. Individual members of the family may be motivated albeit on a very limited and short-term basis.

3 User-friendly family therapy recognizes that the structure of the therapist–user relationship is unbalanced and that successful therapy is at least partly dependent on the therapist's discharging her responsibility to create a context which facilitates change.

This guideline is really a corollary of the second one. As we have pointed out in earlier chapters, first-order systems theorizing tended to render users invisible and, as a result of the same process, also rendered the therapist invisible. The therapist tended to become an appendage of the all-powerful team that delivered therapy to, and at, a passive family which was expected to follow the directives of the experts behind the screen. A curious spin-off from this model was that the issue of matching therapist and user evaporated – such matching became a non-issue. A model that stresses the importance of the therapeutic alliance naturally rediscovers the significance of the therapist as a person but at the same time it takes a realistic attitude to what a therapist can bring to therapy in terms of personal resources.

Windy Dryden and Laurence Spurling's book *On Becoming a Psychotherapist* (1989) is a particularly valuable contribution to the growing literature on the significance of the person of the therapist in determining the successful outcome of therapy. Charles Kramer's earlier book *Becoming a Family Therapist – Developing an Integrated Approach to Working with Families* (1980) also makes a useful contribution to this literature, since it stresses the need for family therapists to be aware of the personal changes they must make in order to become therapists who can effectively work with the range of problems that families bring to therapy. However, it is Dryden and Spurling's work which really challenges therapists to come to terms with the process that has propelled them into becoming therapists in the first place. In their book, the different therapists give very thoughtful accounts of the personal journeys they took in becoming psychotherapists.

In the opening chapter of the book, Paul Gilbert, William Hughes and Windy Dryden succinctly summarize the significance of therapist factors in influencing the process of psychotherapy:

> We believe that in common with much anecdotal evidence the person of the therapist matters. Therapists require a certain kind of interpersonal intelligence and to be able to apply science. But like musicians or artists, technique will carry a person so far. Those therapists who are probably the more successful are able to marry pragmatically different sets of styles and approaches which are not a mish-mash of eclecticism but a carefully considered application of approaches to suit different clients at different points on their journey. Therapists who are themselves heavily defended will tend to focus on what they are doing and on their techniques. There will, of course, always be some clients who will be helped even by the most defended of therapists. Nevertheless many clients and professionals have expressed the view that the success of a therapy depends on finding the right person (i.e. therapist) as much as finding the right school of therapy. . . .
>
> In regard to therapy, therefore, it is as important to focus on the style of the therapist as it is on the techniques of therapy; we need both the singer and the song.
>
> (Dryden and Spurling, 1989, p. 12)

Through our eyes, the metaphor of the singer and the song is decidedly problematic because users are excluded from the metaphor, but nevertheless we can accept the emphasis on the role that the therapist needs to play. We personally believe that since therapists are paid for their role in the relationship they are ethically bound to do their best to ensure that the therapeutic relationship is built. Clearly they also have to ensure that the energy and skill they bring to the task is not disempowering, but to expect users to make an equal contribution to the process, particularly initially, is to misunderstand the nature of the therapeutic relationship.

If a therapist's training has been successful then she can bring real resources to the therapeutic encounter. A whole range of abilities, including the ability to listen, to empathize, to contain and to challenge supportively can be mobilized in order to create a facilitative environment for the user. But, of necessity, the contract does not demand that the user should reciprocate. Of course there will be some elements of reciprocation – a therapist who is able to use a facilitative level of self-disclosure as part of a therapeutic alliance-building approach will often experience genuine support, interest and empathy from users but it would obviously be self-defeating if therapy sessions became focused on the needs of the therapist.

A user-friendly approach, because it is suspicious of many aspects of professionalism, adopts a stance towards the therapist which is essentially humanistic. It stresses the responsibilities of the therapist but it also acknowledges that there are limits to any therapist's resources. Strupp's view of the therapist as polymath needs to be firmly challenged. A more realistic approach stresses that every therapist has both vulnerabilities and strengths. Every therapist will inevitably form weak alliances with some of the users on her caseload despite her best efforts. Rather than turning this into a discussion of therapist deficiency it is better, and more humane, to create a context in which a notion of potential failure is in-built and treated as a fact of life. Therapists are not superhuman and cannot succeed with all families despite supervisory and team support. Transferring a family to a colleague is no dishonour and can be handled respectfully (and in a user-friendly way) if the therapist acknowledges her inability to be helpful to the family.

4 User-friendly family therapy recognizes that therapists generally fail to understand the stress and distress that users experience, particularly on contacting an agency for the first time.

Family therapists, like all psychotherapists, tend to live in professional bubbles that make them insensitive to the fact that the majority of users find coming to therapy very difficult. A user-friendly approach to therapy focuses a great deal of its thinking on how every aspect of the technological and institutional super-structure of therapy can be made more user-friendly. In practice this means that every aspect of therapy needs to be put under the microscope. For example, a simple exercise that gives food for thought is as follows. Pretend one day that you are a user and then imagine entering your own building. How will you be received by the receptionist, if you have one? How friendly is the waiting room? How long will you wait? What are the messages implicit in the furniture and pictures that have been chosen for the waiting room? Is there information about how to find the loos? Are the magazines tatty and irrelevant to you?

The string of questions that could be asked is very long but it is clear from user surveys that such issues are important. As professionals we visit other agencies and often sit in their waiting rooms because we have arrived early. It is a salutary experience and gives us an immediate experience of the agency's user-friendliness. The role that receptionists play in creating user-friendliness cannot be underestimated and we welcome Shaw's article (1992) which provides some interesting ways of training receptionists to be more helpful to users.

But, of course, the first impact that an agency has on its users is not dependent on its reception and waiting room facilities. First contacts with agencies usually take place via letters or phone calls or through home visits by workers. Home visiting is, of course, an important issue as far as user-friendliness is concerned but unfortunately we cannot give it the attention it deserves. Fortunately a review article by David Cottrell (1994) fills the gap for us. We have also included in Appendix 3 a bibliography of papers that are relevant to home visiting (which is, of course, particularly relevant for users who are disabled). Referrers also play an important part in influencing initial contacts, because they may or may not create helpful messages that enhance the engagement process. Most agencies notoriously fail to brief their referrers adequately and also fail to develop a system which enables them to monitor effectively how their referrers present the agency to users. A user-friendly approach to therapy insists that referrer-friendliness is crucial to effective user-friendliness.

Andy has discussed this issue (the so-called 'agency' triangle – between user, referrer and agency) in a previous book (Carpenter and Treacher, 1989) at some length but the essence of a user-friendly approach is to insist that time spent informing referrers about what the agency offers is time well spent. In our experience, there is no substitute for actually meeting referrers and creating a workable rapport with them. Users are often very confused by the referral process and may have very complex feelings about being referred, particularly if they have a longstanding relationship with the referrer. (Brian Dimmock's discussion of referrals by GPs (Dimmock, 1993) is a very interesting example of the attention to detail that is required in such situations if the referral of users with complex difficulties is to be undertaken successfully.)

Clearly our discussion at this point could become very tedious because every minute aspect of therapy could be put under the microscope under the terms of this guideline but nevertheless it is important to stress that the basic technology of family therapy, the use of video and screens, has to be tackled from a user-friendly point of view. We will discuss this issue in more detail in Chapter 13 but it is worth pointing out that there is a very simple innovation that can help to make the introduction of the screen and video a very different experience to users. If an agency has a choice of interview rooms, it is often possible to begin an initial interview by meeting the family in an ordinary interview room. The first part of the interview can then focus on introductions and explaining how the therapist would like to work. If the family is happy with the contract negotiated, then the session can transfer to the screen room. An interview that takes place from the beginning in a screen room equipped with video is a very different experience and is, in our opinion, coercive because the implicit message of the interview is, 'we've brought you into this room which is designed for family work – if you refuse to allow us to use our normal methods you are a problem to us'.

A more radical approach to the issue of the use of screens has been taken by Young (1990), who argues that the screen can be equated with Jeremy Bentham's panopticon (a circular prison with cells built round the warders' well, which, through being located at the centre of the circle, enabled warders to keep prisoners under continual observation (see Michael Ignatieff (1978) for a fuller discussion of its role in controlling prisoners). All the metaphors associated with the use of a screen are exactly opposite to the ones that a user-friendly approach normally invokes. Andersen's policy of reversing the process by having the team literally lit up and the family viewing them through the screen (Andersen, 1987) is very interesting, but we remain undecided about whether to be pro or anti screens. As we have seen from our survey, users' opinions are also divided. Perhaps it is best to leave the issue to be negotiated, family by family, but using the non-screen interviewing room policy as the place where the initial contract is negotiated.

The shift in emphasis exemplified by this change of policy needs to permeate all aspects of therapy. As we have pointed out in earlier discussions of both Lorion's work (Lorion, 1978) and the work of Pam Pimpernell (Pimpernell and Treacher, 1990), the essential change is in *providing* users with information about therapy during the contract-making stage of therapy rather than attempting to *extract* information from users about their problem. Users who are engaged in therapy by being adequately informed and by being made aware of their rights (as suggested in a previous guideline) are better able to exert real choices about how therapy will unfold. Lorion's use of preparation techniques for both users and therapists can become an essential and creative part of this process, but therapists need to resist the pressure to rush and work at their pace rather than that of their users. The simple policy change of allowing two hours for a first interview, rather than an hour, can have a dramatic effect on engagement rates because users feel much more comfortable and heard if the therapist can combine the information-giving aspects of the engagement process with the necessary centring on the users' need to ventilate and share their problems.

Interestingly, the scheduling of a two-hour session in a clinic which usually utilizes just an hour can cause timetabling difficulties. But such a difficulty is a perfect illustration of the gap that exists between therapist and user. A skilled therapist can no doubt undertake a skilful and productive interview using an hour as a time base; the felt experience of the users at the receiving end may be that the interview was indeed skilful but their need to ventilate and get things off their chest in their own way and at their own pace may well have run up against the tight scheduling of the therapist.

It is continual attention to such difficulties as these which characterize user-friendly approaches. Even in situations when consultation is being given, it is all too easy for therapists to lose the user's perspective. A useful consultation device can help to prevent this process: having a team member take the role of trying to empathize with the users can be valuable; so is the device of periodically saying to each other, 'and supposing family members had heard this part of our discussion, what would they be saying?'

5 A user-friendly approach to therapy recognizes that family members cannot be treated as though they were identical members of a system. Class, gender, sexual orientation, power, age, disability, ethnic origin, religion and socio-cultural background are some of the more obvious sources of difference which may need to be taken into consideration if successful therapy is to be undertaken with a given family.

In many ways this guideline is a corollary of guideline 2. Clearly a therapist's ability to engage users and to be 'street credible' to them depends on her ability to be sensitive both to their needs and to who they are. Therapists need to have an acute sensitivity to the way that users use language and communicate with one another but the therapist also needs an ability to tune into many facets of family life. But at a deeper level, therapists need to prepare themselves actively when they work with families that clearly differ from themselves, particularly in terms of class origin, ethnicity and religious beliefs. Again Lorion's research (Lorion, 1978; Lorion and Felner, 1986) is important because it clearly demonstrates that therapist preparation programmes which increase therapists' knowledge of their users' lives are valuable in helping therapists avoid stereotyping their users. The work of personal construct family therapists (Rudi Dallos, 1991; Harry Procter, 1984 and in press) is also important in this context. Their conceptualization of family construct systems is particularly valuable because it insists that therapists take a highly phenomenological approach to their users. This demands that they get to understand how family members construe important aspects of their lives. Knowledge of the family construct system enables the therapist to be much more sensitive to the way that users see the world and avoids many of the errors of the objectively expert position which misleads a therapist into thinking that she knows how a family functions – perhaps because she thinks she has seen an apparently similar family before.

The pioneering work of Charles Waldegrave (1990) and his colleagues at the Family Centre, Lower Hutt, New Zealand, also needs to be discussed in this context. Working in a multi-ethnic, multi-cultural context bedevilled by severe socio-economic difficulties, the Lower Hutt team has developed some very well grounded, ethically informed ways of working with users from diverse backgrounds. Unfortunately our own practice (which has been developed in south-west England) has been very weak in terms of developing ways of working with people from different ethnic backgrounds; 99.5 per cent of people living in the south-west are of Caucasian origin but we nevertheless need to develop our practice in this area more consciously.

Jay Lappin's (1983) paper is particularly valuable since it is full of ideas about how to become a culturally conscious family therapist. He stresses the importance of forming a therapeutic alliance based on a discussion of both differences and continuities between the therapist's culture and the user's culture but he warns against the dangers of stereotyping, of going too fast and of using translators. Clearly the pace of therapy needs to be slower because a great deal of mutual accommodation needs to take place. For a further discussion of such issues, see Carpenter and Treacher (1989), especially Chapter 3, and the important texts by Nancy Boyd-Franklin (1989) and Monica McGoldrick, John Pearce and Joseph Giordano (1982).

Another area of neglect by us concerns the issue of religious differences. A recent paper by Prest and Keller (1993) has drawn attention to the fact that many therapists are themselves not actively religious and are therefore very reticent about exploring religious beliefs in family therapy sessions. And yet users' religious beliefs may have an enormous bearing on how they think therapy should proceed. The importance of exploring users' concepts of the causation of problems and how they can be changed necessarily needs also to include questions about the power of prayer and about any religious ideas that could have a bearing on the issues being explored.

In many ways it is very difficult to illustrate adequately the significance of this guideline but fortunately previous chapters of our book have touched on aspects of this issue. As an example of the type of work that a therapist needs to do in preparing to meet different types of users, we will briefly mention how a therapist could prepare herself for working with long-term users of adult mental health services. Viv Lindow, who is very active in the user movement, has kindly agreed to our reproducing a bibliography which she has recently collated (see Appendix 4). The value of such a bibliography is that it enhances therapists' ability to understand the often shattering experiences that users bring to therapy. Often they have been abused by the very services that have been apparently designed to help them. As we know from Masson's work, family therapy may also have contributed to a feeling of being abused, so there is absolutely no grounds for family therapists to assume that somehow family therapy escapes without criticism.

The truth of the matter is that therapists need to find ways of understanding the uniqueness of every family they work with. We have noticed in our own practice that it is precisely when we think we know a lot about a family that we are lulled into a false sense of security. The challenge is to find ways of enabling ourselves to be continually thinking about the uniqueness of the family – its particular ways of communicating and of problem-solving etc. – rather than slotting the family into some category which obscures its uniqueness. John Schwartzman's (1983) discussion of the use of ethnographic techniques as tools that clinicians can use is very relevant to our discussion at this point. Family therapists clearly need to be anthropologists for all the families they meet because each family has its own microculture.

*6 A user-friendly approach to family therapy assumes that it is integrated
models of therapy that can offer users the best deal in terms of actually being
offered ways of working that are likely to suit them.*

We have explored this issue in previous chapters so we can afford to be brief. The
idea that any one model of therapy is so well evolved that it can suit all possible
users seems, to us, to be scarcely worth debating any more. For us, it is the
development of integrated models that seem to be the way forward because such
models are much more likely to address the basic issue that many users require
different inputs from therapy at different times in their careers as users. Andy has
explored this issue in previous work (Treacher, 1985, 1988b, 1992) but we would
also draw attention to Windy Dryden's (1992) book *Integrative and Eclectic
Therapy – a Handbook*, which is a very valuable source book for anybody
interested in developing integrated models.

One model, in particular, is very interesting to us because of our working in
child guidance settings. Ann Jernberg's 'family theraplay' (Jernberg, 1989) seeks
to combine the strengths of structural family therapy with the strengths of child
psychotherapy. The approach draws upon the important work of the Guerneys,
who have developed a form of therapy – Child Relationship Enhancement
therapy (CRE: Guerney and Guerney, 1987) – which is based initially on child-
centred play sessions which are aimed at developing the child's communication
and expressive skills. This work is initiated by a therapist but parents become
involved quite quickly and are supportively coached so that they can take over
from the therapist. This approach is particularly suitable for parent–child
relationships dogged by failure-to-attach issues. Parental involvement is the
critical factor in the approach – skilful child psychotherapy or play therapy by
itself is not user-friendly because it runs the risk of leaving the child and its
parents disconnected.

In many ways, family theraplay is a classic example of a user-friendly, integrated model. It only works if a strong working alliance between the parents and
therapists is established. Parents who feel hopelessly deskilled by their child are
offered a working model of how to relate to their child and a supportive environment in which they can practise new skills which give them a sense of empowerment and competence. The therapeutic work is intense but the model recognizes
that it is basically impossible to ask a parent to behave differently if their own
difficulties are clearly transgenerational in origin. Transgenerational disruptions
in child care skills and the development of attachment bonds necessarily involve
intense but supportive therapeutic work that conversational models of therapy
cannot, in our opinion, possibly deliver.

We would like to extend our discussion to the pros and cons of other integrated
models but space does not allow us to do so. Treacher (1992) contains a brief
bibliography of integrated models, but we would hasten to add that an integrated
model may not necessarily be user-friendly.

7   User-friendly family therapy insists that therapists must adopt a stance of self-reflexivity. Hence they must be willing to accept that if they themselves had difficulties they would willingly attend therapy sessions organized by therapists who utilize a model of therapy similar to their own.

Some psychiatrists we know would happily undertake ECT if they became depressed but we wonder whether strategic therapists would actually accept that strategic therapy was a way of solving any family problems they might need to take to therapy? We know of no study that has actually investigated therapists' needs in this way but our own informal studies of therapists attending our training workshops concerning user-friendliness have revealed just how complex the answers to this question can be. The following list of needs was generated by 13 therapists (9 women and 4 men) attending a recent workshop. We have slightly edited this list so that each need is expressed in the same grammatical form (the exact wording in the original list would make reading rather more complicated).

Therapists as users: a list of the characteristics they would want their family therapist to have

Able to control
Being aware of particular needs
   of family members
Being consistent
Being challenging
Listening but then moving into action
Being practical
Sharing clients' views
Being able to contain
Avoiding being expert
Being understanding
Providing reassurance
Giving advice
Being available when needed
Able to clarify roles
Self-disclosing
Being non-judgemental
Providing advocacy
Not backing off critical issues

Being fallible
Being flexible
Being facilitating
Providing family therapy in a
   structured way
Not making assumptions
Involving the wider family
Observing confidentiality
Providing a parental figure
Looking competent
Creating self-worth
Providing friendship
Not being aloof
Being real
Being responsive
Being expert
Empowering
Being sensitive
Support-giving

This list records the collective needs of the therapists as a group. Unfortunately we did not collect the data in such a way that we could rate the importance of these needs but the list does illustrate just how complex and contradictory such needs can be. Sadly, we don't know of any accounts of family therapists themselves going to family therapy but recently a Hollywood film has neatly illustrated just how powerful the 'biter-bit' scenario can be. The *Guardian* of 10 April

1992 ran a very moving review of the recent Hollywood film *The Doctor*, written by Jane Martin, a junior hospital doctor who had herself suffered from cancer. In the film William Hurt plays an American surgeon who has everything he wants in life – except compassion for his patients. He gets cancer and is referred to his own hospital for treatment. The plot is about how the experience changes him.

Jane Martin's own comments about the film are very poignant, as the following quotation reveals:

> Producer Laura Ziskin was fascinated by the concept of 'the doctor' as patient. Central to it is the idea that doctors and their patients are on different sides of the track, and that their perspectives on illness are strikingly different. The consequences that follow have profound implications for both players in the charade.
>
> Firstly, as patients, particularly when seriously ill, we may want to believe that our physicians are capable of remaining invulnerable to disease because this would endow them with the strength to take care of us. We project onto our doctors powerful fantasies about being looked after and we need to see the fantasy figure as heroically invincible. But there is another side to this. Because the figure of our fantasy is invincible, he cannot have experienced our suffering, and this can leave us feeling desperately alone and misunderstood.
>
> Secondly, as doctors, we cling to the delusion that we are made of different stuff from mere mortals. This protects us from the intolerable idea that we too might fall victim to the ghastly affliction of our patients. . . .
>
> When you have been on the other side of the sheets, you do indeed know how it feels. You have been as vulnerable as hell. There are positives. I hope I have become a more compassionate doctor and can hold on to the empathy. But the journey doesn't end in the land of the sick. What remains to be negotiated is the return to one's former role, that of the healer, the one who isn't supposed to be sick. And this sets up another conflict, for how do we learn how to stay with the knowledge of the experience of illness and yet at the same time reclaim our former defences?
>
> (Martin, 1992)

Of course, the vast majority of doctors never enter the sick role for a significant period of time, so they never have a shared experience on which to build. Because of their role, and because of their training, they build elaborate defences against their potential (human) vulnerability and hence it is no surprise to find that doctors collectively manage their private lives worse than their patients – they feature prominently in statistics for alcoholism, drug abuse, divorce and suicide. Family therapists who adopt the same technical-cum-scientific stance as doctors (and hence seek to remain aloof and distant in therapy) must surely run the same risks of internalizing the stress that cannot be avoided because it is part and parcel of undertaking the job.

Perhaps the 'technical' structure of family therapy – the screens and the use of teamwork – creates a collective defence which makes the therapist less vulnerable. However (as we have seen from the research we have examined so far), this has the reciprocal effect of leaving many users feeling alienated and less cared for precisely because the technology is so distancing. Our user-friendly approach attempts to confront this issue by insisting that family therapists can learn from the mistakes of the medical profession. If therapists are adequately and supportively trained within a model that emphasizes *the practitioner's right to be cared for* then it is possible to begin to reverse some of the macho, uncaring traditions that have been established within the profession (see guideline 8).

So one crucial spin-off from adopting a user-friendly approach to therapy is the basic and fundamental principle that user-friendliness is only viable *if therapist-friendliness is also a cornerstone of the approach.* Therapist-friendliness is perhaps a very woolly term (even more so than user-friendliness) but the thrust of our argument is clear. Given our stress upon the crucial significance of the therapeutic alliance in providing a context for successful therapy, it is clear that a therapist's contribution to building such alliances is predicated on the flexibility, job satisfaction, level of self-esteem and general *joie de vivre* that the therapist brings to the job. An agency which works well creates enough nurturance and autonomy for its therapists to be able to nurture the users that attend. These are embarrassingly obvious statements but unfortunately there are strong traditions in family therapy that militate against this approach.

For example, the idea of trainee-centred training (paralleling user-centred family therapy) is by no means universally accepted. Judith Mazza, in her chapter on training strategic therapists, in Howard Liddle *et al.*'s *Handbook of Family Therapy Training and Supervision* (1988), is untroubled by advocating covert techniques which are utilized to change trainees' behaviour in ways dictated by the trainer. A trainee-friendly approach would, of course, stress the contractual nature of training and avoid using methods which place the trainer in such a powerful position.

8 A user-friendly approach to family therapy recognizes that research needs to play a crucial role in contributing to the development of theory and practice. This is an ethical issue because therapies that fail to develop a body of research data supporting their efficacy are clearly vulnerable to criticism. Users' experiences of therapy and their satisfaction with therapy must, of necessity form a crucial part of the assessment of the value of any model of therapy.

Again, this is a rather long-winded guideline, but we agree with a number of commentators (including Ian Bennun, 1992 and Glenys Parry, 1992) who have argued that unmonitored practice is difficult to defend from an ethical standpoint. In fact we would argue that the track record of family therapy is weak in terms of trying to provide research backing for different models of therapy. Normally it is efficacy research that is used in such assessments but utilizing efficacy data is itself full of pitfalls from a user-friendly point of view because therapists have a tendency to establish their own criteria for success which may not correlate with users' reports of either success or satisfaction. An interesting example of this type of thinking is summarized by Gurman, Kniskern and Pinsof (1986) in the review we have already mentioned earlier in this chapter. After commenting on the difficulties of using user-satisfaction ratings as a criterion for judging the value of therapy, they add the following rider:

> Sluzki (1984) . . . points out that, beyond all the usual criticisms of using patient satisfaction ratings, such ratings may contain an inherent, though rarely acknowledged, bias in favour of the 'cosier' family therapies which emphasize the therapist's affective connectedness with the family, in comparison to family therapies, such as strategic and brief interactional therapy . . . that allegedly down play the salience of the therapist's personal characteristics. Sluzki argues that, in fact, one might well expect, in such therapies, only a low positive, or even a negative correlation between patient ratings of general satisfaction with treatment and their observable behavioural outcomes.
>
> (Gurman *et al.*, 1986, p. 608)

Clearly, from a user-friendly point of view this extreme example of positivistic thinking is anathema. As Andy has pointed out (with John Carpenter) in an earlier discussion of user-friendliness, this statement can be translated into every- day language in the following way:

> Therapists (because they are scientists) know best, so if they happen to use maverick forms of intervention which produce behavioural change despite users' disliking them that is perfectly okay because change is what the user came for.
>
> (Treacher and Carpenter, 1993, p. 32)

Carlos Sluzki's position is, in our opinion, just a sophisticated version of the 'doctor knows best' arguments that some psychiatrists use to justify the use of ECT. A user-friendly approach insists on worrying about therapy outcome findings which demonstrate a discordance between user satisfaction and therapist-derived data which indicates that positive behavioural change has occurred. The crude pragmatic position which argues that the end justifies the means is a formula for disaster in psychotherapy. We prefer to adopt the classical Hippocratic stance of *primum non nocere* rather than be involved in forms of therapy which users find problematic. Theories of therapy which give therapists permission to ignore users' experiences are, in practice, self-defeating because they fail to solve what for us is the sixty-four-thousand-dollar question: Can alternative, ethically justifiable, user-friendly approaches be developed which are both effective in solving or alleviating the problems that users bring to therapy and are experienced by them as respectful and acceptable?

Our discussion of efficacy is but one example of the basic issue that is posed by this guideline. Ignoring users' experiences is an ethical, not a rational-scientific issue, but an ethically grounded theory of therapy needs to develop not only a comprehensive ethical code, but a viable way of enforcing the code. This takes us back to the point we argued in relation to our first guideline. Therapists cannot be left to monitor their own work – an independent body needs to take on this role. What is required of therapists is a willingness to reconstrue the role of research and audit in relation to therapy. Since it is straightforwardly unethical not at least to audit the work we undertake as therapists, it is essential to see the whole issue of feedback from users as an ethical, not a scientific, issue.

The task that faces contemporary practitioners is to develop therapist-friendly measures – so-called 'dirty' research – which can readily be used on a day-to-day basis to collect meaningful data about what is happening to users as they move through therapy. Pinsof's 'Intersession Report' instrument (1982) is a good example of such a measure. It takes two minutes to complete with the user rating nine areas of his or her life (work, physical health, relationships with parents, etc.) on a five-point scale which estimates whether life has improved, stayed the same or deteriorated.

Clearly a measure like this can be invaluable to both user and therapist in providing a snapshot of how therapy is proceeding. Perhaps some user fatigue will be experienced if it is used too often and too mechanically, but if users are involved well and the discussion of the use of the measure is made really meaningful to them, then it is likely that the measure contributes to the building of the therapeutic alliance. Its use clearly communicates to the user the therapist's concern about the user and the necessity to keep a sharp eye on whether therapy is contributing gains to the user's life or not.

Elsewhere Andy has pointed out that the scientist-practitioner (associated perhaps most strongly with the profession of clinical psychology), has proved a singular failure in influencing the day-to-day activities of practitioners. (For further discussion of this issue, see Pilgrim and Treacher, 1992, especially Chapter 4, entitled 'The scientist-practitioner model – problems and paradoxes'.) There is no claim of originality in making this point but we believe that the scientist-practitioner model does not realistically address the basic facts of life that practitioners have to face within work contexts which are continually beleaguered by long waiting lists and inadequate resources.

Donald Schön's discussion of an alternative, reflective-practitioner model (Schön, 1983) is a useful antidote to the unrealistic demands of the scientist-practitioner model. It is a model that requires a practitioner to reflect continually on the unfolding processes in which she is involved. Family therapists, particularly when working with colleagues, are actively engaged in such reflective processes but our user-friendly stance insists that users' experiences must be incorporated into this process – not just through the process of questioning and sharing ideas but by utilizing other means (diaries, questionnaires, self-report checklists) which contribute much more information to the reflective process. Clearly, busy clinicians are limited by time constraints in what they can do but there are very real possibilities for unleashing the energies of users who may have more time to devote to such projects.

Needless to say, the changed context of the NHS with its emphasis on audit, patient charters and 'value for money' creates a new sense of urgency for practitioners. Many see such developments as undermining the autonomy of professional workers but we believe that excessive autonomy is the enemy of good practice. In order to survive, professionals need to demonstrate actively that their work is ethical, effective and creates user satisfaction. Needless to say, no professional claims concerning these three dimensions will hold water unless users are deeply involved in establishing whether their experiences of therapy overlap with their therapists' experiences.

Finally, it should be pointed out that family therapists have recently shown an increased interest in auditing procedures which can be developed in user-friendly ways. Ian Wilkinson (1992), J. Chase and Jeremy Holmes (1990) and Peter Bruggen and Sharon Pettle (1993) have contributed important and practical ideas which can be very useful to busy practitioners. There is not much evidence of genuine user involvement in these audits but we would be optimistic that audit measures can be modified on a user-friendly basis.

9 A user-friendly approach to therapy stresses the crucial importance of training and professional development in influencing therapists' attitudes. Just as family therapy needs to be user-friendly, family therapy training needs to be trainee-friendly. Basically this means that training for therapists also needs to be based on ethically sound principles.

This is a theme that we have touched upon several times elsewhere in our book, so we can again afford to be brief. The crux of the matter, from our point of view, is that the authoritarian stances of many of the original family therapy models tend to permeate training programmes. The original models neglected user perspectives and perpetuated the problem by training the next generation of therapists to neglect users also. Apprenticeship models of training unfortunately tended to produce conformist trainees who followed the directions of their powerful, hands-on trainers.

Interestingly, as Tamara Kaiser (1992) has pointed out in a very important paper, ethical issues concerned with the relationship between the trainer and trainee were largely ignored. Kaiser insists, and we agree with her, that training models need to develop very well worked out ethical codes which reflect the trainee's right to be respected and to be offered a training environment in which a relationship of trust can be built up.

Training models that respect the skills and person of the trainee and seek to help her develop her skills and abilities on a clearly contractual basis naturally mirror therapy models which offer users the same sort of contract. In a previous section of this chapter we drew attention to a different model of training which felt able to intervene covertly to change trainee behaviour. Needless to say, we take exception to such a model on ethical grounds. As user-friendliness basically espouses a position of do-as-you-would-be-done-by, it is impossible for us to support a model which gives a trainer such a maverick and powerful role.

Interestingly, our notion that trainee–supervisor relationships need to be built on a co-operative basis gains some support from a study by Barbara Frankel and

Fred Piercy (1990), who have been able to demonstrate that when supervisors and trainees both demonstrated effective 'Support' and 'Teach' behaviours (as defined on a number of scales), users tended to remain co-operative or become co-operative more frequently than when both such behaviours were not present. This finding implies that modelled co-operativeness has a clear spin-off.

Apart from espousing a position of co-operativeness between trainer and trainee, a user-friendly approach also necessarily espouses the idea that trainees need to undertake personal work of many kinds and to enter therapy. Since the person of the therapist emerges as such a crucial factor in determining the outcome of therapy, it is important that therapists gain the widest possible experience that equips them for the role. Stuart Lieberman (1979) has offered some useful exercises for exploring therapists' unfinished business but the stress on the value of experience which is central to the notion of user-friendliness also means that the model invites trainees (and therapists for that matter) to undertake personal work. Any therapist who has never had the experience of herself going to a therapist is vulnerable to a criticism which simply says 'but you have no idea of the experience' – empathy is not enough.

Harry Aponte (1992) has recently explored the implications of personal train- ing as far as structural family therapy is concerned. He argues that the model needs a method of training that integrates the existential, human mutuality of the therapeutic relationship with its more technical aspects. This requires therapists to be trained in the use of the self – of being able to utilize aspects of their personal history and personal style to help create new therapeutic possibilities for their users. Interestingly, the structural therapy model has always invited therapists to explore such possibilities but there was little recognition in its associated training model of how to help trainees become more flexible and more personal in their approach to their clients.

10 A user-friendly approach to family therapy recognizes that therapy has crucial limitations in helping users. It recognizes that some families also need their therapist to play a supportive role in gaining access to material resources that can be crucial to their well-being.

This guideline attempts to address an important issue that can be central to therapy. A pure therapeutic approach that eschews trying to help users solve problems of living (such as inability to pay fares to the sessions, housing prob- lems that impinge on family life, victimization by neighbours, and so on) cannot possibly succeed in helping users become empowered and in control of their lives. There are times, therefore, when part of the therapist's role in developing a therapeutic alliance with her users hinges around her ability to utilize her pro- fessional network to attempt to create changes that are important to the family. Obviously we are not advocating that the therapist should become the family's welfare officer but a willingness to help the family make gains on such fronts is crucially important.

The Automobile Association advertising campaign which hinges around the catch-phrase 'but I know a man who can' is unfortunately sexist, so we need immediately to change it to 'but I know someone who can'. But it is nicely apposite to situations often faced by therapists. In other words, the therapist's task is to help the family find advocates and allies who can help them in their battles to secure the basic necessities of life without which they are vulnerable.

Needless to say, the role of self-help organizations is very significant. Unfortunately, many therapists remain aloof from such organizations, perhaps on the basis that they create dependency or give messages that are counter-therapeutic in their eyes. We would argue that it is necessary to build up working relationships with such organizations whether we like it or not. If we do not, we place ourselves in the unfortunate position of acting as gatekeepers by default, that is, we fail to inform users of possibilities that may indeed help them.

Clearly we have touched upon an important issue here which needs further elaboration by us. We are very aware of possible pitfalls in our position. For example, Athena McLean (1990), in a very important article analysing the impact of the American user movement, the National Alliance for the Mentally Ill (NAMI), has pointed out how alarmingly powerful such an organization may become in terms of influencing government policies and the allocation of research funds. However, we believe, nevertheless, that family therapists need to explore the possibilities of collaborating with such organizations, particularly at a local level where networking contacts can create flexible arrangements that would be impossible at a national or regional level.

11 A user-friendly aproach to therapy is not simplistically user-centred. It recognizes that at times statutory, ethical and clash-of-values issues may make it essential that the therapist challenges users' attitudes and behaviour.

Last, but not least, this guideline recognizes the complexity of the therapist role and acknowledges that there may well be, at times, a clash between the therapist and her users which is apparently unbridgeable. Rachel Hare-Mustin and her colleagues (1979) have written an important article which addresses the possible gap between the rights of clients and the responsibilities of therapists. Clearly there are times when the therapist must necessarily relate to users not as a therapist but as a statutory worker who must report aspects of the family's behaviour to the appropriate agency. Paradoxically, such reporting can, nevertheless, be undertaken in ways that are still user-friendly, i.e. that are respectful, pay meticulous attention to family members' rights and maintain the message: 'I am still available to you as your therapist; if you want to continue working with me, I will do so. If you want to fire me then, of course, I understand but I want to make clear that I am not rejecting you. I am doing what I am doing because I am legally bound to do so'.

Clashes of values may take other forms and can equally cause enormous difficulties, and it is essential that we do not argue for a utopian position that insists that a therapist should be able to work with anybody. Albert Ellis (the American originator of Rational Emotive Therapy) is notorious for saying that he would have gladly worked with Hitler in therapy but we find his position ludicrous. Debbie Luepnitz (1988) has interestingly discussed a very different example of the psychiatrist Franz Fanon refusing to work with a French police-man who was effectively a professional torturer, viciously interrogating FLN members in Algeria. He complained to Fanon about being anxious and having sleepless nights. Needless to say, Fanon refused to work with him unless he gave up his job.

People who have seriously transgressed major societal rules, behaving crimin-ally or irresponsibly, obviously still have the right to have services provided for them. Fortunately, the voice of such users is now being heard through research projects and other avenues. Coral Brown's study of child-abusing parents (Brown, 1985) is an important step in the right direction because it records the complexity of feelings that such parents have, but clearly Lorion's ideas about therapist preparation are very useful once again because they offer a model for how therapist training can be utilized in helping professionals be positive to users that are so easy to reject.

Needless to say, therapist support systems play a decisive role in helping professionals working with users who seemed to have behaved so inhumanly. Only an intensely therapist-friendly system can possibly help therapists cope with the stresses and strains of working with such users. So we return once again to a previous guideline which insists that user-friendliness is predicated on therapist-friendliness.

CONCLUSION

It will be clear from the way we have presented our guidelines that some are more clearly elaborated than others. This reflects the state of our knowledge and experience at this time but we freely admit that a great deal of extra work needs to be undertaken if these guidelines are to have real flesh on their bones. We hope they do provide a good enough starting framework for guiding user-friendly practice but, obviously, there is an invitation to you as a reader to see whether they make sense to you. In our next, and final, chapter, Sigurd will attempt to illustrate several facets of his user-friendly informed practice. We hope these examples will provide some flesh to the bones that we have outlined in this chapter.

Chapter 13

Bringing it back home

Putting a user-friendly perspective into practice

Sigurd Reimers

In Chapter 12 we attempted to draw the threads together from the previous chapters by discussing a series of guidelines which help translate our ideas about user-friendliness into a framework for practice. In this chapter we carry this process a step further by looking at several facets of therapy which we have attempted to change using our user-friendly framework. What we shall be describing is not a new model of therapy: it is more a shift in emphasis – a new stance which seeks to place the user–therapist alliance at the centre of therapeutic work.

PLANNING FIRST MEETINGS

Before planning therapy with a particular family, therapists are confronted by problems of defining what constitutes the 'family' for the purposes of therapy. In individual therapy it may be relatively easy to define who the user is, but in family therapy we are likely to be working from our own definitions of the 'family' before we even begin the convening process. For example, we have already seen that the ideal of the nuclear family, consisting of two parents caring for their own 'natural' children, is still a strong one. It is an ideal towards which many people, who feel that they have failed in establishing a 'proper' family, still aspire.

A user-friendly family therapist who is planning to start work with a new family needs to face these delicate issues early on if she is to be able to form a sensitive therapeutic alliance with the family. There is also, of course, a question of anti-discriminatory practice. If a therapist's assumptions about the 'family' are too limited (perhaps by being determined by a professional middle-class point of view), she may impose a practice which undermines the confidence of already vulnerable people, and which may be insensitive to the values of the family's wider community.

When I was working as part of a family therapy team in South Wales, a colleague was about to start working with the Morgan family, where Robert, aged 8, was referred because of behaviour problems. Robert was living with his father and stepmother and it seemed obvious to invite the household to attend the first session, and to bear in mind the possibility of at some stage contacting Robert's mother who had left the home some years earlier. We nearly overlooked the importance of grandmothers within Welsh culture, and it later turned out that Robert's paternal grandmother was a central figure in this family, even though she did not live in the same house. In fact, Robert had spent a significant part of his childhood living with his grandparents, and his father deferred to and depended on his own mother as far as many domestic matters were concerned.

My example is a fairly obvious one, but it is easy to undermine people by overlooking the definitions of 'family' which users themselves hold.

Although she needs to be keenly in tune with users' own definitions of the 'family', there may be times when the therapist feels she needs to argue in favour of excluding some members from family interviews (e.g. fathers who have sexually abused their children), or to include others (e.g. parents who, following divorce and remarriage, are no longer part of their children's family life, but are still sorely missed by them). A user-friendly family therapist has constantly to check her own assumptions about family life, particularly if her own background is different from that of the users with whom she is working.

WHO SHOULD COME TO THE MEETING? ISSUES IN CONVENING

Theories of family therapy commonly assert that problems occur and are defined within certain systems. The definition of these systems themselves may change over time, and the composition of therapeutic interviews may reflect this process. It is usual to invite the 'family' to the first meeting, but initial conversation with the convened family members often opens up the possibility of discussing who it would make most sense to work with subsequently.

Users can therefore be immediately included in the process of defining and planning the therapy from the start. What has tended to happen in family therapy is that therapists have often restricted their interviews to certain conventional combinations, whilst ignoring other unconventional ones which might open very different therapeutic possibilities. A particular difficulty arises when certain problems become seen as related to, or a property of, particular types of family. Terms like 'enmeshment', 'conflict avoidance' and 'disengagement' have been useful within structural family therapy in helping to make sense of family problems, but have had the disadvantage of stereotyping families, as both feminists and second-order therapists have pointed out. Indeed Anderson and Goolishian (1988) have gone so far as to suggest that there is no natural or obvious system for treatment – it is something that must be negotiated and renegotiated throughout therapy. The problem-determined system, as they call it, is viewed as a constantly changing system. Conceptually, the term has the advantage of reducing the risk of typecasting families because it insists on including a variety of both family and professional systems within its remit. So how do we know or decide which is the appropriate system to be working with? We can start in a fairly standard way, by inviting the users' household and begin the discussion with whoever turns up.

We can write an open invitation, suggesting that whoever would like comes to the first session. I have found that, when possible, telephoning can be a particularly good way of starting the discussion about the most appropriate system to be working with, despite the limitations of the telephone in only being able to talk to one person at a time.

> Harry, aged 4, was referred by his mother because she was worried about his angry and withdrawn behaviour following his parents' separation. One of my hunches was that Harry was responding to the disruptiveness and competition in the adults' relationship. I thought it might be helpful to bring the adults together in order to discuss how they could handle their child care arrangements in a more harmonious way. When I raised this possibility with Harry's mother on the phone, she said that she preferred to come on her own. When asked whether she was willing to bring the children, she replied that they already had enough worries without having to come to the Centre. Some years ago I would probably have regarded this as a sign of over-protectiveness on the part of the mother, but I went along with her idea. In due course I did meet the father, and Harry's mother later asked that the children come along for a meeting as well.

Varying the interview composition can also give family members and the therapist opportunities to have a greater variety of experiences, and this variety in itself can contribute to the process of change. Harry's mother, for example, had come across as a dignified and rather aloof person in her individual sessions, but had seemed much more uncertain when her children were present. This difference later formed a useful basis for further discussion with her. As we saw in our research, users are frequently appreciative of variations in interview composition. More often than not I will now interview family members in different combinations – sometimes a child alone, parents on their own, separated parents, the whole household, as well as occasionally friends and extended family. Users seem to enjoy the possibilities generated by these variations, and they seem to like reflecting about earlier types of interview. In particular I have found that a feedback session is often a good way of making links between individual work with children, sessions with parents, and family sessions. I have many good experiences of feedback sessions with parents about issues which their children have raised in individual sessions and are willing for me to share with their parents.

Using material from earlier individual sessions is, of course, a way of working with which educational psychologists are familiar. Because their work is largely concerned with the assessment of children, it is important that, if they use a family approach, they are clearly seen by users to be operating within clear agency boundaries and focusing on the child. Robert Ziffer (1985) found that 'peripheral' fathers became more willing to attend test sessions when they were unwilling to attend therapy sessions. He goes on to say that he uses the feedback session, and not the test report, as the major vehicle for discussing assessments and plans. This would seem to have an added empowering effect in that it involves users more actively as participants in a discussion, rather than forcing them into the role of bemused bystanders.

As a footnote to my discussion, it is worth adding that Andy's practice is slightly different. Working mostly with adolescents, he shares my policy of trying to phone the family at first point of contact, but he usually suggests that parents of the adolescent are present at the first interview (which can be at a clinic or at home). Meeting the parent or parents alone creates a different message from meeting the family for the first time. It helps to build the therapeutic alliance with the parents and creates a much safer place for a basic discussion of the difficulties the family faces. Many parents feel either guilty about, or beleaguered by, their children, so a supportive interview aimed at exploring possible contracts usually helps to engage the parent(s) more successfully.

Such a policy has its disadvantages in that there is a risk that the children in the family will feel that the therapist is too much aligned with the parents but, if staffing allows, another therapist can be assigned in order to undertake sessions with the adolescent (and his or her siblings). This therapist can then act as the advocate for the children in conjoint sessions – helping create a model of working which relies on a great deal of negotiation between parents and adolescents, facilitated by the therapists.

ENGAGING WITH THE FAMILY

It is rare for therapists to be the first port of call when families have difficulties, so it is very important that we acknowledge the part played by other professionals. Family members are likely to approach family therapy with assumptions based on experiences of other types of help and on the accounts of other people about what constitutes family therapy. Even in agencies where referrals are only accepted if they are made with the consent of users, many users feel pushed into accepting help.

> In Chapter 7 we looked at the responses from Mr and Mrs Jones, who were foster carers and had been referred by their social worker because of the difficulties they had been having with their foster son Tom.
>
> The social worker had worried that Mr and Mrs Jones might be handling Tom inappropriately, and they had reluctantly agreed to the referral. They had felt unable to tell their social worker that they did not want any help, and they explained this to the therapist. They said that, although they were indeed having difficulties with Tom, they did think that they could handle him without any outside help. This basic difference of opinion might have taken longer to surface, if at all, had the therapist not explored carefully with the foster carers what they had thought of the referral and what earlier experiences they had had of professional help.

We have had many experiences where such exploratory first sessions have turned out to be the only ones, because the users were not really wanting help at the time.

Some of these users, having had their reluctance respected, would later return of their own accord. As Diana Merrington and John Corden found in their own consumer study: 'On the basis of the recollection of these families, the weakest link seems to be the referring agent' (Merrington and Corden, 1981, p. 258). Even where users do not have a major concern about the referral, I would always try and ask them what sense they had made of the referral and what picture they had been given of the agency by the referrer.

I assume that users – no less than therapists – hypothesize both about their problems and about therapy, and I like to ask them what their particular theories or hunches are about the problem. It is not unusual for me to arrive at roughly similar hypotheses to those of users. Sometimes when we do not, we can discuss the relative merits of our different hypotheses. It is not often that I hold a hypothesis that I would find it hard to share with a user, and so I enter my hypotheses in the case notes, knowing that these are available for users to see, should they wish to.

I think that the traditional brief therapy format is a neat way of validating users' own accounts of their difficulties. It is a good way of starting from where the users are, particularly by asking the four basic questions:

> What does each of you think the problem is?
> For whom, and in what way, is it a problem?
> What have you tried to do about the problem?
> What were the results of these attempts?

I often then go on to ask about other experiences of help:

> What advice or help have friends or relatives offered you?
> What has been your experience of other agencies?

As a result of the discussion which follows we may agree that other people should be invited to subsequent meetings. Often, as we have seen, users come with clear ideas about what kind of help they are seeking, but sometimes these ideas develop later. I therefore like to ask in the first session whether there is a particular type of help they are seeking, and in later sessions I may ask what thoughts they are now having about the kind of help they would like.

> This was particularly important for Mrs Wilford, who had been referred by her ex-husband because of Jonathan's misery at home. Jonathan lived with his mother, and although she did not feel that there really was a problem, she agreed to the referral. A plan for working together was agreed upon, but it became clear to me after one session that Mrs Wilford was unhappy about the arrangements. When asked about what thoughts she had had since last time about what she wanted from therapy, she replied that she had come to realize how disappointed she was in therapy, and how she had felt manipulated into it by her ex-husband. It now became important to discuss her expectations about therapy fully enough for her to feel comfortable about returning in the future should she wish to.

Users' experiences of therapy vary very markedly, as our research has demonstrated, so it is crucial to keep monitoring these experiences. I therefore like to ask users before the end of the first interview, as well as at other times, what their experience of the session has been like. Again, the question is intended to convey the idea that this is an important issue for me. The answers can also provide feedback about whether to change the format of therapy. Therapy does not necessarily finish when the session ends, and I like to use as a resource any discussions about therapy which may have taken place at home. I often ask users what conversations they have had at home about the last session, what they talk about in the car going home, who reminds the rest of the family that it is time to come to the Centre, and so on.

> The sessions with Angela, aged 16 (who suffered from anorexia nervosa), her mother and younger brother, Mark, were becoming stale, and Angela was quietly angry with my co-therapy colleague and me for making a lot of fuss about her weight loss. Both Angela and her mother seemed to be wondering what the point of having family sessions was, and there seemed to be an unbridgeable gulf between us and the family members.
>
> I commented that we didn't seem to be getting very far and wondered what they used to say about therapy after the sessions. Quick as a flash, Angela commented, 'We talk about the colour of your socks, actually, and wonder which jazzy pair you will be wearing next time.'
>
> The focus on the therapist–user relationship contributed to a different atmosphere and to a more open discussion of the problems which the family were facing in attending the sessions.

QUESTIONS AND ANSWERS

Questions form a central feature of most therapies, and in family therapy they have been developed, as we have seen, to a very refined level, particularly under the influence of the Milan and post-Milan approaches. Karl Tomm reminds us that a therapist's questions may not be as open as they seem:

> To ask a particular question, then, is to invite a particular answer. The kinds of questions a therapist chooses to ask depend on what kinds of answers the therapist would like to have heard.
>
> (Tomm, 1988, p. 14)

A user-friendly isssue is: what sense does the user make not just of the particular questions being asked, but also of the questioning process itself? A member of one of the families we were recently working with summarized our approach as 'nothing but questions, bloody questions'. As Merrington and Corden claim, users also want something else:

> Some families would have liked clearer information about how the workers themselves viewed the problem . . . could clearer feedback be given without

undermining the family's responsibility? . . . Most families . . . seemed to have assumed that the worker had a hidden purpose which she would share with them afterwards, and a few families felt 'cheated' when this did not happen.

(Merrington and Corden, 1981, p. 259)

Custom-building therapy may therefore involve a subtle combination of questions, comments, reflections and advice, and we will now look at some of these in greater detail.

Future perspectives

An essential part of forming and sustaining the therapeutic alliance is to focus on here-and-now issues and concrete behaviour. However, an exclusive focus on detailed problems and continually going over the same ground can contribute to defensiveness, a sense of blame and despondency. A future orientation can, by contrast, help both users and therapists develop new and creative ideas, providing users do not feel lost in the process. As Luigi Boscolo and Paolo Bertrando explain:

Clients undergoing therapy almost always have a linear conception of time, a 'historical' conception according to which the past determines the present and imposes insuperable constraints on the future. We, on the contrary, look first at the meanings and actions created in the present; after that, we may work on their past. The relations between past and present start to change because they are seen from a different point of view. Once the norms of necessity are relaxed, it is possible to introduce the future as hypothesis, possibility, eventuality.

(Boscolo and Bertrando, 1992, p. 121)

Some questions which I find particularly helpful to use are, 'Can you tell me what life might be like once you have dealt with this problem?' 'Would it take a while before anyone noticed any improvements – would you all know at once?' and 'Supposing you were to look back on this difficult episode in a few years' time, what might you think?' This last question can be useful where children are concerned since it is a reminder to us all that maturation plays its own part in bringing about changes.

Mrs Harris had been having enormous problems with her teenage children Shaun and Maria since she divorced her husband many years earlier. They were disobedient, stayed out late, and occasionally threatened her with violence. During therapy sessions family members continually disagreed about who was responsible for what, and there was a strong sense that nothing would ever change.

Eventually Mrs Harris described a dream she had had for many years about how they should be as a family. After the divorce she had always wanted to sit down with the children for Sunday lunch. This would confirm for her that they were still a family. Following further discussions about how a future involving

Sunday lunch together might look, relationships improved enough for both Mrs Harris and her children to feel that they had made an important achievement, despite all their other problems.

By extending the conversation beyond the immediate problem, family members were able to find a different way of relating to each other and look to the future.

Exceptions to the rule

Another way of helping users out of a narrow portrayal of their problems can be to look for the exception to the rule. Brief solution-focused therapists like Steve de Shazer (1991) encourage users to identify those – possibly very few – occasions where an existing solution has worked, and to build on these successes.

> Julie and Ron had been having marital problems for many years, and Julie had been diagnosed as depressed following the birth of their first child. Their day-to-day conflicts had become so predictable to them that they would frequently yawn with boredom as each recounted the other's latest faults.
>
> The one spark of hope for Julie seemed to occur on the rare occasions when Ron accurately guessed how she might be feeling, and for Ron when she was more explicit about what was on her mind. They had hardly been aware of these exceptions until they were talked about in therapy. They turned out to be important beginnings to change, because previously Julie had insisted that Ron's concern for her was only valid if he was willing to guess without being told. By the same token Ron would only be sympathetic if Julie told him clearly what was troubling her. Further discussion of what had been a strongly gendered way of relating enabled them for the first time in years to see each other in a different light.

Whilst such a focus on positives clearly has its user-friendly aspects, if applied routinely, it runs the risk of not seeming to take the user's problems or concerns seriously.

Externalizing the problem

The Australian family therapist Michael White (1989) has helped pioneer the idea of 'externalizing' the problem. This process involves attributing to the identified problem a separate existence which enables people to blame each other less and instead to join forces and form a coalition against the problem 'out there' and so reduce a sense of blame.

Michael White and David Epston (1990) and Terry Heins (1988) give many delightful examples of children and their parents fighting together against 'Sneaky Poo', 'Slippery Mouth', 'Tricky Wee' and other mythical creatures which burden the lives of parents and children who are struggling with each other over troubles like soiling, swearing, bedwetting and so on.

This approach requires users to be willing to make a playful leap in their imagination at the same time as feeling that both they and their concerns are being taken seriously by the therapist. However, it would be inadvisable to use this approach where, as in child abuse or marital violence, it is important to help users take more (and not less) personal responsibility for their own behaviour. Nevertheless, there are many ways in which externalizing of the problem can also be helpful in work with adults.

> Rita was diagnosed as suffering from occasional psychotic outbursts and these would sometimes lead to hospitalization. She was also strongly rejecting her 10-year-old son Luke, because she had always wanted a girl. After seeing a video recording of an earlier session, she suddenly came to realize that the legacy of this rejection went back to seeing her own mother on her death-bed. Her mother had told Rita, who was pregnant with Luke at the time, that she was going to give birth to a daughter. After this dramatic recollection, she began to place this previously forgotten, but overwhelming, event at a greater distance as something she could with some effort keep 'out there' and separate from the rest of herself.

Reflecting processes

As Judy Davidson and her colleagues have pointed out, using a reflecting team is less of a method of working and more a different way of thinking about systems. It is also a rather particular way of thinking: 'Rather than providing a framework for clinical neutrality, the reflecting team highlights an awareness of personal subjectivity' (Davidson *et al.*, 1988, p. 76). One principle behind the therapist's offering her subjectivity is to encourage careful listening, on the part of the therapeutic team as well as family members. This is why the team members do not directly address the therapist and family, or vice versa. It is rather like the effect of sending a letter. There is a time lag, there can be no immediate response, what has been said cannot be unsaid, but neither does it have to be commented on. For this reason team members choose their words carefully, especially as they will not have conferred with each other behind the one-way screen before coming into the room. The emphasis on listening and on avoiding direct conversation between the team and the therapist-plus-family is designed to allow for sufficient, but not too much, difference to develop. In this way new ideas can emerge at a pace and in a way decided by family members. These ideas may in turn result in therapeutic change. Tom Andersen (1987) stresses that the format of the session is explained to the family by two members of staff before the session starts, and this allows for family members to ask for a different approach if they wish.

Clearly this is not only a way of thinking. It is also a way of relating to users. From a user-friendly position we are particularly interested in the common description of the method as non-competitive, non-hierarchical, collaborative, and respectful to users. However, for some families the reflecting team will be too 'different', despite its aim at a greater degree of equality. In place of the therapeutic term 'different', we could sometimes substitute more robust words like alarming, intimidating, funny or plain crazy – people's experiences of 'respectfulness' can be very varied.

Despite some personal scepticism, however, I have found the method at times to be both refreshing and creative. Classically (see Andersen, 1987) it involves using a team, a one-way screen with reversible lighting and sound systems. The team and the therapist-plus-family comment on each other's conversations at various points in the session. There are also many other variations. The team may remain in the interview room throughout the session, there may be a single supervisor (see Davidson *et al.*, 1988), or the therapist may work entirely on her own (see Finn Wangberg, 1991), thinking aloud at various points or talking to no one in particular. The reflecting team or reflecting process allows for users to receive feedback from their therapists or, as one user said to Tom Andersen's team: 'We were wondering what you behind the screen were thinking about us. Now we know.'

For my own part I tend to use a reflecting process as part of live supervision in the room. This allows the session to flow with fewer disruptions and possibly makes it easier for family members to ask directly for our opinions. It also allows for the demystification of the supervisor, who can occasionally relate directly to family members, and at the end allows us to ask questions such as, 'What has it felt like talking with us like this today?'

I usually work as part of a male-female twosome, and I have also found other varieties of reflective processes useful.

Norma and Martin had been coming to therapy sessions for some time. Norma had a severe alcohol problem, and Martin, who was a transport driver, never felt that he could trust Norma to be alone at home, and made sure that one of their children was always at home with her. We had been using live super-vision in the room, including reflecting back to each other and to the family members. We suspected that Martin was occasionally violent to Norma, and we knew that Norma had been beaten up by their 18-year-old son Paul, apparently with the connivance of his father. Norma was largely silent during the sessions, and seemed to feel very blamed. My female colleague suggested to Norma that they both go and sit behind the one-way screen whilst I had a conversation with Martin and Paul about violence towards women.

After a period of time the two women returned to the interview room and discussed what they had heard, in the presence of the men. My colleague and I then discussed other aspects of the session, this time in front of the family. This replaced our usual practice of leaving the room for our mid-session discussion. Not surprisingly, what had been a stale and predictable session had become much more creative, not least by helping the weakest member, Norma, find her own 'voice'.

Educational approaches

We have already mentioned some of the limitations of the patient management or psychoeducational approach, which involves helping family members, through careful coaching, to avoid expressing feelings of blame and hostility towards the family member who has been labelled 'schizophrenic'. There is, of course, always a risk of stigmatizing the 'identified patient' within this approach, but the method can be an effective way of helping family members create clearer boundaries and deal with negative feelings in a more constructive way. The approach has been extended into other areas, such as adolescent anorexia (le Grange, *et al.*, 1992) and children's behaviour problems (Vostanis *et al.*, 1992). Information giving (and educational techniques in general) have a very clear place in user-friendly practice. Because users easily feel blamed when they are seeking help, a supportive educational approach can sometimes work best.

A fair percentage of my caseload involves working with stepfamilies where children are displaying behaviour problems. Such behaviour is commonly explained as a response to difficulties in accepting new, and letting go of old, parent figures. In fact, this and other similar hypotheses are so commonly accepted that the Stepfamilies Association has produced a number of booklets for helping people with the process of making a new family. I frequently lend stepfamilies leaflets or books which can allow them to relate to sometimes challenging ideas without having to feel confronted by a therapist as well. Reading or listening to other people's accounts can feel an acceptable way to many users of normalizing a problem and not feeling blamed, as group workers will testify, and literature or tapes can be used for a wide range of concerns. Similar positive experiences have been noted by families with disabled children, and the Ready to Play booklets, published by the National Toy Libraries Association, are an example of a down-to-earth, non-threatening and non-patronizing approach.

> Mrs Johnson had been lent the book *Stepmothering* (Donna Smith, 1990), and had found it useful in dealing with her very lonely position. In many ways, however, she had found her own situation quite different, and my discussion with her provided a good basis for developing new ideas. She was asked in what way her situation was different from those described in the book, and what ideas she would add if *she* were writing the book.
>
> Did she think that there were other ways of being a stepmother? Did one ever stop being a stepmother? What differences were there in her mind between being a stepmother and being a 'natural' father? I also gave my own comments on the subject, and shared some views which I had heard expressed by other users. As we will see in a later section, questions about gender rarely fail to raise interest and energy.

This last case is perhaps a good example of how a relatively normative, educational approach can be combined with the more open-ended format of circular questioning which allows for users to find and express their own meanings and opinions. The user-friendly aspect of this is constantly to search for, even experiment with, ways of helping users make sense of what is happening to them and which allow a strong sense of co-working to emerge.

Using authority

So far I may have painted a picture of a user-friendly therapy as a respectful venture, where the therapist is careful always to work co-operatively with the family. This does not mean that the therapist will always agree with family members. Indeed, there may well be times when she has to act in clear opposition to their stated wishes. The challenge in such situations is to try and relate in a way that allows for the therapeutic alliance to be maintained.

> I was working the Walton family because Mary and Keith were concerned about Simon's sleeping problems and bedtime routine. Simon was 8 and had a sister Penny, aged 6, and a brother Kenneth, 2. Keith had been unemployed for a few years and was being treated for depression. Most of the day-to-day parenting fell to Mary. Both the management of the problem and the communication between family members were improving, when Mary mentioned that on one occasion recently Keith had been heavy-handed with Simon, and this had resulted in Simon's being thrown across a room and hitting the wall. It was only later in the session that I reacted to this statement, largely thanks to my supervisor, and explained that I would have to inform the Social Services. The parents were understandably alarmed at this, and we spent the rest of the session discussing how we could best continue working together once the incident had been investigated.
>
> I posed a number of questions:
>
> Would they ever trust me again?
> What would Keith say to Mary after they had returned home?
> What were their worst fears now?
> How could they now find confidence to deal firmly with bedtime routines?
>
> After the episode had been promptly and efficiently investigated I made sure to have an immediate telephone conversation with Keith to emphasize my opinion about the importance, as I saw it, of our continuing our work together. Mary and Keith did return for further work, and the therapeutic relationship continued, if anything on a more realistic basis than before. Violence was now clearly on the agenda, and our discussions included Mary's previously unacknowledged fear of Keith.

This example is quoted as an antidote to the understandable concern therapists sometimes have about damaging the relationship with users by challenging them about socially unacceptable behaviour. Quite apart from the enormous risks of keeping information about dangerous situations to oneself, we doubt whether a therapeutic alliance based on collusiveness is any alliance at all.

Women, men and children

In Chapter 11 we argued that as family therapists, we need to 'bring power into the room' (see Williams and Watson, 1988) by considering the effects of gender, age, race, class, sexuality, disability and other inequalities in power within relationships. We can do this by referring to 'power' in our hypotheses, in our questions and statements, and in any representations we make to other agencies.

Power affects therapy both directly and indirectly. When it is indirect, it is often invisible and taken for granted. We can help to make power more visible if we as therapists become more aware of how it is manifested at various levels. These may be listed as follows:

1 Inequalities based on dominant discourses (powerful and widely held beliefs)
2 Inequalities based on the practice of agencies
3 Inequalities within families
4 Inequalities amongst family members in therapy sessions
5 Inequalities between therapist/team members and family members

The therapeutic alliance always contains some imbalance in power, and for family therapists it is further complicated by the fact that there is seldom one user and also because the 'membership' of the user-system can change in the course of therapy. Having worked within a mixed gender team in various child-focused agencies, I have become impressed by how hard it is for us, even as sophisticated and sensitive therapists, to achieve a gender and generation balance in our thinking when we are dealing with a number of users at the same time. Superficially it would understandable if female therapists spent more time listening to female users and showed more interest in 'women's issues' and if male therapists did the same with men. But the reality is not so simple. Even when speaking to men, male therapists are likely to show more interest in 'women's issues' in the questions they ask and the comments they make. Also, many female therapists, aware of some men's tenuous links with therapy and eager to make *family* therapy work, may bend over backwards to give men positive attention and make them comfortable in therapy. Either way it is easy for us to lose that delicate balance, and be seen as taking sides. A user-friendly perspective may encourage us to deal with these dilemmas by bringing them into the open. I will give four brief case examples of situations which have brought therapist and users together in considering gender issues within therapy.

> Jonathan was 14, and his arguments with his mother were becoming more acrimonious, resulting in threats of violence towards her. Mrs Thompson, who was a single mother, saw 12-year-old Patricia as much easier to relate to, although there was a magnetic quality to the arguments between mother and son which tended to leave Patricia on the sidelines. In a family session, following a particularly heated but predictable exchange between Jonathan and his mother, I asked Patricia, 'Do you think it makes a difference whether you are a man or a woman in your family?' At this point Patricia, who had

been largely silent during the two family sessions, turned on her mother and brother and accused them of always leaving her out of important discussions because they thought the views of girls were less important than those of boys.

In a later individual session, Mrs Thompson and I were looking back at our work together, and I asked Mrs Thompson, 'Do you think there is a woman's point of view in all this?' She replied, 'I think it is easier for a woman to understand. But it was good to see you and Rose [the consultant in the family sessions] disagree – that clinched it for me.'

A similar question was posed to the Macmillan family:

Dorothy and Helen were a lesbian couple, who were concerned about Helen's son John, aged 12, who was constantly stealing at home. Helen's teenage daughters, Gemma and Tina, also attended a family session. The situation had been so bad that John had spent a short period with foster carers. Gemma and Tina sat looking glum as John's latest thefts were being recounted. I asked, 'What's the difference between being a woman and a man in this situation?' Both girls immediately sat up and joined in the conversation. It was as if gender could be discussed as a common, even unifying theme, whereas the theft was John's problem.

Addressing gender, then, helps the therapist move from very specific to more global issues.

Frank suffered from repeated episodes of manic-depressive psychosis. Carol, his wife, had a mild learning disability and was said to have difficulties controlling their 4-year-old daughter Karen. During a couples session following a recent hospital stay, I was talking to Frank:

Therapist:	Why did your wife suggest that you should be discharged from hospital?
Frank:	She needed help with Karen.
Therapist:	Why else do you think?
Frank:	Because she couldn't cope.
Therapist:	Frank, why else might a woman want her husband discharged?
Frank:	Because she missed me.

Frank had come across as a man who was locked in his view of women as not competent at disciplining children, and afraid to admit his need for affection. The move to a more global approach allowed these issues to be addressed.

In a case of suspected sexual abuse I was talking with Mr and Mrs Appleby (who had brought their two boys and two girls to the session) about 14-year-old Hilary's recent tendency to mix with much older boys and to stay out late at night. They had just talked about 17-year-old Bernadette, who used to do the same but had now stopped, and I then asked a question which produced an unexpected answer:

> *Therapist:*   Is it a coincidence that when Hilary took over the disruptive
> role from Bernadette, as Mrs Appleby has just explained, it was
> a case of girl following girl, rather than the two boys?
> *Mr Appleby:*   Are you suggesting that I sexually abused them?
> *Mrs Appleby:* I have been told I've failed so many times.

This striking interchange illustrates – perhaps in an extreme way – some fairly classic
differences between men and women which may emerge when sexual abuse is even
hinted at. Put simply, the man feels accused, and the woman feels a failure.

What do these brief episodes have in common? They all occurred at a point
where therapy was progressing in a conventional manner. There had been a
substantial focus on the fine details of the problem which had brought the users
to therapy. The discussion about gender had the effect of a surge of energy
flowing into family relationships which were in many ways unequal, strongly
gendered and, not least, taken for granted. Therapy can, of course, never totally
rely on moments of inspiration, but it is striking how much interest in these
gender issues I have found even amongst users where I would not have expected
to find it.

In Chapter 11 we saw how feminist authors have challenged family therapy
practice by highlighting some of the difficulties women experience, not only at
home, but also in therapy. These difficulties may relate to being overlooked,
being held responsible for home and family, and feeling a failure when problems
occur. The problems for men in therapy tend to be different. Many men feel
uncomfortable in what they see as a woman's world, have difficulties in expressing themselves in words, and feel superfluous at home. A user-friendly therapist
who is aware of these issues will want to connect with both women and men by
understanding the particular gendered vulnerabilities and strengths of each. For
men, an emphasis on their strengths could involve greater attention to the world
of work, sport and hobbies, and the personal relationships that are linked (or not
linked) with these, although many men (and women) will have poor experiences
of work, either because of unemployment or because their work is menial or
demeaning. It seems to us that being user-friendly involves focusing on the
unique as well as on the universal in each situation. This means that our own
assumptions about gender differences, however subtle, should be checked by
discussing them with our users.

Children and adolescents also present challenges to do with power because of
their vulnerable position in the family. Family therapy, like most therapies, relies
heavily on words, and a user-friendly therapist will need to pay careful attention
to conducting sessions involving children in such a way that children can be
helped both to understand and contribute to therapy in their own particular way.

This is where using a variety of interview compositions may be helpful. We
know that parents often want to be seen on their own, partly because they feel
protective of their children and self-conscious about talking about problems in

front of them, and partly because young children can easily become bored and distracting during adult conversations. When meeting with parents on their own, numerous writers, including notably Ellen Wachtel (1987, 1990), warn against too readily making hypotheses that assume marital problems 'underlying' a child's behaviour problem. Similarly she urges therapists to avoid usurping the position of parents when interviewing children on their own. Nevertheless she sees great value in having some individual sessions with children. Ron Taffel (1991) suggests that some children will not talk about their anxieties in family sessions as readily as when they are seen on their own.

> Nine-year-old Daniel had been referred because of spiteful behaviour towards his younger sister Sarah. His mother suffered from multiple sclerosis, and his father was frantically busy both at home and at work. A family session revealed that Daniel was regarded by his parents as having few redeeming features, and he was largely silent throughout. In an individual session he talked readily about his shock at finding his grandmother dead on the floor some years earlier, and he thought that there was something he should have done to save her life. Daniel was happy for this to be discussed with his parents during a feedback session with them. His parents initially saw Daniel's account as overdramatized, and I had to restrain myself with difficulty from simply becoming Daniel's ally and arguing with the parents.
>
> In a later family session, which used drawings to show how children can understand and express feelings, the parents became more sympathetic as they saw for themselves how much thought Daniel had given to the problems they were experiencing as a family.

Children of all ages can make major contributions to family sessions, but Wachtel (1987) argues that family therapists may unwittingly be guilty of child neglect in their attitude to children's problems.

Joan Zilbach claims that the reason family therapists often feel discomfort at involving children in therapy may be the fact that 'few family therapy training programs actually teach or even discuss playing with children in family therapy'. She continues:

> Play is regarded as 'serious business' by family therapists who do include children in their family therapy sessions. When children are included in family sessions, therapists watch carefully, join, and, through the observation of play, drawing, bodily movement, and other actions, gain further understanding of children and their families which becomes therapeutically useful.
>
> (Zilbach, 1986, pp. 16–17)

In my own practice I try to start as I wish to continue, by making sure that children have some understanding, either from their parents if possible, or from myself, of why they have been brought and what they may expect of therapy. I will also try and bridge the adult and child world, as the following example illustrates.

Kevin Evans, aged 8, had been referred because he had twice hit his sister so hard that she had to be seen at the Accident and Emergency department. Mrs Evans, who was a single mother, felt responsible for these incidents, and thought that Kevin's behaviour was caused by the divorce, which she had initiated.

She regarded him as an unexpressive boy, just like the other men in her family. Kevin sat impassively as his mother continued to talk about how she was trying to understand his behaviour. Both Kevin and Sian came alive when I started drawing faces and asking the children what feelings the faces expressed. As the faces became more ambiguous, some guessing was called for as well as some discussion of the differences of opinion. In due course the children were urged to draw their own faces and to guess what feelings the other had intended to convey. At various points I turned to Mrs Evans to check what her perception of the whole process was, and to seek help from her in making connections back to the problem which had brought them to therapy.

Sometimes I will go on to discuss possible alternative scenarios for the future, or, if the subject seems too provocative, I may use the FIAT (Family Interaction Apperception Test) pictures to start a discussion. These are a series of drawings of ambiguous family situations devised by Salvador Minuchin *et al.* (1967), originally for assessment purposes, but which are equally suitable as a safe method for starting a family conversation about emotive subjects.

Structural family therapists have, of course, used action-based techniques like genograms, sculpts and circularity drawings, which can help family members, both children and adults, explore new ways of looking at old problems. Similarly, therapists like Lee Combrinck-Graham (1991), who follow a more Milan-systemic approach, have refined circular questioning to relate to children's natural curiosity. In the end, what makes any of this user-friendly is not child-centredness in itself, since this can alienate the adults, but a careful regard for the experiences of the therapy on the part of all the family members at various times, including a consideration of power issues. We can then help custom-build the therapy on the basis of these experiences and considerations.

Cameras, teams and screens

The use of the video and one-way screen has been the cause of so much criticism and suspicion from users that one may wonder what scope there still is left for a user-friendly therapist to continue using them. Indeed the criticism does not only come from users. Ben Furman (1990) refers to the one-way screen as a barrier and a *cordon sanitaire*.

As we have seen in Chapter 9 Mashal *et al.* (1989) summarized some users' views about the 'impenetrability of the group behind the mirror', and Jay Efran and Leslie Clarfield (1992) wondered whether this and other technical procedures may be regarded by future generations as quaint practices akin to blood-letting. Kristen Diethelm *et al.* (1992) describe the more authentic encounter with the family they experience when the team remains in the interview room. Perhaps such a backlash is to be expected in view of the rather remote and controlling legacy of family therapy, epitomized by the notable advocate of the one-way screen, Peggy Papp, who argued that the team should remain 'at a distance, an invisible eye, an anonymous voice, lending the impact of objectivity' (Papp, 1980, p. 49).

Yet the argument is not a simple one from a user-friendly point of view. Jeffrey Kassis and William Matthews, who themselves have considerable reservations about the use of the screen, remind us of its benefits, for the therapist of having a safe learning environment which provides an important meta-position, and for the user of having his or her need for maintaining stability validated. Taking as their starting point – in their words – the therapeutic alliance, they claim that the risk of using the one-way screen is that it can be invasive in cases of sexual abuse, and also difficult for other people who feel particularly victimized or powerless. As they conclude, 'our clients who have had these experiences view the mirror as symbolic of having little control over their lives' (Kassis and Matthews, 1987, p. 39).

The authors recognize that there are advantages and disadvantages, and make a habit of asking users the simple question, 'How do you feel about our using the one-way mirror?' Some of their users prefer to proceed without it, but others say that they want the team to remain behind the screen, some even saying that they do not want to meet the team. If we accept that users do not always quite confirm our favourite theories, we should avoid the enthusiastic but extravagant one-sidedness of Furman, who will at times have between 20 and 50 observers in the room with the family. He makes the staggering claim that, 'A crowd makes no noticeable difference in the clients' reactions to the sessions' (Furman, 1990, p. 62).

In my own practice, I will explain to family members, before asking for consent, that in my view an advantage of the screen can be that it is often more effective if the supervisor or team is thinking about our conversation but in another room. With children I will sometimes draw the distinction between the 'talking room' and the 'thinking room'. In fact, children (and their parents) often want to see the observation room and meet the team, and this is usually suggested by the therapist anyway. I highlight the personal nature of supervision whether it involves the screen or not. The mixed gender nature of the team encourages us to reflect closely amongst ourselves and with our users about gender variables within the family and the team. Also, if a member of the team has a child of a similar age to one in the family, this may be mentioned as part of exploring similarities and differences.

There have also been times when it has been extremely helpful for a member of the team to join in the session with the therapist. On a few occasions when I have been acting as supervisor to a female colleague, I have been introduced to the family and later conducted individual sessions with a teenage boy who is finding it hard relating to a woman. There are, of course, many other possible useful variations which can make sensitive use of the team, but it is important in such cases to maintain clear communications with one's colleague and not create a competitive or confusing situation.

The attitude of the team is a crucial one, and is one which must be carefully checked. Tom Andersen issues a warning: 'The screen (the process of observing) tends to magnify criticisms of the "why-did-they-do-this-or-that" category' (Andersen, 1987, p. 424).

Kassis and Matthews (1987) found that team members were more empathic when they were in the interview room, and, in a similar vein, Diethelm *et al.* claimed that, 'Since we are all in the same room at the same time, there is an opportunity to more genuinely feel the pain and the perspective of the family' (Diethelm *et al.*, 1992, p. 50). We may debate whether feeling other people's pain is always the most important task of the team, but a user-friendly therapist need not make a once-and-for-all decision about the use of the screen. Rather, she bears in mind that users' experiences of therapy may change radically with time, and methods of work may need to be openly reviewed at various times.

Many of the considerations that we have referred to in relation to the one-way screen also apply to the video. The use of video has been criticized as intrusive and threatening, as we can understand from a strategy advocated by Peggy Papp of 'leaving the video camera running [during the session break] to record the family interaction' (Papp, 1980, p. 51). A more open practice need be no less effective therapeutically, but raises the question of our reasons for observing the tapes. If we regard families and therapists less as parties to a struggle and more as people with whom we are co-constructing new realities, narratives or solutions, then the purpose behind the use of video is likely to be different. Why not make the recording part of the process of co-construction? There are a number of ways I currently attempt to do this. The first is to discuss video excerpts which I have reviewed between sessions with family members. I might say that I was struck, moved or confused by part of the previous session and asked family members whether they had any thoughts about it. I might also share some thoughts of mine about it – rather in the style of a reflecting team.

The second approach involves suggesting to the family members that we review a piece of tape together. Sometimes the effect can be emotional, as in the case of Rita on p. 230, amusing or thought-provoking. As the idea of co-construction is an important one for me, I may discuss my own part in the process being reviewed, unless this seems intrusive, and ask for comments. The tape can sometimes be embarrassing for the therapist, as it can be for users, but the learning points, as Nancy Boyd-Franklin (1989) suggests in relation to the development of an anti-racist practice, can be very immediate and lead to a greater sense of levelling with family members.

Members of the Thompson family were interested in seeing some excerpts from earlier sessions before concluding therapy. At the end of seeing the episode described on p. 234, there was a long silence before Mrs Thompson, who was not in the habit of praising anyone, said slowly that she had never realized how wise her children were and wished she could show the excerpt to other family members.

A third way I use video feedback is to start a recording with the shared intention of reviewing it later in the same session. This can be particularly useful for users who are practising new ways of relating to each other in the session, and can help the therapist avoid quick interpretations and taking sides.

> Joan and Peter had come back together after a period of separation, but were finding it difficult to talk about their continuing problems. Joan, in particular, found Peter's way of dealing with her children 'frankly pathetic', but was unsure about what to say next, as was Peter. As an experiment, they tried a couple of different ways of talking together. They then looked at the video recording and continued their discussion about a joint problem that now had an aspect of being 'out there' as well as being deeply personal.

In this chapter I have looked at some of the issues to do with the use of the one-way screen and video from a user-friendly point of view, but I would not want to conclude without considering working in a simpler way since, as Efran and Clarfield suggest, this 'encourages therapy to go ahead without a clinical cast of thousands, using a therapist, a room, and one or more individuals with problems on their minds' (Efran and Clarfield, 1992, p. 210). I am particularly thinking of home visiting as distinct from the use of screens and video. Although arguments about pressure of time, motivation, distractions, intrusiveness and control of sessions are both familiar and relevant, I have no doubt that there is a case for home visiting as a way of connecting with people whom we might otherwise never meet at an office. Through home visiting, a therapist can gain a completely different view of the family, but most importantly from a user-friendly perspective it can, if acceptable to family members, help towards equalizing the power imbalance between therapist and users. We would not want to draw any general conclusions about the relative merits of office- and home-based interviews, but rather suggest that therapists take the question seriously, and if in doubt, ask the users.

EPILOGUE

In this chapter Sigurd has explored many examples of how his family therapy practice has developed in a user-friendly direction. As a reader you may find this chapter a little frustrating because of its limited comprehensiveness. However, we have been prevented from tackling all the topics we would like because of lack of space and, to be frank, lack of first-hand experience in a number of areas. We are aware that we have not looked in any great detail at a number of issues, such as sexual abuse, violence and suicidal behaviour, which create very testing situations for therapists. We have also only made limited attempts to explore working with families from ethnic minorities.

Clearly our user-friendly ideas need to be elaborated in a number of important areas like these, but we are relatively confident that further work could prove productive in extending this stance, so that it does provide useful and practical ideas that are of benefit to both users and therapists.

Perhaps our book reflects too much the child- and adolescent-focused settings in which we work but we hope its usefulness is not confined to these settings. We are certainly aware that workers in different agencies need to custom-build their work to suit the users who participate in the services they offer. We hope that our user-friendly stance can encompass all settings because it is based on principles which are universal, but we would be the first to acknowledge that the acid test of this statement is in your hands. We would hope that if you have found our ideas interesting and convincing, then you will want to experiment with them yourself. We would be delighted if you would then communicate to us what happens. Writing a book is a frustratingly linear process which forces the reader into adopting a relatively passive position. Hearing from you would be most rewarding for us, so if you have the energy we would like you to contact us at the addresses below. Needless to say, we would welcome your feedback, irrespective of whether you agree with us or not, and irrespective of whether you are a therapist or not.

Contact addresses

Andy Treacher
3 Perkins Village
Farringdon
Exeter
Devon EX5 2JF

Sigurd Reimers
179 Cheddon Road
Taunton
Somerset TA2 7AH

Interview schedule for the Western Wiltshire user study

FIRST SURVEY

Q.1   I know you have had contact recently with the Child and Family Guidance Centre. Can you tell me a little about it?

Q.2   Before you went, can you remember what your feelings were about going?

Q.3   Did anything worry you about going? What was your worst fear?

Q.4   In what ways were you expecting to be helped?

Q.5   Looking back now, how would you describe your feelings about going?

Q.6   Was your experience different from what you expected? Could you say in what ways?

Q.7   Can you say which aspects of going to the Centre were the most valuable?

Q.8   Can you say which aspects of going to the Centre were the least valuable?

Q.9   During the time you attended the Centre, can you remember one thing that was said that was helpful? What was it?

Q.10 During the time you attended the Centre, can you remember one thing that was said that was unhelpful? What was it?

Q.11 Were there times when you felt that the therapy was particularly helpful? Can you give an example?

Q.12 Were there times when you felt that the therapy was particularly unhelpful? Can you give an example?

Q.13 Were you able to let your therapist know if things were going badly? If so, how did you do it?

Q.14 Was the video used during any of your meetings? If so, how was its use explained to you?

Q.15 Why did you think it was being used? How did it make you feel?

Q.16 In what ways, if any, did it seem helpful to use the video?

Q.17 In what ways, if any, did it seem unhelpful to use the video?

Q.18 What are your feelings about the video now?

Q.19 Was the one-way screen used during any of your sessions? If so, how was its use explained to you?

Q.20 Why did you think it was being used? How did it make you feel?

Q.21   In what ways, if any, did it seem helpful to use the one-way screen?

Q.22   In what ways, if any, did it seem unhelpful to use the one-way screen?

Q.23   Can you say briefly what was the problem that brought you to the Centre?

Q.24   Was there another service involved with you over your problem?

Q.25   Who suggested you went to the Centre?

Q.26   How long did you have to wait for your first appointment?

Q.27   Would you have felt able to contact your therapist between appointments if you had needed to?

Q.28   What was happening in your family life at that time which might have affected the problem?

Q.29   Did you feel that your therapist understood your problem?

Q.30   Did you feel that your therapist understood how you felt about your problem?

Q.31   Did your therapist understand how you thought the problem could be helped?

Q.32   Can I ask you about the sex of your therapist? Was the person male or female? Would it have made any difference? Would you have liked to choose your therapist?

Q.33   How did the problem change during the time you were going to the Centre?

Q.34   If a similar problem occurred in your family now, where would you go to get help?

Q.35   Would you recommend the service to anyone else?

Q.36   If so, under what circumstances?

SECOND SURVEY

Most of the same questions were asked, although the wording may have been changed a little, the grouping of questions altered, and some questions were asked in a different order. The numbering of the questions is therefore different.

Some questions had turned out to be repetitive, or to have produced few interesting answers. Because we wanted to ask some new questions we decided, in the interest of brevity, to omit questions 1, 5, 9, 10, 11, 12, 23, 24, 25, 27, 31 and 32 from the subsequent surveys.

The additional questions were:

Q.1   How did you feel when you first spoke to [the referrer] about the problem?

Q.2   Would you have found it easier or more difficult to have contacted the Centre directly?

THIRD SURVEY

No further questions were omitted, but several were added:

Q.8   Were all the family seen together at the Centre?

Q.9a   Were you expecting to be seen together or not?

Q.9b   What did it feel like being seen together as a family?

Q.9c   Did being seen together affect how you saw the problem?

Q.34   How many times did you come to the Centre?

Q.35   Did that seem enough or not enough appointments?

Q.36   What do you feel about the way in which your contact with the Centre ended?

This interview schedule may be used without further permission, but please acknowledge its origin when results are written up.

Appendix 2

Child and family guidance information leaflet

The
Child and Family
Guidance Service

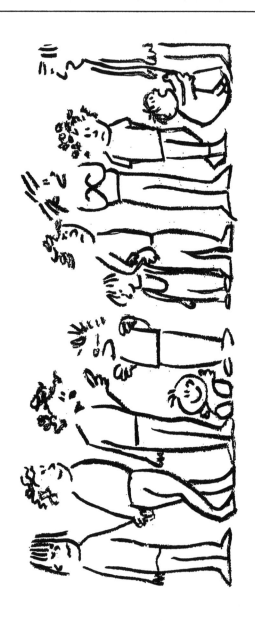

Information

All families have difficulties from time to time. Often a family can cope when things stop running smoothly, but sometimes they need outside help.

The Child and Family Guidance Service is free of charge: it is paid for through rates and taxation.

What kinds of families come to the Centre?

We see all kinds of families – families with two parents, families with divorced parents, single-parent families, families where relatives are bringing up children, or families where children are adopted or fostered.

How old must the children be?

Any age from 0–18 years

What kinds of problems do you help with?

Parents usually come and see us if they are worried about their child's behaviour or feelings, or about their family.

What can you do to help?

We listen to what people have to say about what is worrying them. We don't claim to have any magic cure, but we do have a lot of experience and a range of qualifications within the team. It can be useful for parents simply to talk to someone from outside the family. Some people want to discuss ideas about how to tackle the problem, others want straight advice. We try not to blame anyone because we believe that bringing up children is a difficult task.

Is it confidential?

We keep records to remind us of the details of our work and to help us to plan ahead. You may want to see these records and this is usually possible. You can always discuss this with us. Should we need to contact other agencies, we would always speak to you first.

How do we get an appointment?

Sometimes GPs, Health Visitors or Teachers will contact us on the parents' behalf, when the parents have given their permission. Parents often make direct contact, so please write to us or phone at one of the addresses below.

How long must we wait for an appointment?

We can usually give you an appointment within a couple of weeks after being contacted.

Who do we need to bring?

At some point we usually like to meet the whole family. This way we get more people working with us (even young children can be helpful), and this gives us a better understanding of the problem. Sometimes parents want to talk without the child being present. We are always willing to discuss this. Sometimes we work with one member of the family.

How often will we need to come?

Problems don't go away immediately, especially if they have been around for a long time. We usually suggest you come regularly for a number of appointments. These last for about an hour.

Appendix 3

Home visiting references

Acworth, A. and Bruggen, P. (1985) 'Family therapy when one member is on the death bed', *Journal of Family Therapy* 7: 379–385.

Carr, A. (1986) 'Three techniques for the solo family therapist', *Journal of Family Therapy* 8: 373–382.

Clark, T. *et al.* (1982) *Outreach Family Therapy*, New York: Jason Aronson.

Falloon, I., Boyd, J. and McGill, C. (1984) *Family Care of Schizophrenia*, New York: Guilford.

Friedmann, A. (1962) 'Family therapy as conducted in the home', *Family Process* 1: 132–140.

Herbert, M. (1988) 'Behaviour modification of children with aggressive conduct disorders: the use of triadic model interventions in home settings', *Issues in Criminological and Legal Psychology* 12: 46–57.

Kingston, P. and Smith, D. (1983) 'Preparation for live consultation and live supervision when working without a one-way screen', *Journal of Family Therapy* 5: 219–233.

Lindsey, C. (1979) 'Working with rage and anger – the establishment of a therapeutic setting in the homes of multiproblem families', *Journal of Family Therapy* 1: 117–124.

Messent, P. (1992) 'Working with Bangladeshi families in the East End of London', *Journal of Family Therapy* 14: 287–304.

Pottle, S. (1984) 'Developing a network-orientated service for elderly people and their carers', in A. Treacher and J. Carpenter (eds) *Using Family Therapy*, Oxford: Blackwell.

Smith, D. and Kingston, P. (1980) 'Live supervision without a one-way screen', *Journal of Family Therapy* 2: 379–387.

Zarski, J. *et al.* (1991) 'The invisible mirror: in-home therapy and supervision', *Journal of Marital and Family Therapy* 17: 133–143.

Mental health service users: some national addresses and reading list

Compiled by Viv Lindow

Survivors Speak Out 34 Osnaburgh Street, London NW1 3ND tel. 071 916 5472: network of mental health system survivors, user groups and allies.

Mindlink 22 Harley Street, London W1N 2ED (MIND's consumer network: free membership).

Hearing Voices Network c/o MACC, Swan Buildings, 20 Swan St, Ancoats, Manchester M4 5JW tel. 061 834 9823 (network of people who hear voices).

UK Advocacy Network (UKAN) Premier House, 14 Cross Burgess Street, Sheffield.

Scottish Users' Network 40 Shandwyck Place, Edinburgh.

Voices c/o London Advisory Centre, 197 King's Cross Road, London WC1X 9BX (affiliated to the National Schizophrenia Fellowship).

BOOKS

Ahmed, Tanzeem, Naidu, Bablu and Webb-Johnson, Amanda (eds) (1992) *Concepts of Mental Health in the Asian Community*, Confederation of Indian Organisations (UK), Westminster Bridge Road, London SW1 7XW.

Barker, Ingrid and Peck, Edward (eds) (1987) *Power in Strange Places: User Empowerment in Mental Health Services*, London: Good Practices in Mental Health.

Beeforth, M. *et al.* (eds) (1990) *Whose Service is it Anyway? Users' Views on Co-ordinating Community Care*, Lewisham: RDP.

Bell, S. (1990) *Hearing Voices*, Littlemore Hospital, Oxford OX4 4XN: Oxford Survivors' Publishing.

Boyle, Mary (1990) *Schizophrenia: A Scientific Delusion?* London and New York: Routledge.

Breggin, Peter (1991) *Toxic Psychiatry. Drugs and Electroconvulsive Therapy: The Truth and Better Alternatives*, London: Fontana.

Browne, D. (1990) *Black People, Mental Health and the Courts*, London (169 Clapham Road SW9 0PU): Afro-Caribbean Mental Health Association, CRE and NACRO.

Chamberlin, Judi (1988) *On Our Own*, London: MIND.

Cohen, David (ed.) (1990) *Challenging the Therapeutic State: Critical Perspectives on Psychiatry and the Mental Health System*, New York: *Journal of Mind and Behaviour.*

Fernando, Suman (1991) *Mental Health, Race and Culture*, London: Macmillan/ MIND.

Frame, Janet (1980) *Faces in the Water*, London: Women's Press.

Frederick, J. (1991) *Positive Thinking for Mental Health: Black people in Lewisham Give Their Views on Local Mental Health Services*, London: The Black Mental Health Group (The Playtower, Ladywell Road SE13 7UW (send £3.50)).

Gordon, Barbara (1979) *I'm Dancing as Fast as I Can*, New York: Bantam.

Green, Hannah (1964) *I Never Promised You a Rose Garden*, London: Pan.

Hutchinson, M., Linton, G. and Lucas, J. (1990) *User Involvement Information Pack*, MIND.

Johnstone, Lucy (1989) *Users and Abusers of Psychiatry: A Critical Look at Traditional Psychiatric Practice*, London: RKP.

Laing, Jimmy and McQuarrie, Dermot (1992) *Fifty Years in the System*, London: Corgi.

Leech, Mark (1992) *A Product of the System*, London: Gollancz.

McNeill, Pearlie, McShea, Marie and Parma, Pratibha (eds) (1986) *Through the Break: Women in Personal Crisis*, London: Sheba.

Masson, Jeffrey Moussaieff (1988) *Against Therapy*, London: Fontana/Collins.

Millett, Kate (1990) *The Loony Bin Trip*, London: Virago.

Pembroke, Louise Roxanne (ed.) (1992) *Eating Distress: Perspectives from Personal Experience*, London: Survivors Speak Out (34 Osnaburgh Street, NW1 3ND).

Podvoll, Edward (1990) *The Seduction of Madness*, London: Century.

Read, Jim and Wallcraft, Jan (1992) *Guidelines for Empowering Users of Mental Health Services*, London: COHSE/MIND Publications.

Read, Sue (1989) *Only for a Fortnight: My Life on a Locked Ward*, London: Bloomsbury.

Riley, Joan (1992) *A Kindness to the Children*, London: The Women's Press.

Rose, S., Lewontin, R. C. and Kamin, L. J. (1984) *Not in Our Genes*, Harmondsworth: Penguin.

Showalter, Elaine (1987) *The Female Malady*, London: Virago.

Survivors' Poetry (1992) *from dark to light*, London: Survivors' Press.

Warner, Richard (1985) *Recovery from Schizophrenia*, London: RKP.

Webb-Johnson, A. (1991) *A Cry for Change: An Asian Perspective on Developing Quality Mental Health Care*, Confed. of Indian Organisations, 5 Westminster Bridge Road, London SE1 7XW.

JOURNALS

Asylum: a magazine for democratic psychiatry, c/o Prof. F. A. Jenner, Manor Farm, Brightonholmlee Lane, Wharncliffe Side, Sheffield S30 3DB.

Mindwaves: journal of MIND's service user network, see Mindlink address on
p. 247, free for Mindlink members, sub for others.

Openmind: MIND's journal has user-friendly and user-written articles (address
below).

Hearing Voices Newsletter c/o Manchester Hearing Voices Network, address on
p. 247.

VIDEOS

We're Not Mad We're Angry
From Anger to Action

Many of the items on this list can be obtained from MIND publications, 1st floor,
Kemp House, 152–160 City Road, London EC1V 2NP; they will send a
catalogue.

Bibliography

Aghassy, G. and Noot, M. (1990) *Seksuele kontakten binnen psychotherapeutische hulp-verleningrelasies*, 's-Gravenhage: VUGA.

Albronda, H., Dean, R. and Starkweather, J. (1964) 'Social class and psychotherapy', *Archives of General Psychiatry* 10: 276–283.

Alexander, J. and Parsons, B. (1982) *Functional Family Therapy*, Monterey, CA: Brooks/Cole.

Alexander, J. *et al.* (1976) 'Systems – behavioural intervention with families of delinquents', *Journal of Consulting and Clinical Psychology* 44: 656–664.

Alger, I. and Hogan, P. (1971) 'Enduring effects of video feedback experience on family and marital relationships', in J. Haley (ed.) *Changing Families – A Family Therapy Reader*, New York: Grune and Stratton.

Andersen, T. (1987) 'The reflecting team: dialogue and meta-dialogue in clinical work', *Family Process* 26: 415–428.

Anderson, C. (1986) 'The all-too-short trip from positive to negative connotation', *Journal of Marital and Family Therapy* 12: 351–354.

Anderson, C., Hogarth, G. and Reiss, D. (1980) 'Family treatment of adult schizophrenic patients: a psycho-educational approach', *Schizophrenia Bulletin* 6: 490–505.

Anderson, H. and Goolishian, H. (1988) 'Human systems as linguistic systems: preliminary and evolving ideas about the implications for clinical theory', *Family Process* 27: 371–393.

Aponte, H. (1992) 'Training the person of the therapist in structural family therapy', *Journal of Marital and Family Therapy* 18: 269–281.

Armstrong, D. (1982) 'The doctor–patient relationship', in P. Wright and A. Treacher (eds) *The Problem of Medical Knowledge*, Edinburgh: Edinburgh University Press.

Armsworth, M. (1989) 'Therapy of incest survivors: abuse or support?', *Child Abuse and Neglect* 13: 549–562.

Atkinson, B. and Heath, A. (1990) 'Further thoughts on second-order family therapy – this time it's personal', *Family Process* 29: 145–155.

Barofsky, I. (1978) 'Compliance, adherence and the therapeutic alliance', *Social Science and Medicine* 12: 369–376.

Baruch, G. and Treacher, A. (1978) *Psychiatry Observed*. London: Routledge and Kegan Paul.

Bateson, G. (1972) *Steps to an Ecology of Mind*, London: Paladin.

Baum, O. and Felzer, S. (1964) 'Activity in initial interviews with lower-class patients', *Archives of General Psychiatry* 10: 345–353.

Bennun, I. (1986) 'Evaluating family therapy: a comparison of Milan and problem-solving approaches', *Journal of Family Therapy* 8: 225–242.

Bennun, I. (1988) 'Treating the system or the symptom: investigating family therapy for alcohol problems', *Behavioural Psychotherapy* 16: 165–176.

Bennun, I. (1989) 'Perceptions of the therapist in family therapy', *Journal of Family Therapy* 11: 243–256.

Bennun, I. (1992) 'Some reflections on family therapy', *Clinical Psychology Forum* 48: 22–25.

Bennun, I. (1993) 'Family management and psychiatric rehabilitation', in J. Carpenter and A. Treacher (eds) *Using Family Therapy in the 90s*, Oxford: Blackwell.

Benson, M., Schindler-Zimmerman, T. and Martin, D. (1991) 'Accessing children's perceptions of their family: circular questioning revisited', *Journal of Marital and Family Therapy* 17: 363–372.

Birch, J. (1990) 'The context-setting function of the video "consent" form', *Journal of Family Therapy* 12: 281–286.

Bjørgo, M. and Due-Tønnessen B. (1992) 'Dette sier klientene! Brukerundersøkelse ved et familierådgivningskontor' (This is what clients say: a study of users of a family counselling service), *Fokus på Familien* 4: 219–226.

Bordin, E. (1979) 'The generalizability of the psychoanalytic concept of the working alliance', *Psychotherapy: Theory, Research, and Practice* 16: 252–260.

Bordin, E. (1983) 'Myths, realities and alternatives to clinical trials', paper delivered at the International Conference on Psychotherapy, Bogota, Columbia.

Boscolo, L. and Bertrando, P. (1992) 'The reflexive loop of past, present, and future in systemic therapy and consultation', *Family Process* 31: 119–130.

Boscolo, L. *et al.* (1987) *Milan Systemic Therapy: Conversations in Theory and Practice*, New York: Grune and Stratton.

Boszormenyi-Nagy, I. and Spark, G. (1983) *Invisible Loyalties*, Hagerstown, Maryland: Harper and Row.

Boszormenyi-Nagy, I. and Ulrich, D. (1981) 'Context and Family Therapy', in A. Gurman and D. Kniskern Vol. 1, *Handbook of Family Therapy*, New York: Brunner/Mazel.

Bowen, M. (1972) 'Toward the differentiation of self in one's own family', in J. Framo (ed.) *Family Interaction*, New York: Springer Publishing Company.

Boyd-Franklin, N. (1989) *Black Families in Therapy*, New York: Guilford.

Brannen, J. and Collard, J. (1982) *Marriages in Trouble: the Process of Seeking Help*, London: Tavistock.

Brock, G. and Coufal, J. (1989) 'Ethics in practice', *Family Therapy Networker* March/April: 27.

Brody, M. (1959) *Observations on Direct Analysis: The Therapeutic Techniques of Dr John N. Rosen*, New York: Vantage Press.

Brown C. (1985) *Child Abuse – Parents Speaking*, University of Bristol Social Work Department.

Bruggen, P. and Pettle, S. (1993) 'RUMBASOL: audit in practice', *Journal of Family Therapy* 15: 87–92.

Brunning, H. (1992) 'Auditing one's work – what do clients think about therapy?' *Clinical Psychology Forum* 40: 7–10.

Burck, C. (1978) 'A study of families' expectations and experiences of a child guidance clinic', *British Journal of Social Work* 8: 145–158.

Burnham, J. (1986) *Family Therapy – First Steps towards a Systemic Approach*, London: Tavistock.

Calof, D. (1984) 'An exchange of identities', *Family Therapy Networker* March/Apr: 42–46.

Campbell, D., Draper, R. and Huffington, C. (1989) *Second Thoughts on the Theory and Practice of the Milan Approach*, London: Karnac Books.

Carpenter, J. (1993) 'Working together', in J. Carpenter and A. Treacher (eds) *Using Family Therapy in the 90s*, Oxford: Blackwell.

Carpenter, J. and Treacher, A. (1989) *Problems and Solutions in Marital and Family Therapy*, Oxford: Basil Blackwell.

Carr, A. (1991) 'Milan systemic family therapy: a review of ten empirical investigations', *Journal of Family Therapy* 13: 237–264.

Carter, E. and McGoldrick, M. (1980) *The Family Life Cycle. A Framework for Family Therapy*, New York: Gardner Press.

Cecchin, G. (1987) 'Hypothesizing, circularity, and neutrality revisited: an invitation to curiosity', *Family Process* 26: 405–413.

Cecchin, G., Lane, G. and Ray, W. (1993) 'From strategizing to non-intervention: toward irreverence in systemic practice', *Journal of Marital and Family Therapy* 19: 125–136.

Chase, J. and Holmes J. (1990) 'A two-year audit of a family therapy clinic in adult psychiatry', *Journal of Family Therapy* 12: 229–242.

Clare, P. (1988) *Informing the Public – Making Videos about Social Services. Bristol Papers in Applied Social Studies* No. 6, Bristol: School of Applied Social Studies, University of Bristol.

Combrinck-Graham, L. (1991) 'On technique with children in family therapy – how calculated should it be?' *Journal of Marital and Family Therapy* 17: 373–377.

Conn, J. and Turner, A. (1990) 'Working with women in families', in R. Perelberg and A. Miller (eds) *Gender and Power in Families*, London: Routledge.

Coote, A., Harman, H. and Hewitt, P. (1990) *The Family Way – A New Approach to Policy-Making*, London: Institute for Public Policy Research.

Cottrell, D. (1994) 'Family therapy in the home', *Journal of Family Therapy* 16 (in press).

Crane, R., Griffin, W. and Hill, R. (1986) 'Influences of therapist skills on client perceptions of marriage and family therapy outcome: implications for supervision', *Journal of Marital and Family Therapy*, 12: 91–96.

Cronen, V. and Pearce, B. (1985) 'Toward an explanation of how the Milan method works: an invitation to a systemic epistemology and the evolution of family systems', in D. Campbell and R. Draper (eds) *Applications of Systemic Family Therapy*, London: Grune and Stratton.

Dallos, R. (1991) *Family Belief Systems, Therapy and Change*, Milton Keynes: Open University Press.

Dare, C. and Lindsey, C. (1979) 'Working with rage and anger – the establishment of a therapeutic setting in the homes of multi-problem families', *Journal of Family Therapy* 1: 117–124.

Dare, C. *et al.* (1990) 'The clinical and theoretical impact of a controlled trial of family therapy in anorexia nervosa', *Journal of Family Therapy* 12: 39–57.

Davidson, J., Lax, W., Lussardi, D., Miller, D. and Ratheau M. (1988) 'The reflecting team', *Family Therapy Networker* Sept/Oct: 44–76.

Diethelm, K., Fentress, D., London, M. and McCarthy, J. (1992) 'Out from behind the mirror', *Journal of Strategic and Systemic Therapies* 11: 46–52.

Dimmock, B. (1993) 'Developing family counselling in General Practice', in J. Carpenter and A. Treacher (eds) *Using Family Therapy in the 90s*, Oxford: Basil Blackwell.

Doherty, W. and Boss, P. (1991) 'Values and ethics in family therapy', in A. Gurman and D. Kniskern (eds) *Handbook of Family Therapy* Vol. 2, New York: Brunner/Mazel.

Douglas, J. (1981) 'Behavioural family therapy and the influence of a systems framework', *Journal of Family Therapy* 3: 327–340.

Drane, J. (1982) 'Ethics and psychotherapy: a philosophical perspective', in M. Rosenbaum (ed.) *Ethics and Values in Psychotherapy: A Guidebook*, New York: Free Press.

Dryden, W. (ed.) (1992) *Integrative and Eclectic Therapy – a Handbook*, Milton Keynes: Open University Press.

Dryden, W. and Hunt, P. (1985) 'Therapeutic alliances in marital therapy', in W. Dryden (ed.) *Marital Therapy in Britain* Vol. I, London: Harper and Row.

Dryden, W. and Spurling, L. (1989) *On Becoming a Psychotherapist*, London: Tavistock/Routledge.

Efran, J. and Clarfield, L. (1992) 'Constructionist therapy: sense and nonsense', in S. McNamee and K. Gergen (eds) *Therapy as Social Construction*, London: Sage.

Efran, J. and Lukens, M. (1985) 'The world according to Humberto Maturana', *Family Therapy Networker* May/June: 23–75.

Falloon, I., Boyd, J. and McGill, C. (1984) *Family Care of Schizophrenia*, New York: Guilford.

Fine, M. and Turner, J. (1991) 'Tyranny and freedom: looking at ideas in the practice of family therapy', *Family Process* 30: 307–320.

Fisher, L., Anderson, A. and Jones, J. (1981) 'Types of paradoxical interventions and indications/contraindications for use in clinical practice', *Family Process* 20: 25–36.

von Foerster, H. (1981) *Observing Systems*, Seaside, CA: Intersystems.

Ford, D. and Hearn, J. (1988) *Studying Men and Masculinity. A Sourcebook in Literature and Materials*, Bradford: Department of Social Studies, University of Bradford.

Frank, J. (1971) 'Therapeutic factors in psychotherapy', *American Journal of Psychotherapy* 25: 350–361.

Frankel, B. and Piercy, F. (1990) 'The relationship among selected supervisor, therapist, and client behaviours', *Journal of Marital and Family Therapy* 16: 407–421.

Frude, N. and Dowling, E. (1980) 'A follow-up analysis of family therapy clients', *Journal of Family Therapy* 2: 149–162.

Furman, B. (1990) 'Glasnost therapy', *Family Therapy Networker* May/June: 61–70.

Furman, B. and Ahola, T. (1988) 'Return of the question "why"; advantages of exploring pre-existing explanations', *Family Process* 27: 395–409.

Garfield, S. (1973) 'Basic ingredients of psychotherapy', *Journal of Consulting and Clinical Psychology* 41: 9–12.

Gergen, K. (1991) 'The saturated family', *Family Therapy Networker* Sept/Oct: 27–35.

Gilbert, P., Hughes, W. and Dryden, W. (1989) 'The therapist as a crucial variable in psychotherapy', in W. Dryden and L. Spurling (eds) *On Becoming a Psychotherapist*, London: Tavistock/Routledge.

Gill, O. (1988) 'Integrated work in a neighbourhood family centre', *Practice* 2: 243–255.

von Glaserfeld, E. (1984) 'An introduction to radical constructivism', in P. Watzlawick (ed.) *The Invented Reality*, New York: W. W. Norton.

Goldner, V. (1985) 'Feminism and family therapy', *Family Process* 24: 31–47.

Goldner, V. (1991) 'Essay book review', *Journal of Family Therapy* 13: 341–345.

Goolishian, H. and Anderson, H. (1992) 'Strategy and intervention versus non-intervention: a matter of theory', *Journal of Marital and Family Therapy* 18: 5–15.

Goolishian, H. and Winderman, L. (1988) 'Constructivism, autopoiesis, and problem determined systems', *Irish Journal of Psychology* 9: 130–143.

le Grange, D., Eisler, I., Dare, C. and Hodes, M. (1992) 'Family criticism and self-starvation: a study of expressed emotion', *Journal of Family Therapy* 14: 177–192.

Guerney, L. and Guerney, B. (1987) 'Integrating child and family therapy', *Psychotherapy* 24: 609–614.

Gurman, A. and Kniskern, D. (1978) 'Research on marital and family therapy: progress, perspective and prospect', in S. Garfield and A. Bergin (eds) *Handbook of Psychotherapy and Behavior Change: an Empirical Analysis*, 2nd edition, New York: John Wiley.

Gurman, A. and Kniskern, D. (1981) *Handbook of Family Therapy* Vol. 1, New York: Brunner/Mazel.

Gurman, A. and Kniskern, D. (1991) *Handbook of Family Therapy* Vol. 2, New York: Brunner/Mazel.

Gurman, A., Kniskern, D. and Pinsof W. (1986) 'Research on marital and family therapies', in S. Garfield and A. Bergin (eds) *Handbook of Psychotherapy and Behavior Change*, 3rd edition, New York: Wiley.

Haley, J. (1973) *Uncommon Therapy – The Psychiatric Techniques of Milton H. Erickson MD*, New York: Norton.

Haley, J. (1976) *Problem Solving Therapy*, San Francisco: Jossey Bass.

Hare-Mustin, R. (1978) 'A feminist approach to family therapy', *Family Process* 17: 181–194.

Hare-Mustin, R. (1986) 'The problem of gender in family therapy theory', *Family Process* 26: 15–27.

Hare-Mustin, R. *et al.* (1979) 'Rights of clients, responsibilities of therapists', *American Psychologist* 34: 3–16.

Heatherington, L. and Friedlander, M. (1990) 'Couple and family therapy alliance scales – empirical considerations', *Journal of Marital and Family Therapy* 16: 299–306.

Heins, T. (1988) 'Relearning childthink', *Australian and New Zealand Journal of Family Therapy* 9: 143–149.

Heubeck, B. *et al.* (1986) 'Father involvement and responsibility in family therapy', in M. Lamb (ed.) *The Father's Role: Applied Perspective*, New York: Wiley.

Hoehn-Saric, R. *et al.* (1964) 'Systematic preparation of patients for psychotherapy, 1. Effects of therapy, behaviour and outcome', *Journal of Psychiatric Research* 2: 267–281.

Hoffman, L. (1981) *Foundations of Family Therapy: A Conceptual Framework for Systems Change*, New York: Basic Books.

Hoffman, L. (1985) 'Beyond power and control: toward a "second-order" family systems therapy', *Family Systems Medicine* 3: 381–396.

Hoffman, L. (1990) 'Constructing realities: an art of lenses', *Family Process* 29: 1–12.

Hoffman, L. (1991) 'A reflexive stance for family therapy', *Journal of Strategic and Systemic Therapies* 10: 4–17.

Hoffman, L. and Long, L. (1969) 'A systems dilemma', *Family Process* 8: 211–234.

Holroyd, J. and Brodsky, A. (1977) 'Psychologists' attitudes and practices regarding erotic and non-erotic physical contact with patients', *American Psychologist* 32: 843–849.

Howe, D. (1980) 'Inflated states and empty theories in social work', *British Journal of Social Work* 10: 25–32.

Howe, D. (1989) *The Consumers' View of Family Therapy*, London: Gower.

Hudson, P. (1980) 'Different strokes for different folks: a comparative examination of behavioural, structural and paradoxical methods in family therapy', *Journal of Family Therapy*, 2: 181–190.

Hunt, P. (1985) *Clients' Responses to Marriage Counselling*, Rugby: National Marriage Guidance Council.

Ignatieff, M. (1978) *A Just Measure of Pain – The Penitentiary in the Industrial Revolution 1750–1850*, London: Macmillan.

Illich, I. (1975) *The Limits of Medicine: Medical Nemesis – the Expropriation of Health*, London: Calder and Boyars.

Illich, I. *et al.* (1977) *Disabling Professions*, London: Marion Boyars.

Inger, I. (1993a) Workshop address at the Dartington Event, Dartington Hall, July 1993.

Inger, I. (1993b) 'A dialogic perspective for family therapy: the contribution of Martin Buber and Gregory Bateson', *Journal of Family Therapy* 15: 293–314.

Inger, I. and Inger, J. (1992) *Co-constructing Therapeutic Conversations: A Consultation of Restraint*, London: Karnac.

Jackson, S. (1986) 'Therapeutic change and anorexia nervosa: views of a family and a therapist', *Australian and New Zealand Journal of Family Therapy*, 7: 69–74.

Jacobson, N. and Margolin, G. (1979) *Marital Therapy: Strategies Based on Social Learning and Behavior Exchange Principles*, New York: Brunner/Mazel.

Jenkins, J. *et al.* (1982) 'Failure: an exploration and survival kit', *Journal of Family Therapy* 4: 307–320.

Jernberg, A. (1989) 'Training parents of failure-to-attach children', in C. Schaefer and J. Briesmeister (eds) *Handbook of Parent Training. Parents as Co-Therapists for Children's Behavior Problems*, New York: Wiley.

Johnson, T. (1972) *Professions and Power*, London: Macmillan.

Johnstone, L. (1992) 'Family management in "schizophrenia": a critical review', *Clinical Psychology Forum*, 47: 3–9.

Jones, E. (1988) 'The Milan method – quo vadis?' *Journal of Family Therapy* 10: 325–338.

Jones, E. (1993) *Family Systems Therapy: Developments in the Milan-Systemic Therapies*, Chichester: Wiley.

Jordan, B. (1979) *Helping in Social Work*, London: Routledge.

Jordan, B. (1981) 'Family therapy – an outsider's view', *Journal of Family Therapy* 3: 269–280.

Kaffman, M. (1987) 'Failures in family therapy: and then what?', *Journal of Family Therapy* 9: 307–328.

Kaiser, T. (1992) 'The supervisory relationship: an identification of the primary element in the relationship and application of two theories of ethical relationships', *Journal of Marital and Family Therapy* 18: 283–296.

Kardener, S., Fuller, M. and Mensh, I. (1973) 'Sex and the physician–patient relationship', *American Journal of Psychiatry* 131: 1134–1136.

Kardener, S., Fuller, M. and Mensh, I. (1974) 'A survey of physician attitudes and practices regarding erotic and non-erotic contact with patients', *American Journal of Psychiatry* 130: 1077–1081.

Kassis, J. and Matthews, W. (1987) 'When families and helpers do not want the mirror: a brief report of one team's experience', *Journal of Strategic and Systemic Therapies* 6: 33–43.

Kelly, G. (1955) *The Psychology of Personal Constructs*, New York: Norton.

Kerr, M. and McKee, L. (1981) 'The father's role in child health care', *Health Visitor* 54: 47–51.

Kierkegaard, S. (1974) *Sickness unto Death*, Princeton: Princeton University Press.

Kingston, P. (1979) 'The social context of family therapy', in S. Walrond-Skinner (ed.) *Family and Marital Psychotherapy – A Critical Approach*, London: Routledge.

Koziarski, M. *et al.* (1986) 'Family therapy in a mother and toddler project', *Journal of Family Therapy*, 8: 207–234.

Kraemer, S. (1983) 'Why I am not a family therapist', *Changes*, 2: 8–10.

Kraemer, S. (1988) Letter to the editor, *Journal of Family Therapy* 10: 412–414.

Kramer, C. (1980) *Becoming a Family Therapist – Developing an Integrated Approach to Working with Families*, New York: Human Sciences Press.

Kuehl, B., Newfield, N. and Joanning, H. (1990) 'A client-based description of family therapy', *Journal of Family Psychology* 3: 310–321.

Lappin, J. (1983) 'On becoming a culturally conscious family therapist', *Family Therapy Collections* 6: 122–136.

Leff, J., Berkowitz, R., Shavit, N., Strachan, A., Glass, I. and Vaughn, C. (1989) 'A trial of family therapy v. a relatives group for schizophrenia', *British Journal of Psychiatry* 154: 58–66.

Lieberman, S. (1979) *Transgenerational Family Therapy*, London: Croom Helm.

Lishman, J. (1978) 'A clash in perspective? A study of worker and client perceptions of social work', *British Journal of Social Work* 8: 301–311.

Lorion, R. (1978) 'Research on psychotherapy and behavior change with the disadvantaged', in S. Garfield and A. Bergin (eds) *Handbook of Psychotherapy and Behavior Change*, 2nd edition, New York: Wiley.

Lorion, R. and Felner, R. (1986) 'Research on psychotherapy with the disadvantaged', in S. Garfield and A. Bergin *Handbook of Psychotherapy and Behavior Change*, 3rd edition, New York: Wiley.

Luepnitz, D. (1988) *The Family Interpreted: Feminist Theory in Clinical Practice*, New York: Basic Books.

McGoldrick, M., Pearce, J. and Giordano, J. (1982) *Ethnicity and Family Therapy*, New York: Guilford Press.

MacKinnon, L., Parry, A. and Black, R. (1984) 'Strategies of family therapy: the relationship to styles of family functioning', *Journal of Strategic and Systemic Therapies* 3: 6–22.

McLean, A. (1986) 'Family therapy workshops in the United States: potential abuses in the production of therapy in an advanced capitalist society', *Social Science and Medicine* 23: 179–189.

McLean, A. (1990) 'Contradictions in the social production of clinical knowledge: the case of schizophrenia', *Social Science and Medicine* 30: 969–985.

Mahoney, M. (1978) 'Cognitive and self-control therapies', in S. Garfield and A. Bergin (eds) *Handbook of Psychotherapy and Behavior Change*, 2nd edition, New York: Wiley.

Maluccio, A. (1979) *Learning from Clients – Interpersonal Helping as Viewed by Clients and Social Workers*, New York: Free Press.

Markovitz, L. (1992) 'Crossing the line', *Family Therapy Networker* November/December: 24–31.

Martin, J. (1992) 'Doctors need a taste of their own medicine', the *Guardian* Friday 10 April.

Mashal, M., Feldman, R. and Sigal, J. (1989) 'The unraveling of a treatment paradigm: a follow-up study of the Milan approach to family therapy', *Family Process* 28: 457–470.

Mason, B. and Mason, E. (1990) 'Masculinity and family work', in R. Perelberg and A. Miller (eds) *Gender and Power in Families*, London: Routledge.

Masson, J. (1990) *Against Therapy*, London: Fontana.

Masson, J. (1992) *The Assault on Truth: Freud and Sexual Abuse*, New York: Farrar, Straus and Giroux.

Maturana, H. (1983) 'What is it to see?' *Archives of Biology and Medicine*, 16: 255–269.

Maturana, H. and Varela, F. (1980) *Autopoiesis and Cognition: The Realization of the Living*, Dordrecht: Reidl.

Maturana, H. and Varela, F. (1987) *The Tree of Knowledge*, Boston: Shambhala.

Mayer, J. and Timms, N. (1970) *The Client Speaks: Working Class Impressions of Casework*, London: Routledge and Kegan Paul.

Mazza, J. (1988) 'Training strategic therapists: the use of indirect techniques', in H. Liddle *et al.* (eds) *Handbook of Family Therapy Training and Supervision*, New York: Guilford Press.

Mendez, C. *et al.* (1986) 'The bringing forth of pathology', *Journal of Marital and Family Therapy* 12: 2.

Merrington, D. and Corden, J. (1981) 'Families' impressions of family therapy', *Journal of Family Therapy* 3: 243–261.

Minuchin, S. (1974) *Families and Family Therapy*, Cambridge MA: Harvard University Press.

Minuchin, S. and Fishman, C. (1981) *Family Therapy Techniques*, Cambridge MA: Harvard University Press.

Minuchin, S., Montalvo, B., Guerney, B. and Schumer, H. (1967) *Families of the Slums: An Exploration of Their Structure and Treatment*, New York: Basic Books.

Minuchin, S. *et al.* (1978) *Psychosomatic Families*, Cambridge MA: Harvard University Press.

Mitchell, M. and Fowkes, F. (1985) 'Audit reviewed: does feedback on performance change clinical behaviour?' *Journal of the Royal College of Physicians of London* 19: 251–254.

Montalvo, B. and Haley, J. (1973) 'In defense of child therapy', *Family Process* 12: 227–244.

Murray, E. and Jacobson, L. (1978) 'Cognition and learning in traditional and behavioural psychotherapy', in S. Garfield and A. Bergin (eds) *Handbook of Psychotherapy and Behavior Change*, 2nd edition, New York: Wiley.

Napier, A. and Whitaker, C. (1978) *The Family Crucible*, New York: Harper and Row.

Nash, E. *et al.* (1965) 'Systematic preparation of patients for short-term psychotherapy II: relation to characteristics of patient, therapist and psychotherapeutic process', *Journal of Nervous and Mental Disease* 140: 374–383.

Newfield, N., Kuehl, B., Joanning, H. and Quinn, W. (1990) 'A mini-ethnography of the family therapy of adolescent drug abuse: the ambiguous experience', *Alcoholism Treatment Quarterly* 7: 57–79.

di Nicola, V. (1984) 'Road map to schizophrenia: Mara Selvini Palazzoli and the Milan model of systemic family therapy', *Journal of Strategic and Systemic Therapies* 4: 50–62.

O'Brien, A. and Louden, P. (1985) 'Redressing the balance – involving children in family therapy', *Journal of Family Therapy* 7: 81–98.

Orlinsky, D. and Howard, K. (1978) 'The relation of process to outcome in psychotherapy', in S. Garfield and A. Bergin (eds) *Handbook of Psychotherapy and Behavior Change*, 2nd edition, New York: Wiley.

Orne, M. and Wender, P. (1968) 'Anticipatory socialization for psychotherapy: method and rationale', *American Journal of Psychiatry* 124: 88–98.

Osborne, K. (1982) 'Women in families: feminist therapy and family systems', *Journal of Family Therapy* 5: 1–10.

Overton, A. (1960) cited by Carolyn White.

Palazzoli, M. (1974) *Self-Starvation*, London: Human Context Books.

Palazzoli, M. (1984) 'Behind the scenes of the organization: some guidelines for the expert in human relations', *Journal of Family Therapy* 6: 229–307.

Palazzoli, M. (1986) 'Toward a general model of psychotic family games', *Journal of Marital and Family Therapy* 12: 339–349.

Palazzoli, M. *et al.* (1978) *Paradox and Counterparadox*, New York: Jason Aronson.

Palazzoli, M. *et al.* (1980) 'Hypothesizing – circularity – neutrality. Three guidelines for the conductor of the session', *Family Process* 19: 3–12.

Papp, P. (1980) 'The Greek chorus and other techniques of paradoxical therapy', *Family Process* 19: 45–57.

Parry, G. (1992) 'Improving psychotherapy services: applications of research, audit and evaluation', *British Journal of Clinical Psychology* 31: 3–19.

Parsons, T. (1951) *The Social System*, Chicago: Free Press.

Patterson, G. and Forgatch, M. (1985) 'Therapist behavior as a determinant for client non-compliance: a paradox for the behavior modifier', *Journal of Consulting and Clinical Psychology* 53: 846–851.

Paul, N. and Paul, B. (1986) *A Marital Puzzle*, New York: Gardner Press.

Penn, P. (1982) 'Circular questioning', *Family Process*, 21: 267–280.

Perelberg, R. (1990) 'Equality, asymmetry, and diversity: on conceptualizations of gender', in R. Perelberg and A. Miller (eds) *Gender and Power in Families*, London: Routledge.

Piercy, F., Sprenkle, D. and Constantine, J. (1986) 'Family members' perceptions of live observation/supervision: an exploratory study', *Contemporary Family Therapy* 8: 171–187.

Pilalis, J. (1984) 'The formalization of family therapy training', *Journal of Family Therapy* 6: 35–46.

Pilalis, J. and Anderton, J. (1986) 'Feminism and family therapy – a possible meeting point', *Journal of Family Therapy* 8: 99–114.

Pilgrim, D. and Treacher, A. (1992) *Clinical Psychology Observed*, London: Routledge.

Pimpernell, P. and Treacher, A. (1990) 'Using a videotape to overcome clients' reluctance to engage in family therapy', *Journal of Family Therapy* 12: 59–72.

Pinsof, W. (1982) 'The Intersession Report', unpublished instrument, Centre for Family Studies/The Family Institute of Chicago, Institute of Psychiatry, Northwestern Memorial Hospital.

Pinsof, W. and Catherall, D. (1984) 'The Integrative Psychotherapy Alliance Scale', unpublished paper, Centre for Family Studies/Family Institute of Chicago, Institute of Psychiatry, Northwestern Memorial Hospital.

Pinsof, W. and Catherall, D. (1986) 'The integrative psychotherapy alliance: family, couple, and individual scales', *Journal of Marital and Family Therapy* 12: 137–151.

Pirotta, S. (1984) 'Milan revisited: a comparison of the two Milan schools', *Journal of Strategic and Systemic Therapies* 3: 3–15.

Prest, L. and Keller, J. (1993) 'Spirituality and family therapy: spiritual beliefs, myths and metaphors', *Journal of Marital and Family Therapy* 2: 137–148.

Procter, H. (1984) 'A construct approach to family therapy and systems intervention', in E. Button (ed.) *Personal Construct Theory and Mental Health*, Beckenham, Kent: Croom Helm.

Procter, H. (in press) 'The family construct system', in D. Kalekin-Fishman and B. Walker (eds) *The Construction of Group Realities: Culture and Society in the Light of Personal Construct Theory*, Haifa, Israel: Krieger.

Raskin, N. and van der Veen F. (1970) 'Client-centred family therapy', in J. Hart and T. Tomlinson (eds) *New Directions in Client Centred Therapy*, Boston: Houghton Mifflin.

Reichelt, S. (1990) 'Virker familieterapi?' (Does family therapy work?) *Fokus på Familien* 18: 3–11.

Reimers, S. and Dimmock, B. (1990) 'Mankind and kind men: an agenda for male family therapists', *Journal of Family Therapy* 12: 167–182.

Reiss, D. (1980) *The Family's Construction of Reality*, Cambridge MA: Harvard University Press.

Rogers, A., Pilgrim, D. and Lacey, R. (1993) *Experiencing Psychiatry – Users' Views of Services*, London: Macmillan/Mind.

Russell, J. and Leyland, M. (1986) 'Families' opinions on their experience of family meetings/therapy in a child guidance centre', *Association for Family Therapy Newsletter* 6: 5–9.

Saraga, E. (1993) 'The abuse of children', in R. Dallos and E. McLaughlin (eds) *Social Problems and the Family*, London: Sage Publications.

Schön, D. (1983) *The Reflective Practitioner: How Professionals Think in Action*, Hants: M. T. Smith.

Schön, D. (1991) *The Reflective Practitioner – How Professionals Think in Action*, New York: Basic Books.

Schonfield, J. *et al.* (1969) 'Patient–therapist convergence and measures of improvement in short-term psychotherapy', *Psychotherapy: Theory, Research and Practice* 6: 267–272.

Schwartz, R. and Breunlin, D. (1983) 'Research: why clinicians should bother with it', *Family Therapy Networker* March/Apr: 23–27, 57–59.

Schwartzman, J. (1983) 'Family ethnography: a tool for clinicians'. *Family Therapy Collections* 6: 137–149.

Seligman, P. (1989) Book review, *Community Care*, 20 July.

Selvini, M. (1991) Comment, *Journal of Family Therapy* 13: 265–266.

Selvini, M. and Selvini Palazzoli, M. (1991) 'Team consultation: an indispensable tool for the progress of knowledge', *Journal of Family Therapy* 13: 31–52.

Shapiro, R. (1974) 'Therapist attitudes and premature termination in family and individual therapy', *Journal of Nervous and Mental Disease* 159: 101–107.

Shapiro, R. and Budman, S. (1973) 'Defection, termination and continuation in family and individual therapy', *Family Process* 12: 55–67.

Shaw, E. (1992) 'The training of receptionists', *Australian and New Zealand Journal of Family Therapy* 13: 37–42.

Shaw, I. (1976) 'Consumer opinion and social policy – a research review', *Journal of Social Policy* 5: 19–32.

Shaw, I. (1984) 'Literature review. Consumer evaluations of personal social services', *British Journal of Social Work* 14: 277–284.

de Shazer, S. (1985) *Keys to Solution in Brief Therapy*, New York: W. W. Norton.

de Shazer, S. (1991) *Putting Difference to Work*, New York: W. W. Norton.

Shields, C. *et al.* (1991) 'Anatomy of an individual interview – the importance of joining and structural skills', *American Journal of Family Therapy* 19: 3–18.

Shoham-Salomon, V. and Rosenthal, R. (1987) 'Paradoxical interventions: a meta-analysis', *Journal of Consulting and Clinical Psychology* 55: 22–28.

Sigal, J. *et al.* (1976) 'Problems in measuring the success of family therapy: impasse and solutions', *Family Process* 15: 409–422.

Slipp, S. and Kressel, K. (1978) 'Difficulties in family therapy evaluation', *Family Process* 17: 409–422.

Sloane, R. *et al.* (1970) 'Role preparation and expectancy of improvement in psychotherapy', *Journal of Nervous and Mental Diseases* 150: 18–26.

Sluzki, C. (1984) Personal communication to Gurman, Kniskern and Pinsof.

Smith, D. (1990) *Stepmothering*, Hemel Hempstead: Wheatsheaf Harvester.

Smith, D. and Kingston, P. (1980) 'Live supervision without a one-way screen', *Journal of Family Therapy* 2: 379–387.

Speck, R. and Attneave, C. (1974) *Family Networks*, New York: Vintage Books.

Stanton, M. and Todd, T. (1979) 'Structural family therapy with drug addicts', in E. Kaufman and P. Kaufman (eds) *The Family Therapy of Drug and Alcohol Abuse*, New York: Gardner Press.

Stone, A. *et al.* (1966) 'The role of non-specific factors in short-term psychotherapy', *Australian Journal of Psychology* 18: 210–217.

Street, E. (1994) *Counselling for Family Problems*, London: Sage.

Strømnes, H. (1991) 'Tanker om familieterapi fra en pasients synsvinkel' (Thoughts about family therapy from a patient's point of view), *Fokus på Familien* 19: 155–164.

Strupp, H. (1973) 'The interpersonal relationship as a vehicle for therapeutic learning', *Journal of Clinical and Consulting Psychology* 41: 13–15.

Strupp, H. (1978) 'Psychotherapy research and practice: an overview', in S. Garfield and A. Bergin (eds) *Handbook of Psychotherapy and Behavior Change*, 2nd edition, New York: Wiley.

Strupp, H. and Bloxom, A. (1973) 'Preparing lower-class patients for group psychotherapy: development and evaluation of a role induction film', *Journal of Consulting and Clinical Psychology* 41: 373–384.

Taffel, R. (1991) 'How to talk with kids', *Family Therapy Networker*, July/August: 39–70.

Teismann, M. (1980) 'Convening strategies in family therapy', *Family Process* 19: 393–400.

Timms, N. (1973) *The Receiving End – Consumer Accounts of Social Work Help for Children*, London: Routledge and Kegan Paul.

Timms, N. and Blampied, A. (1985) *Intervention in Marriage – the Experience of*

Counsellors and Their Clients, Sheffield: University of Sheffield Joint Unit for Social Services Research.

Tomm, K. (1987a) 'Interventive interviewing, Part 1. Strategizing as a fourth guideline for the therapist', *Family Process* 26: 3–13.

Tomm, K. (1987b) 'Interventive interviewing, Part 2. Reflexive questioning as a means to enable self-healing', *Family Process* 26: 167–183.

Tomm, K. (1988) 'Interventive interviewing, Part 3. Intending to ask lineal, circular, strategic, or reflexive questions?' *Family Process* 27: 1–15.

Treacher, A. (1983) 'On the utility or otherwise of psychotherapy research', in D. Pilgrim (ed.) *Psychology and Psychotherapy*, London: Routledge and Kegan Paul.

Treacher, A. (1985) 'Working with marital partners: systems approaches', in W. Dryden (ed.) *Marital Therapy in Britain, Volume 1. Contextual Therapeutic Approaches*, London: Harper and Row.

Treacher, A. (1986) 'Invisible patients, invisible families', *Journal of Family Therapy* 8: 267–306.

Treacher, A. (1987) 'Der Mailander Ansatz – Eine erste Kritik', *Zeitschrift für Systemische Therapie* 5: 162–169.

Treacher, A. (1988a) 'The Milan method: a preliminary critique', *Journal of Family Therapy* 10: 1–8.

Treacher, A. (1988b) 'Family therapy: an integrated approach', in E. Street and W. Dryden (eds) *Family Therapy In Britain*, Milton Keynes: Open University Press.

Treacher, A. (1992) 'Family therapy: evolving an integrated approach', in W. Dryden (ed.) *Integrative and Eclectic Therapy – a Handbook*, Milton Keynes: Open University Press.

Treacher, A. (1993) 'The case against registration of family therapists', *Context, a News Magazine of Family Therapy* 14 (spring): 7.

Treacher, A. and Carpenter, J. (1982) 'Oh no! not the Smiths again! An exploration of how to identify and overcome "stuckness" in family therapy, part 1', *Journal of Family Therapy* 4: 285–305.

Treacher, A. and Carpenter, J. (eds) (1984) *Using Family Therapy*, Oxford: Blackwell.

Treacher, A. and Carpenter, J. (1993) 'User-friendly family therapy', in Carpenter, J. and Treacher, A. (eds) *Using Family Therapy in the 90s*, Oxford: Blackwell.

Truax, C. and Mitchell, K. (1971) 'Research on certain therapist interpersonal skills in relation to process and outcome', in S. Garfield and A. Bergin (eds) *Handbook of Psychotherapy and Behavior Change*, 1st edition, New York: Wiley.

Tudor-Hart, J. (1971) 'The inverse care law', *The Lancet* 1: 405–412.

Tushen, M. (1977) 'The political ecology of disease', *Review of Radical Political Economics* 9: 45–46.

Vostanis, P., Burnham, J. and Harris, Q. (1992) 'Changes of expressed emotion in systemic family therapy', *Journal of Family Therapy* 14: 15–28.

Wachtel, E. (1987) 'Family systems and the individual child', *Journal of Marital and Family Therapy* 13: 15–25.

Wachtel, E. (1990) 'The child as an individual: a resource for systemic change', *Journal of Strategic and Systemic Therapies* 9: 50–58.

Waldegrave, C. (1990) 'Social justice and family therapy', *Dulwich Centre Newsletter* No. 1, Adelaide: Dulwich Centre Publications.

Walrond-Skinner, S. (1976) *Family Therapy: The Treatment of Natural Systems*, London: Routledge and Kegan Paul.

Walrond-Skinner, S. (ed.) (1979) *Family and Marital Psychotherapy – a Critical Approach*, London: Routledge.

Walrond-Skinner, S. (1984) 'Whither family therapy? Twenty years on', *Journal of Family Therapy* 6: 1–16.

Walrond-Skinner, S. (1989) 'Spiritual dimensions and religious beliefs in family therapy', *Journal of Family Therapy* (spring edition).

Walrond-Skinner, S. (1990) Book review, *Journal of Family Therapy* 12: 91–92.

Walrond-Skinner, S. and Watson, D. (1987) *Ethical Issues in Family Therapy*, London: Routledge and Kegan Paul.

Walters, M., Carter, B., Papp, P. and Silverstein, O. (1988) *The Invisible Web. Gender Patterns in Family Relationships*, New York: Guilford.

Wangberg, F. (1991) 'Self-reflection: turning the mirror inward', *Journal of Strategic and Systemic Therapies* 10: 18–29.

Warren, N. and Rice, L. (1972) 'Structuring and stabilizing of psychotherapy for low-prognosis clients', *Journal of Consulting and Clinical Psychology* 39: 173–181.

Weitzman, J. (1985) 'Engaging the severely dysfunctional family in treatment: basic considerations', *Family Process* 24: 473–485.

Whan, M. (1983) 'Tricks of the trade: questionable theory and practice in family therapy', *British Journal of Social Work* 13: 321–337.

Whitaker, C. (1967) 'The growing edge', in J. Haley and L. Hoffman: *Techniques of Family Therapy*, New York: Basic Books.

White, C. (1988) 'Asking clients: people's experiences of attending a child and family guidance clinic', discourse for the degree of B.Sc. in sociology, University of Bath.

White, M. (1989) 'The externalizing of the problem', *Dulwich Centre Newsletter*, summer 1988/89, Adelaide: Dulwich Centre Publications.

White, M. and Epston, D. (1990) *Narrative Means to Therapeutic Ends*, New York: W. W. Norton.

Wilkinson, I. (1992) 'Developing an audit system for child and family work', *Clinical Psychology Forum* 48: 11–17.

Williams, J. and Watson, G. (1988) 'Sexual inequality, family life and family therapy', in E. Street and W. Dryden (eds) *Family Therapy in Britain*, Buckingham: Open University Press.

Woodhead, R. (1993) 'Reflections on responses to Masson', *Clinical Psychology Forum* 38: 25–26.

Woodward, C. *et al.* (1978) 'Aspects of consumer satisfaction with brief family therapy', *Family Process* 17: 399–407.

Wright, P. and Treacher, A. (1982) *The Problem of Medical Knowledge*, Edinburgh: Edinburgh University Press.

Young, J. (1990) 'A critical look at the one-way screen', *Dulwich Centre Newsletter*, summer 1989/90: 5–11, Adelaide: Dulwich Centre Publications.

Ziffer, R. (1985) 'The utilization of psychological testing in the context of family therapy', in R. Ziffer (ed.) *Adjunctive Techniques in Family Therapy*, Orlando: Grune and Stratton.

Zilbach, J. (1986) *Young Children in Family Therapy*, New York: Brunner/Mazel.

Zimmerman-Tansella, C. and Colorio, C. (1986) 'Early drop out and clients' experience of family therapy', *International Journal of Family Psychiatry* 7: 203–220.

Zygmond, M. and Boorhem, H. (1989) 'Ethical decision-making in family therapy', *Family Process* 28: 269–280.

Index

Milton Keynes UK
Ingram Content Group UK Ltd.
UKHW040444071024
449327UK00020B/992

9 780415 074315